M. Sofue, N. Endo (Eds.)

Treatment of Osteoarthritic Change in the Hip

Joint Preservation or Joint Replacement?

M. Sofue, N. Endo (Eds.)

Treatment of Osteoarthritic Change in the Hip

Joint Preservation or Joint Replacement?

With 198 Figures, Including 12 in Color

Springer

Muroto Sofue, M.D.
Director of Nakajo Central Hospital
Chairman of the Orthopaedic Division
12-1 Nishihon-cho, Tainai, Niigata 959-2656, Japan

Naoto Endo, M.D.
Professor and Chairman
Division of Orthopedic Surgery
Niigata University Graduate School of Medical and Dental Sciences
1-757 Asahimachi-dori, Niigata 951-8510, Japan

Library of Congress Control Number: 2006938396

ISBN-10 4-431-38198-8 Springer Tokyo Berlin Heidelberg New York
ISBN-13 978-4-431-38198-3 Springer Tokyo Berlin Heidelberg New York

Springer is a part of Springer Science+Business Media
springer.com

Printed in Japan

Typesetting: SNP Best-set Typesetter Ltd., Hong Kong
Printing and binding: Shinano, Japan

Printed on acid-free paper

Preface

The 32nd Japanese Hip Society (JHS) Congress was held November 6–8, 2005, in Niigata, Japan. Guest speakers from many countries and specialists for hip disease presented papers that focused on joint preservation for osteoarthritis of the hip, joint preservation for aseptic necrosis of the femoral head, treatment for epiphyseolysis capitis femoris, and up-to-date information and knowledge on joint arthroplasty. Altogether, there were many important presentations about joint preservation and replacement. This book covers the main themes of the congress.

The starting point for the treatment of hip disease depends on how we can preserve the natural hip joint and on steps leading to regeneration of the diseased, injured, or destroyed joint. Preservation and regeneration treatments following traditional and theoretical methods do not need to use expensive materials, such as the artificial joints used in arthroplasty. On the other hand, preservation and regeneration treatments are difficult to perform and require a lengthy rehabilitation period.

Recently, too much attention has been paid to these demerits, resulting in a yearly decrease in the number of cases receiving joint-preserving treatment. This move away from traditional methods denies the surgeon the experience and knowledge of the benefits associated with the most biologically appropriate treatment. As the president of JHS and a hip surgeon, I believe there is a need to halt this tendency, to promote the benefits of histological treatment, and to allow the young surgeon insight into joint-preservation surgery. Also, as a hip surgeon I am not neglecting joint replacement as a treatment for hip disease. I, myself, perform total hip arthroplasty for patients with severely damaged hip joints and those who have no other therapeutic choice than joint-replacement surgery.

As an editor of this book, I am very hopeful that readers gain insight into the proper treatment of hip disease.

Muroto Sofue
President of the 32nd Japanese Hip Society

Contents

Part III: Osteoarthritis of the Hip: Joint Preservation or Joint Replacement?

Part IV: Total Hip Arthroplasty: Special Cases and Techniques

List of Contributors

Part I
Slipped Capital Femoral Epiphysis (SCFE)

Retrospective Evaluation of Surgical Treatments for Slipped Capital Femoral Epiphysis

Hideki Fujii, Takuya Otani, Seijin Hayashi, Yasuhiko Kawaguchi, Hideaki Tamegai, Mitsuru Saito, Nobutaka Tanabe, and Keishi Marumo

Summary. The summary of our treatment strategy for SCFE is presented. Acute/unstable SCFE in which epiphyseal mobility is observed under fluoroscopy is treated by manual reduction as early as possible, followed by internal fixation with two screws. Chronic/stable SCFE with posterior tilt angle (PTA) less than 40° is treated by in situ single-screw fixation with the dynamic method. For those with PTA of 40° and more, it is important to comprehend the pathology using a CT scan for accuracy, and intertrochanteric flexion osteotomy seems to be one of the simplest and most predictable treatment modalities.

Key words. Slipped capital femoral epiphysis, Stable type, Unstable type, Manual reduction, Chondrolysis

Introduction

We report the outcomes of surgical treatments for slipped capital femoral epiphysis (SCFE) at our department. The treatment strategies for various types of SCFE are reviewed.

Materials and Methods

Our review includes 26 cases, 28 hips, with SCFE that were treated at our university hospital and affiliated hospitals. There were 19 male and 7 female patients. Age at onset ranged from 5 to 31 years, with an average of 12.7 years. The average follow-up period was 3 years and 7 months. Onset modes included 2 hips of acute type, 8 hips of acute on chronic type, and 18 hips of chronic type.

As for treatment method, 10 unstable SCFE that consisted of acute type and acute on chronic type were treated by manipulative reduction followed by internal fixation. Eleven stable/chronic SCFE with posterior tilt angle (PTA) 40° and less were treated

---

Department of Orthopedic Surgery, The Jikei University School of Medicine, 3-25-8 Nishi-Shinbashi, Minato-ku, Tokyo 105-8461, Japan

by in situ fixation. Among the hips of chronic type with PTA more than 40°, 6 were treated by trochanteric osteotomy and 1 by subcapital femoral neck osteotomy.

The evaluated items were as follows. Preoperatively, PTA was measured on Laurenstein X-ray to determine the degree of slippage. We examined MRI for two cases to check contralateral hip for preslip evidence to discuss the need for preventive fixation [1]. Postoperatively, PTA was measured for assessment. Hip function was assessed using Japanese Orthopaedic Association (JOA) hip score and range of motion. Postoperative complications such as femoral necrosis and chondrolysis were also examined.

Results

The average PTA for ten acute/unstable type hips that were treated by manipulative reduction was 51° before reduction and 22° after. There was no case of femoral necrosis, but chondrolysis was observed in one hip. Preoperative PTA was 70° for this case, and narrowing of joint space was observed within a year after the surgery, which was considered to be attributable to chondrolysis. After 2 years postoperative, however, radiographic joint space was improved. At postoperative 4 years and 7 months (Fig. 1), the clinical outcome was good, although some formation of osteophytes was observed [2].

The outcomes for 18 hips of chronic/stable type included that the average postoperative PTA for 11 hips after in situ fixation was 31°. For 7 hips that were treated by osteotomy, preoperative PTA was 51° and postoperative PTA was 25°. There were no complications for the chronic/stable type group.

The PTA measured at the last follow-up was found to be improved by 7° on average for this series of cases when compared with immediate postoperative angle. This

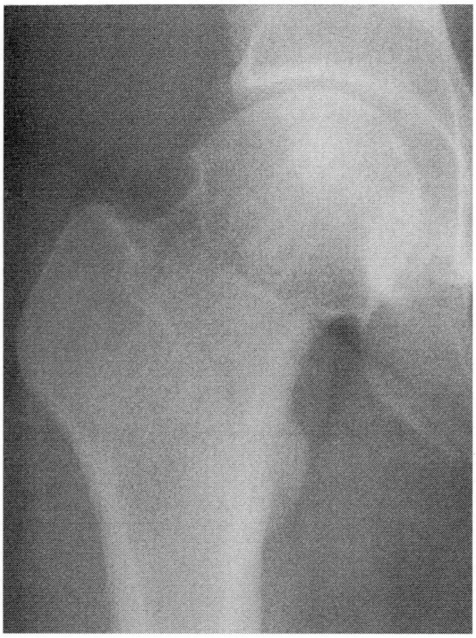

FIG. 1. Case 1. An 11-year-old girl (at time of operation). At 4 years and 7 months after operation, the joint space was improved

change was considered to be an effect of remodeling, as was reported by Bellemans et al. [3].

Clinical results at the last follow-up were generally good. There were no complaints of hip pain. The average Japanese Orthopedic Association (JOA) hip score was 98. Good range of motion was confirmed for flexion, abduction, and external rotation, whereas mild restriction was observed for internal rotation.

Discussion

After reviewing these results as well as the literature, our current treatment strategy has been determined as follows.

Theory and Indication of Manipulative Reduction

The case that is classified as acute/acute on chronic type, clinically classified as unstable type by Loder et al. [4], and is observed to demonstrate obvious mobility at the separated epiphysis under fluoroscopy, should be manually reduced as early as possible, and then internally fixed with two screws (Fig. 2a,b).

The manual reduction technique that we use for the hip with physeal instability is not a forceful manipulation, but rather a quiet and gradual flexion, abduction, and

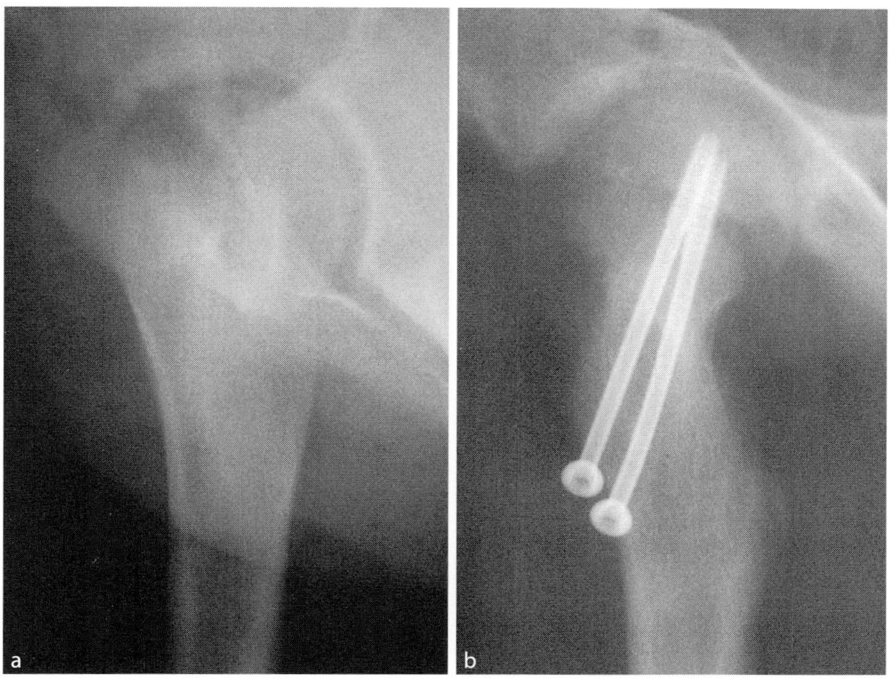

Fig. 2. Case 2. An 11-year-old girl. **a** Posterior tilt angle (PTA) (at time of the injury): 70°. **b** PTA (after reduction): 18° (contralateral PTA, 9°). Note that only the acute portion of the slippage was reduced, and overreduction was avoided

internal rotation of the joint to find a good position of the leg under fluoroscopy [2,5]. Also, it is important to reduce only the acute portion of the slippage and not to overreduce [6].

Morphological improvement gained by manual reduction would lead to functional improvement of the hip and lower the risk of arthritis in the future. Although the possibility is undeniable that blood circulation in the femoral head may be compromised, the opposite possibility does exist, that is to say, manual reduction could improve blood circulation, as indicated by Kita et al. [7]. Taking these considerations into account, we believe our treatment policy is well justified. Both Peterson et al. [8] and Gordon et al. [9] reported that the improvement of blood flow in the vessels supplying nutrients in the epiphysis that was provided by anatomical reduction prevented necrosis of the femoral head. Their reports recommended early reduction for unstable SCFE, which was proved by good clinical results.

Dynamic Single-Screw Fixation

Chronic/stable type slippage with PTA less than 40° is treated by in situ fixation. In the past, we used multiple devices for internal fixation; however, we have been using single-screw fixation recently, which is reported to have a lower complication rate than fixation with multiple screws [5]. We also have tried the dynamic method, reported by Kumm et al. in 1996, in which a screw is inserted to protrude from the lateral cortex to prevent premature physeal closure [10].

A 5-year-old girl and a 12-year-old boy were treated with this dynamic method and are presently being followed (Fig. 3). For the former patient, several screw replacements are anticipated before physeal closure occurs.

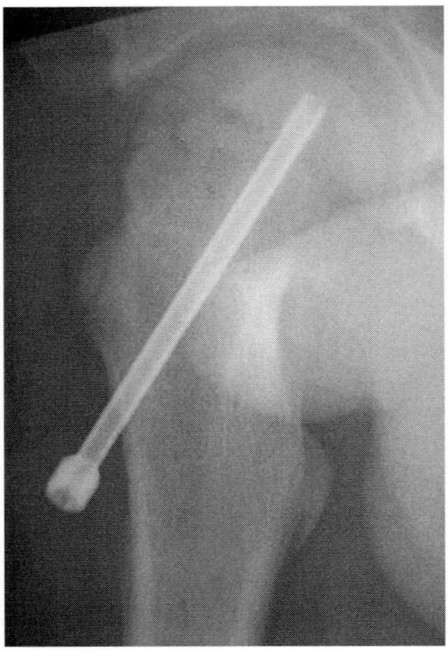

Fig. 3. Case 3. A 12-year old boy with PTA (at injury) 35°. Dynamic single-screw fixation was used

Osteotomy

Chronic/stable type with PTA of 40° and more has been treated by trochanteric and subcapital osteotomy. We employed the Southwick procedure in the past for the chronic/stable type with PTA of 40° to 70°. This procedure is relatively technically demanding, yet does not always seem to be successful in achieving the intended correction. Thus, we are now trying to understand the pathology using computed tomography (CT) scan for accuracy, and also to consider simple flexion osteotomy, depending on the situation (Fig. 4) [11].

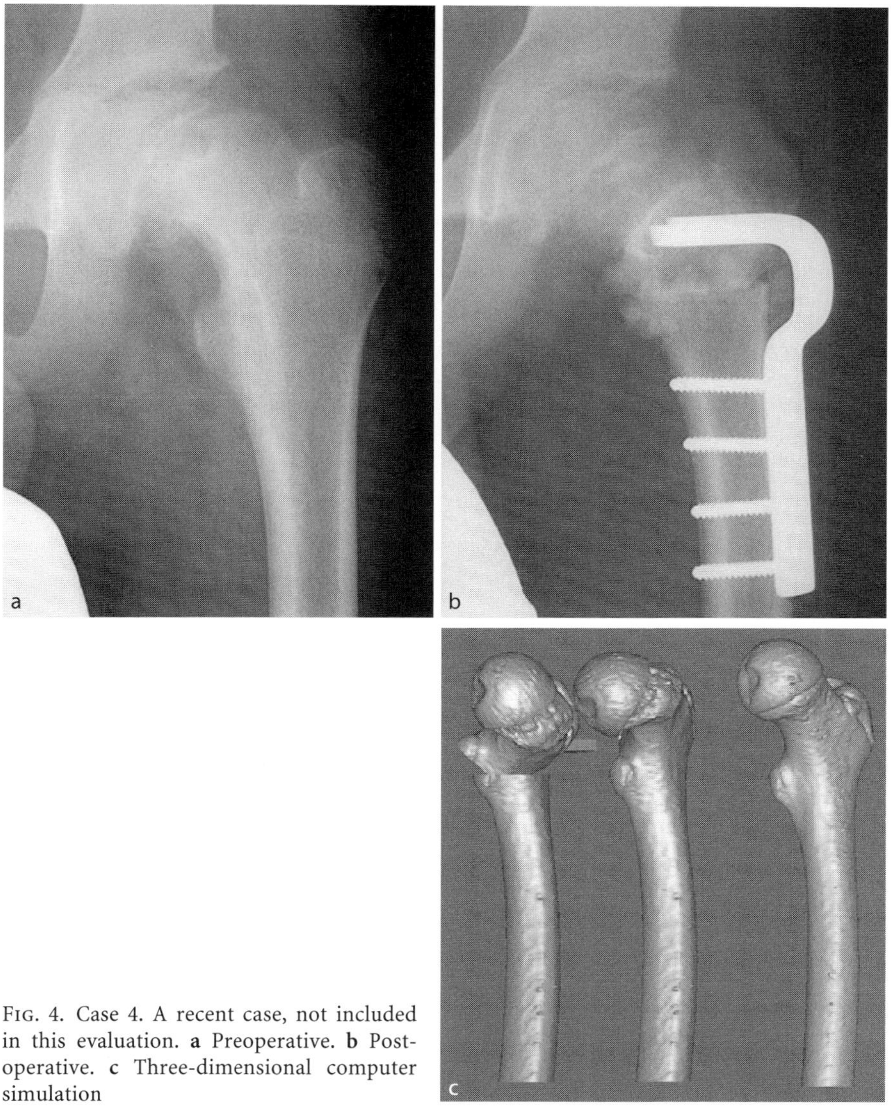

Fig. 4. Case 4. A recent case, not included in this evaluation. **a** Preoperative. **b** Postoperative. **c** Three-dimensional computer simulation

References

1. Lalaji A, Umans H, Schneider R, et al (2001) MRI features of confirmed "pre-slip" capital femoral epiphysis: a report of two cases. Skeletal Radiol 31:362–365
2. Otani T, Suzuki H, Kato A, et al (2004) Clinical results of closed manipulative reduction for acute-unstable slipped capital femoral epiphysis. Seikeigeka 55:771–777
3. Bellemans J, Farby G, Molenaers G, et al (1996) Slipped capital femoral epiphysis: a long-term follow-up, with special emphasis on the capacities for remodeling. J Pediatr Orthop (B) 5:151–157
4. Loder RT, et al (1993) Acute slipped capital femoral epiphysis: the importance of physeal stability. J Bone Joint Surg 75A:1134–1140
5. Aronsson DD, Lorder RT, et al (1996) Treatment of the unstable (acute) slipped capital femoral epiphysis. Clin Orthop Relat Res 322:99–110
6. Casey BH, Hamilton HW, Bobechko WP (1972) Reduction of acutely slipped upper femoral epiphysis. J Bone Joint Surg 54B:607–614
7. Kita A, Morito N, Maeda S, et al (1995) Indication and procedure of manual reduction and subcapital osteotomy for slipped capital femoral epiphysis. Seikei-Saigaigeka 38:631–638
8. Peterson MD, Weiner DS, Green NE, et al (1997) Acute slipped capital femoral epiphysis: the value and safety of urgent manipulative reduction. J Pediatr Orthop 17: 648–654
9. Gordon JE, Abrahams MS, Dobbs MB, et al (2002) Early reduction, arthrotomy, and cannulated screw fixation in unstable slipped capital femoral epiphysis treatment. J Pediatr Orthop 22:352–358
10. Kumm DA, Lee SH, Hackenbroch MH, et al (2001) Slipped capital femoral epiphysis: a prospective study of dynamic screw fixation. Clin Orthop Relat Res 384:198–207
11. Kamegaya M, Saisu T, Ochiai N, et al (2005) Preoperative assessment for intertrochanteric femoral osteotomies in severe chronic slipped capital femoral epiphysis using computed tomography. J Pediatr Orthop B 14:71–78

Treatment of Slipped Capital Femoral Epiphysis

Motoaki Katano, Naonobu Takahira, Sumitaka Takasaki, Katsufumi Uchiyama, and Moritoshi Itoman

Summary. Slipped capital femoral epiphysis (SCFE) is a comparatively rare disorder with various new treatment modalities. Twenty-nine hips (27 patients) in this study were treated (1971–2004). Mean age was 12.5 years, and mean follow-up period was 54.7 months. Among unilateral SCFE patients, there were 7 acute, 6 acute on chronic, and 16 chronic SCFE. Average posterior tilting angle (PTA) on admission was 47.6°. Pinning was performed on 11, osteotomy on 9, and in situ pinning on 9 hips. Unaffected-side prophylactic fixation was performed on 13 hips (44.8%). Postoperative complications of avascular necrosis of the femoral head were noted in 7 hips (24.1%). Femoral head deformity was noted in 3 hips (10.3%). For acute SCFE, we perform gentle reduction by traction and epiphysiodesis. For chronic slips, we perform epiphysiodesis or osteotomy. Opinions remain divided concerning unaffected-side prophylactic fixation; however, we consider observation sufficient. The postoperative complication rate was higher in acute slips. Femoral head avascular necrosis is caused by failure of the remaining capital nutrient vessels. Anatomical reduction of the epiphysis is necessary. Therefore, prophylaxis is indispensable to prevent avascular necrosis. In future reports, we will include many more cases with these procedures, focusing on improved results and patient benefits.

Key words. Slipped capital femoral epiphysis, Epiphysiodesis, Prophylaxis, In situ pinning, Osteotomy

Introduction

Slipped capital femoral epiphysis (SCFE) is a comparatively rare disorder; however, various new methods for its treatment have been reported. The various treatments offer methods for gentle reduction by traction, manual reduction, internal fixation, and osteotomy. For a slight slip, we perform epiphysiodesis such as in situ pinning. For a moderate slip, we perform an osteotomy and open reduction. We have investigated clinical and radiographic evaluation of the patients suffering from SCFE who have undergone surgical therapy in our hospital.

Department of Orthopaedic Surgery, Kitasato University School of Medicine, 1-15-1 Kitasato, Sagamihara, Kanagawa 228-8555, Japan

Materials and Methods

There were 27 patients (23 males, 4 females) in the present study, with 29 hips treated surgically from 1971 to 2004 in the Kitasato University Hospital. Patient age ranged from 7 to 20 (mean, 12.5) years old. The follow-up period was 9 to 99 (mean, 54.7) months. There were no preslips; however, there were 2 cases of bilateral SCFE. Among the patients with unilateral SCFE, there were 7 acute, 6 acute on chronic, and 16 chronic SCFE. The average posterior tilting angle (PTA) on admission was 47.6°. The underlying disease was Down syndrome; hypothyroidism was seen in 1 hip, eunuchoidism and Frohlich's syndrome were seen in 1 hip, and juvenile rheumatoid arthritis (JRA) with short-stature chronic renal failure was seen in 1 hip.

Clinical evaluations of treatment methods, prophylactic fixation of the unaffected side, rehabilitation, complications, and radiographic evaluation of the PTA were investigated.

Results

Of the surgically treated cases, pinning (cannulated screw fixation) was performed on 11 hips, osteotomy on 9 hips, and in situ pinning on 9 hips. According to the classification of severity, pinning was performed on 6 hips and osteotomy was performed on 1 hip of an acute slip. Pinning was performed on 1 hip, osteotomy on 6 hips, and in situ pinning on 9 hips of chronic slips. Pinning was performed on 4 hips and osteotomy was performed on 2 hips in acute on chronic slips (Table 1). Prophylactic fixation of the unaffected side was performed on 13 hips (44.8%), and there was deformity of the femoral head in 1 hip and a femoral neck fracture after removal of the nail in 1 hip. For rehabilitation, partial weight-bearing started after 6 weeks, and brace support for non-weight-bearing was applied in 6 cases. Postoperative complications of avascular necrosis of the femoral head were noted in 7 hips (24.1%). Joint space narrowing and deformity of the femoral head were also noted in 3 hips (10.3%) (Table 2). According to the classification, the acute type of SCFE was seen in 4 of 7 hips (57.1%), acute on chronic type in 2 of 6 hips (33.3%), and the chronic type in 4 of 16 hips (25%). The

TABLE 1. Clinical classification and treatment methods

Type of slip	Pinning	Osteotomy (ARO, VFO)	In situ pinning
Acute	6	1	0
Chronic	1	6	9
Acute on chronic	4	2	0
Total	11	9	9

ARO, anterior rotational osteotomy; VFO, valgus flexion osteotomy

TABLE 2. Complications

Complication	Males	Females	Number (%)
Infection	0	0	0
Avascular necrosis of femoral head	6	1	7 (24.1%)
Osteolysis	0	0	0
Deformity of femoral head	1	2	3 (10.3%)

surgical methods included pinning in 6 of 11 hips (54.5%), osteotomy in 4 of 9 hips (44.4%), and in situ pinning in 0 of 9 hips. Additional operations using bone grafts were performed for avascular necrosis of the femoral head in 2 hips. The average PTA at the time of the injury was 47.6° (20°–85°), and the average postoperative PTA was 17.9° (0°–40°). The average PTA after pin removal at the final follow-up was 15.9° (0°–31°) (Table 3).

Case 1

A 12-year-old boy suffered from acute SCFE with a PTA of 65° that was reduced to 22° by skeletal traction for 2 weeks. We performed epiphysiodesis by a cancellous bone screw in this position. It was removed 6 months postoperatively. Neither deformity of the femoral head nor necrosis was found in the final follow-up period, and he had an excellent postoperative course (Fig. 1).

TABLE 3. Posterior tilting angle (PTA)

Type of slip	Admission	Postoperative	Final follow-up
Acute	54.4°	16.1°	16.5°
	(33°–85°)	(0°–40°)	(8°–20°)
Chronic	41.8°	20.5°	16°
	(20°–80°)	(0°–35°)	(0°–31°)
Acute on chronic	54.8°	13°	14.7°
	(30°–65°)	(0°–30°)	(14°–15°)
Total	47.6°	17.9°	15.9°
	(20°–85°)	(0°–40°)	(0°–31°)

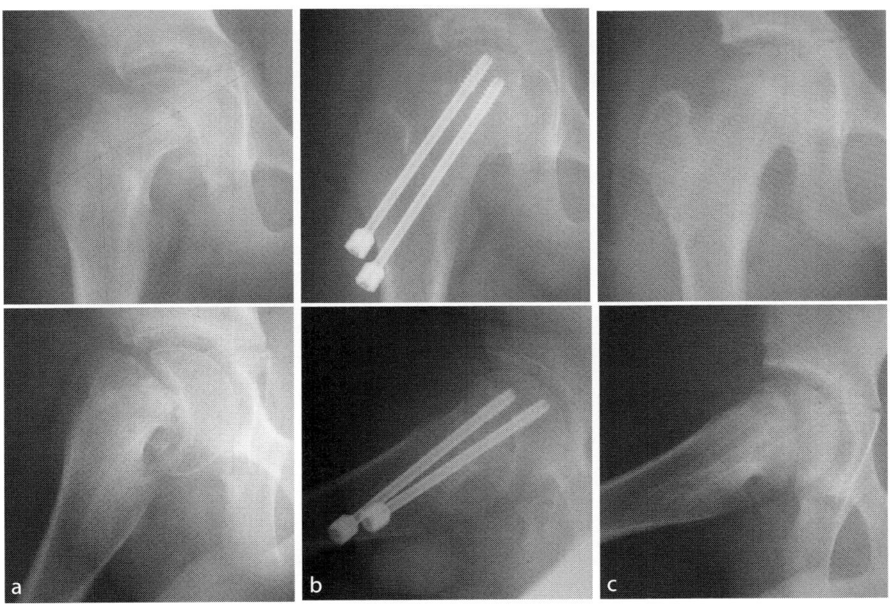

FIG. 1. Case 1. Acute slipped capital femoral epiphysis (SCFE) in a 12-year-old boy with posterior tilting angle (PTA) of 65° on admission (**a**). We performed epiphysiodesis with cannulated screw fixation, PTA was 20° (**b**). At 6 months after epiphysiodesis, the cancellous bone screw was removed with excellent results (**c**)

Case 2

A 13-year-old boy suffered from chronic SCFE with a PTA of 78°. We performed an anterior rotational osteotomy (ARO) of the femoral head using an F-system device. The postoperative PTA was 32°. The patient started partial weight-bearing 6 weeks after the operation. We removed the device 2.5 years postoperatively. A limitation of internal rotation was seen 4 years postoperatively; however, X-rays and clinical examination findings were excellent during the course (Fig. 2).

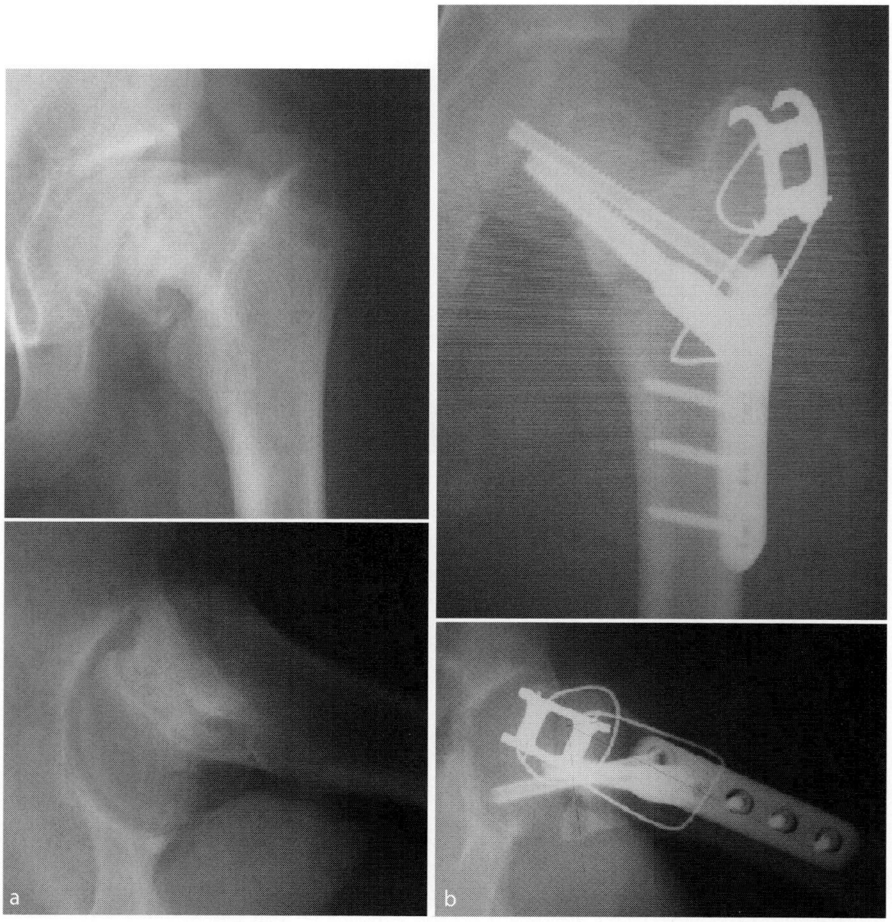

FIG. 2. Case 2. Chronic SCFE in a 13-year-old boy with PTA of 78° (**a**). After anterior rotational osteotomy (ARO) of the femoral head using an F-system device, PTA was 32° (**b**). The device was removed 2.5 years postoperatively (**c**). Limitation of internal rotation was seen 4 years postoperatively (**d**)

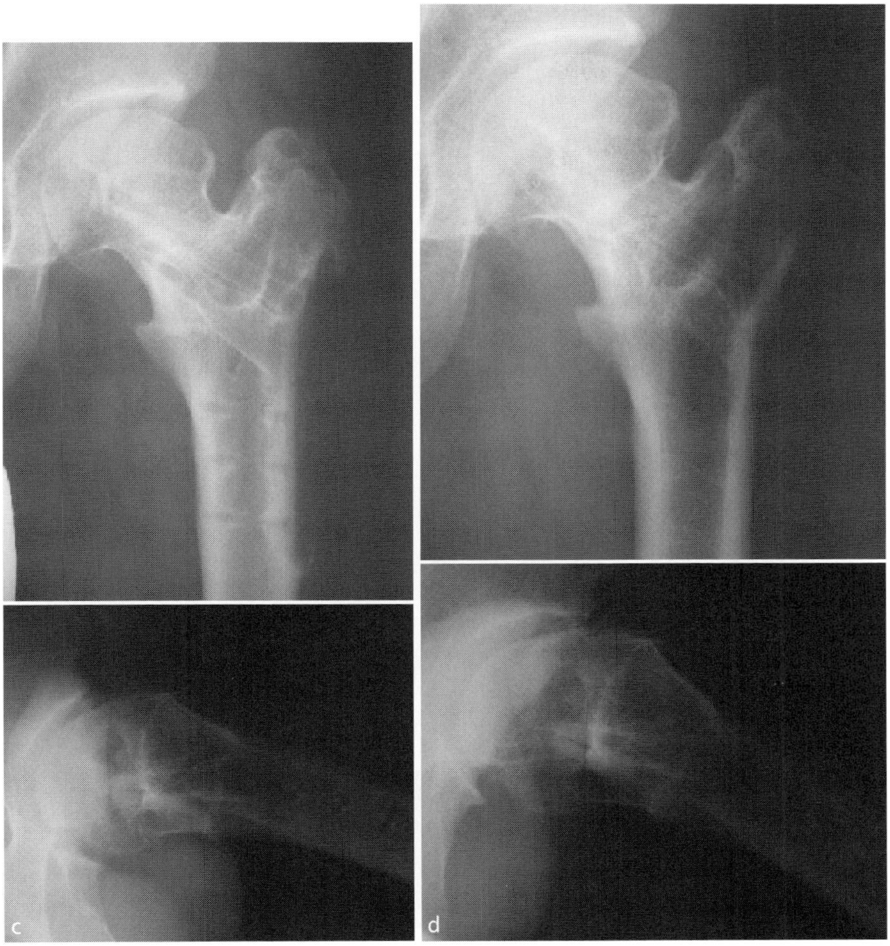

Fig. 2. *Continued*

Case 3

A 13-year-old boy suffered from acute SCFE with a PTA of 85°. We performed epiphysiodesis with cannulated screw fixation because the slip had been reduced by skeletal traction for 10 days. We feared the development of avascular necrosis of the femoral head; therefore, we applied a non-weight-bearing brace and observed the patient's condition. However, we observed flattening of the lateral femoral head after 8 months. We removed the screws 2 years postoperatively and performed strut allograft bone grafting. Twenty years later, the patient was able to walk without pain but had developed a femoral head deformity (Fig. 3).

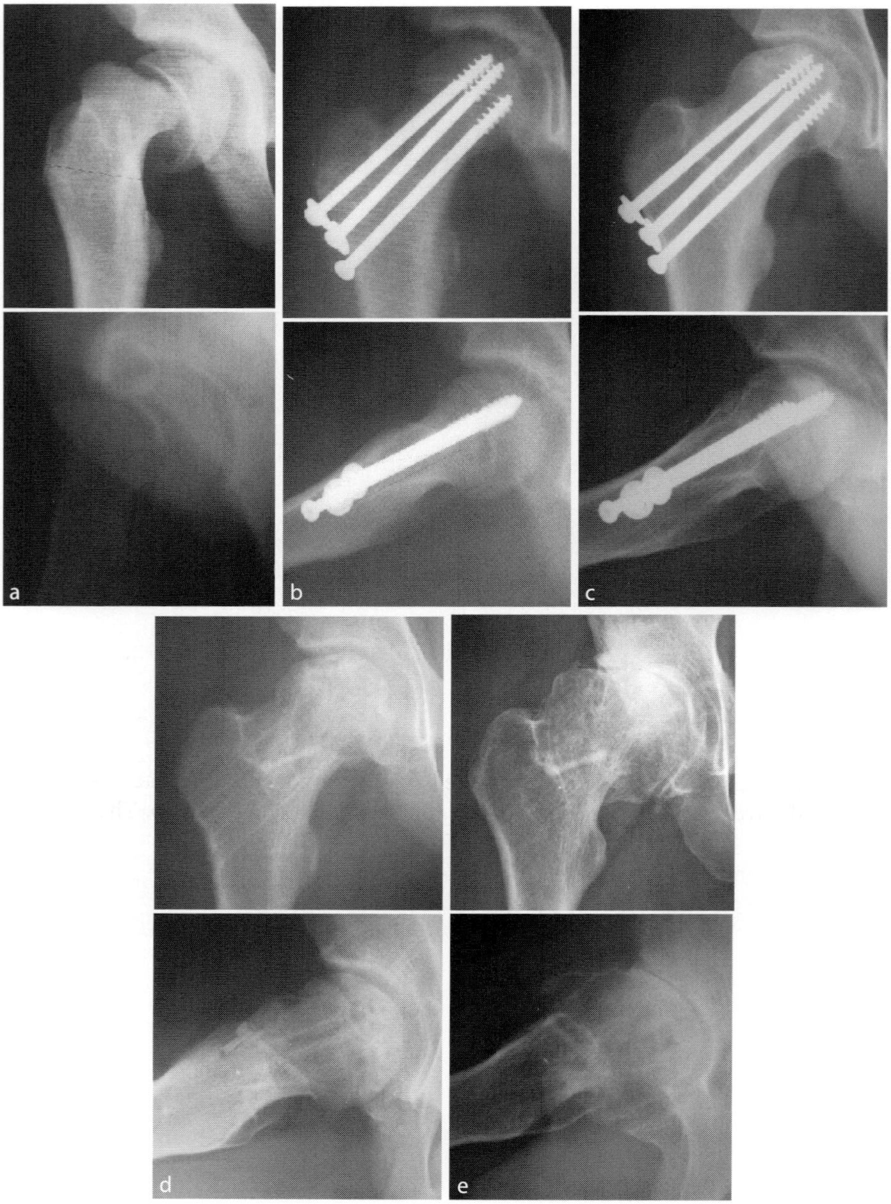

FIG. 3. Case 3. Acute SCFE in a 13-year-old boy with PTA of 85° (**a**). We performed epiphysiodesis with cannulated screw fixation, PTA was 18° (**b**). We observed flattening of the lateral femoral head (**c**). We removed the screws 2 years postoperatively and performed strut allograft bone grafting (**d**). At follow-up at 20 years, he could walk without pain but had developed a femoral head deformity (**e**)

Discussion

For treatment, epiphysiodesis such as in situ pinning was performed for a slight slip of less than 30°. For a more than moderate slip, in situ pinning, rotational Sugioka osteotomy, three-dimensional Southwick osteotomy, Imhauser osteotomy, or a subcapital osteotomy was performed [1–3].

The strategy of treatment for SCFE in our institution for acute or acute on chronic SCFE is to reduce the slip slowly by skeletal traction. After reduction and stabilization, we perform epiphysiodesis by pinning. We do not perform invasive manipulative reduction because that could lead to avascular necrosis of the femoral head. For chronic SCFE, we perform in situ pinning or an osteotomy, depending on the degree of slip. When the preoperative PTA is less than 30° in slip, we perform epiphysiodesis by in situ pinning. When the PTA is 30° to 50°, or moderate slip, we perform a valgus flexion osteotomy, and when the PTA is more than 50° in slip, we perform ARO (Fig. 4) [4].

Regarding prophylactic fixation of the unaffected side, Hotokebuchi and Sugioka [5] and Kato et al. [6] reported that prophylactic nailing is not necessary in the absence of a basal disease such as an endocrine disease, in which case observation alone is sufficient. In addition, Iga et al. [7] showed that unaffected-side fixation should be performed for all cases regardless of the amount of slip, whether acute or chronic. Kita et al. [8] performed internal fixation for prevention for the unaffected side when the affected side was highly suspected of avascular necrosis, or when there was a patient they could not observe sufficiently, or if the patient was suffering from remarkable obesity or endocrinopathy. Castro et al. [9] reported that the risk of iatrogenic chondrolysis and avascular necrosis might outweigh the benefits of prophylactic pinning of the contralateral hip. We have always considered bilateral slip a high risk and have been concerned about the contralateral side of the slip. Therefore, we have performed prophylactic fixation of the unaffected side for all patients since 1985. However, there are not many cases of bilateral slips. Therefore, we have recently changed our strategy to do a cross follow-up with a prophylactic fixation.

As reported by Itoman [4] and Sofue et al. [1], the incidence factors of avascular necrosis of the femoral head involve acute slip, manual reduction, capital osteotomy,

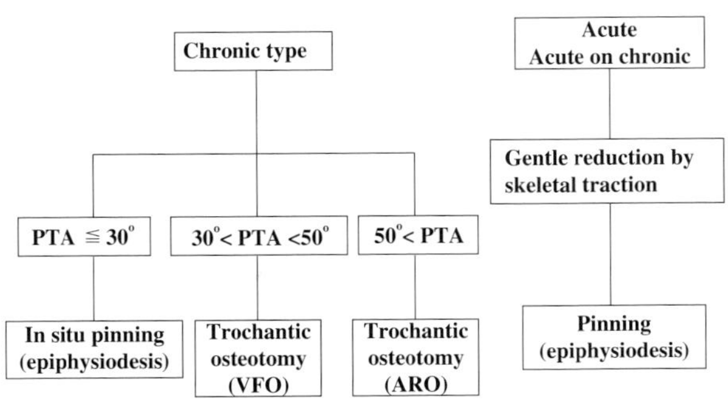

FIG. 4. Strategy of our treatment for SCFE. *VFO*, valgus flexion osteotomy; *ARO*, anterior rotational osteotomy; *PTA*, posterior tilting angle

and open reduction. Reduction could be problematical in that it could damage a nutrient vessel of the femoral head during the procedure or lead to reslipping; however, even manual reduction under general anesthesia is not necessarily a prophylaxis for this risk. Kita et al. [8] reported that it is extremely important to immediately reduce dislocation of unstable persistent nutrient vessels as a prophylactic measure. Manual repositioning may be chosen for cases of femoral head mobility. Otani et al. [10] reported that the necessity of manual reduction is relevant to prophylaxis, which is done to remove pressure and torsion of the epiphyseal nutrient vessels by performing anatomical reduction of the epiphysis in the unstable type of SCFE. In Kitasato University Hospital, avascular necrosis of the femoral head as a postoperative complication was noted in seven hips (24.1%). Even though gentle skeletal traction and fixation were performed to avoid the invasiveness of manual reduction, there was high risk of avascular necrosis of the femoral head. We conjectured that a nutrient vessel to the femoral head had already been damaged before the patient arrived at the hospital. Considering this type of prophylaxis, it may be beneficial to the evaluation to do a cross follow-up using magnetic resonance imaging (MRI), although we did not perform an MRI. If necrosis occurs, we apply a long leg brace and perform a bone graft to reestablish the blood supply, and it is naturally important to prevent a collapse of the femoral head.

Conclusion

For acute SCFE, we perform gentle reduction by traction and epiphysiodesis. For chronic slips, we perform epiphysiodesis or osteotomy. Opinions remain divided concerning prophylactic fixation of the unaffected side; however, we consider observation sufficient. The postoperative complication rate was higher in acute slips. Avascular necrosis of the femoral head is caused by failure of the remaining capital nutrient vessels. It is necessary to perform anatomical reduction of the epiphysis. Therefore, prophylaxis is indispensable to prevent avascular necrosis. In future reports, we will include many more cases with these procedures focusing on improved results and patient benefits.

References

1. Sofue M, Hatakeyama S, Endo N, et al (2005) Imhauser's three-dimensional osteotomy for slipped capital femoral epiphysis. J Joint Surg 24:762–768
2. Southwick WO (1967) Osteotomy through the lesser trochanter for slipped capital femoral epiphysis. J Bone Joint Surg [Am] 49:807–835
3. Sugioka Y, Eguchi M, Kaibara N, et al (1976) Transtrochanteric anterior rotation osteotomy of the femoral head for idiopathic avascular necrosis in adults. Hip Joint 2:23–32
4. Itoman M (1989) Epiphysiodesis for slipped capital femoral epiphysis. J Joint Surg 8:1637–1644
5. Hotokebuchi T, Sugioka Y (1995) Anterior rotational osteotomy for slipped capital femoral epiphysis. Orthop Surg Traumatol 38:639–644
6. Kato Y, Sato M, Umemura M (2002) The study of prophylactic pinning of the contralateral hip in slipped capital femoral epiphysis. Orthop Surg 53:512–516

7. Iga T, Sofue M, Endo N (2003) Slipped capital femoral epiphysis. New Mook of Orthopedics, No 13. Kanehara, Tokyo, pp 77–84
8. Kita A, Maeda S, Funayama K, et al (1995) Indication and procedure of manual reduction and subcapital osteotomy for slipped capital femoral epiphysis. Orthop Surg Trauma 38:631–638
9. Castro FP Jr, Bennett JT, Doulens K (2000) Epidemiological perspective on prophylactic pinning in patients with unilateral slipped capital femoral epiphysis. J Pediatr Orthop 20:745–748
10. Otani T, Fujii K, Tanaka T, et al (2004) Clinical result of closed manipulative reduction for acute-unstable slipped capital femoral epiphysis. Orthop Surg 55:771–777

Indications for Simple Varus Intertrochanteric Osteotomy for the Treatment of Osteonecrosis of the Femoral Head

Hiroshi Ito[1], Teruhisa Hirayama[1], Hiromasa Tanino[1], Takeo Matsuno[1], and Akio Minami[2]

Summary. The purpose of this study was to evaluate the long-term results of simple varus intertrochanteric osteotomy for osteonecrosis of the femoral head. Forty hips in 31 patients were included, with an average age at the time of surgery of 34 years (range, 21–51 years). The mean duration of follow-up was 12.1 years (range, 5–23 years). Osteonecrosis was high-dose-steroid-induced in 20 patients, alcohol-induced in 7 patients, and idiopathic in 4 patients. The amount of varus correction ranged from 15° to 40° (mean, 23°). The JOA hip score increased from a preoperative average of 71 points to 85 points at the most recent follow-up. Thirty (75%) of the 40 hips showed good or excellent results, 10 (25%) hips had fair or poor results, and 4 hips needed prosthetic arthroplasty. In 28 hips with equal to or greater than 25% postoperative lateral head index, 24 (86%) hips showed good or excellent results. Average shortening of leg length was 1.8 cm. Our findings indicate that if necrotic lesions are limited medially and the lateral part of the femoral head remains intact, good long-term results can be obtained by simple varus osteotomy.

Key words. Osteonecrosis of the femoral head, Varus intertrochanteric osteotomy, Long-term clinical results, Lateral head index, Joint-preserving operation

Introduction

The treatment of osteonecrosis of the femoral head is clinically challenging. The extent and location of the necrotic lesion affect the prognosis of osteonecrosis [1–4]. Many studies have shown that the prognosis of this disease without treatment is poor [1–5]. It is important to preserve the hip joint, especially for young and active patients. Total hip arthroplasty in young patients is undesirable because of its limited endurance [6,7]. Joint-preserving procedures include core decompression [8,9], femoral osteotomies [1,8,10–27], and vascularized or nonvascularized bone grafting

[1] Department of Orthopaedic Surgery, Asahikawa Medical College, Midorigaoka Higashi 2-1-1-1, Asahikawa 078-8510, Japan

[2] Department of Orthopaedic Surgery, Hokkaido University School of Medicine, Kita-ku Kita-15 Nishi-7, Sapporo 060-8638, Japan

[8,20,22,28]. The purpose of osteotomy for osteonecrosis of the femoral head is to move the necrotic lesions away from the weight-bearing portions of the hip joint. The lesions of the weight-bearing portions should then be replaced by normal articular cartilage and subchondral bone by osteotomy [1,8,10–27]. Many studies have examined the usefulness of various types of osteotomies for the treatment of osteonecrosis of the femoral head. Results of varus intertrochanteric osteotomies have been reported with various failure rates.

The purpose of this study was to evaluate the long-term results of simple varus intertrochanteric osteotomy for osteonecrosis of the femoral head.

Materials and Methods

From January 1979 we performed simple varus intertrochanteric osteotomies for the treatment of osteonecrosis of the femoral head; 40 hips in 31 patients (20 men and 11 women) were included in this study. Average age at the time of surgery was 34 years (range, 21–51 years), and the mean duration of follow-up was 12.1 years (range, 5–23 years). The diagnosis of osteonecrosis was made based on the clinical history, physical examination, and radiologic evaluation. Osteonecrosis was high-dose-steroid-induced in 20 patients, alcohol-induced in 7 patients, and idiopathic in 4 patients. All 31 patients complained of hip pain while walking at the time of operation. No previous operative treatment was performed in any hips. To be considered for osteotomy, the patients had to show a hip movement range of at least 90° for the flexion-extension arc and 25° for abduction. Ten hips were stage II, 27 hips were stage III, and 3 hips were stage IV according to the Steinberg classification [29]. From 1985 on, we used magnetic resonance (MR) imaging to confirm the diagnosis.

Surgical Technique

The patient was positioned in the lateral decubitus position with the extremity draped free on the table. Using a longitudinal lateral approach, a 15-cm incision was made from the greater trochanter distally along the femur shaft, exposing the lesser trochanter and lateral surface of the femur shaft. Capsulotomy was not performed in any patients. Two Kirschner wires were inserted as osteotomy guides (Fig. 1A); one was placed perpendicular to the femur shaft, the other was placed in the direction for the seating chisel, and intraoperative fluoroscopy was used to confirm the chisel position and the amount of varus correction. From the lateral cortex of the medial lesser trochanter, osteotomy was performed using a power saw (Fig. 1B). A wedge-shaped bony fragment was resected from the proximal fragment (Fig. 1C). For fixation of proximal and distal fragments, an AO 90° double-angle blade-plate was used (Fig. 1D). The amount of varus correction ranged from 15° to 40° (mean, 23°). Flexion and extension correction was not generally taken into account, and only simple varus correction was performed. Osteotomy was designed to gain 25% or more on the postoperative lateral head index (LHI) by radiography (Fig. 2) [18].

Postoperative Treatment

All patients began straight leg-lifting excises from the day after surgery and used wheelchairs for 4 weeks. Partial weight-bearing was started 4 to 6 weeks after the

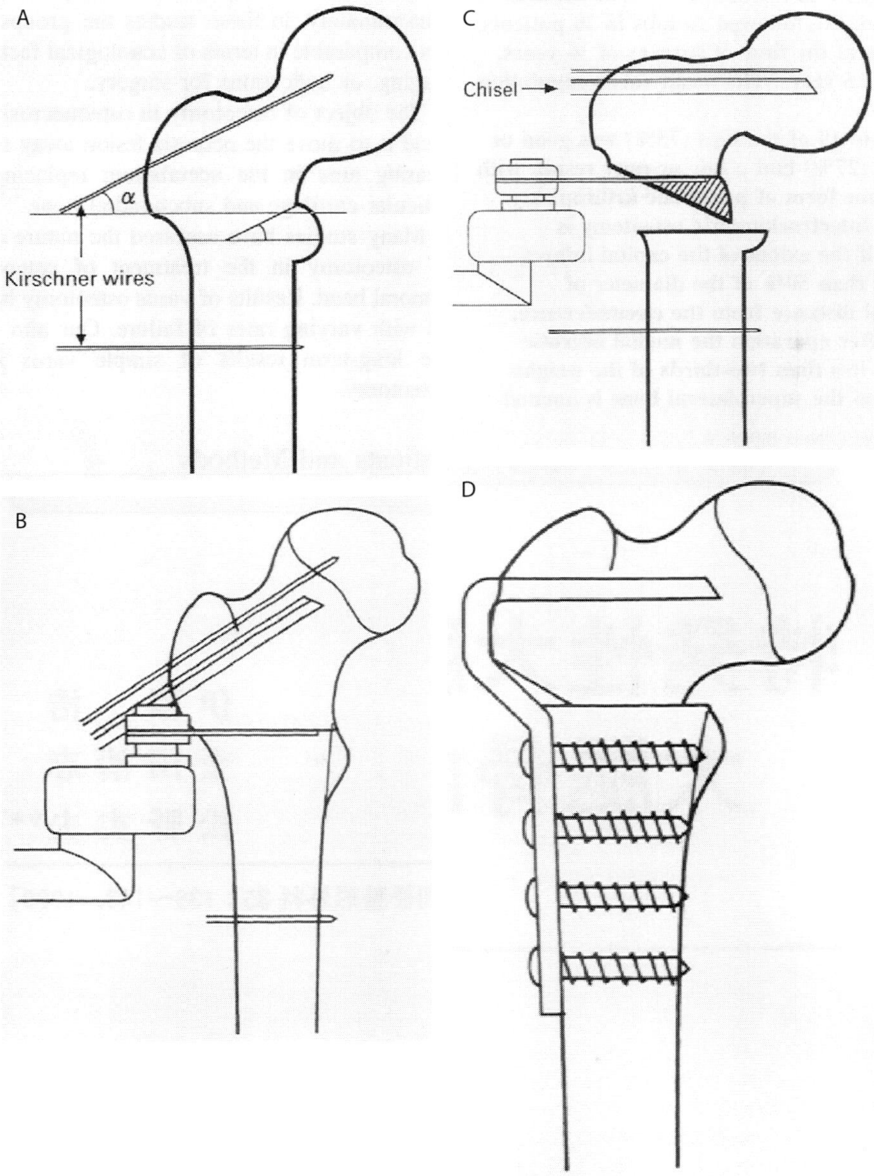

FIG. 1. Technique of simple varus osteotomy using intraoperative radiography or fluoroscopy. **A** Kirschner wires were inserted as osteotomy guides. *Angle* α was the preoperatively planned varus correction angle. **B** After insertion of the *chisel*, perpendicular osteotomy was performed using a power saw from the lateral cortex of the medial lesser trochanter. **C** Proximal osteotomy was performed, by which the half-wedged fragment was resected. **D** An AO 90° double-angle blade-plate was used for fixation of the proximal and distal fragment

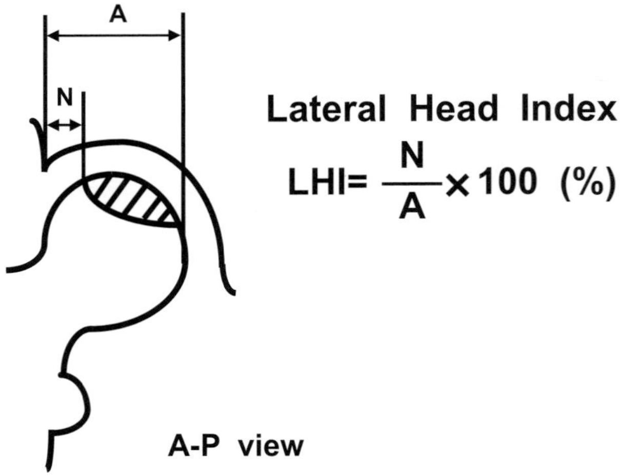

FIG. 2. Lateral head index (*LHI*) value. *A-P*, anteroposterior

operation with two crutches. Full weight-bearing was usually allowed 8 to 12 weeks after the operation. The average hospitalization was 3 months. The patients were encouraged to use two crutches to prevent injury 3 to 4 months postoperatively.

Evaluation

Clinical evaluation was performed according to the Japanese Orthopaedic Association (JOA) hip scoring system. Hips with a score of 90 to 100 points were defined as showing excellent results, 80 to 89 points as good results, 70 to 79 points as fair results, and less than 70 points as poor results. Statistical analysis of the data was performed by the Mann–Whitney *U* test and the Fisher's exact probability test. Probability values less than 0.05 were considered significant.

Results

The result was excellent in 10 hips, good in 20, fair in 6 hips, and poor in 4. Overall, 30 (75%) of the 40 hips showed good or excellent results (Figs. 3, 4). Three hips needed total hip arthroplasty and 1 hip needed hemiprosthetic arthroplasty. The JOA hip score increased from a preoperative average of 71 points (range, 28–78 points) to 85 points (range, 50–100 points) at the most recent follow-up. Progression of collapse was found in 9 (23%) hips. The average postoperative LHI was 48% in the excellent or good groups and 23% in the fair or poor groups (Mann–Whitney *U* test, $P = 0.001$). In 28 hips with equal to or greater than 25% of postoperative LHI, 24 (86%) hips showed good or excellent results.

Complications

There were no intraoperative complications. Two patients showed non-union of the osteotomy site. One patient underwent reoperation 1 year after the initial osteotomy

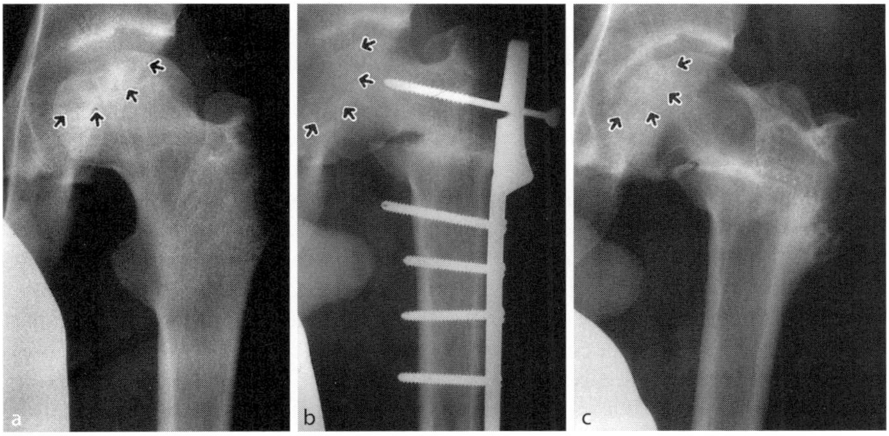

Fig. 3. Radiographic findings of a 47-year-old man with steroid-induced osteonecrosis of the right hip. **a** An anteroposterior view showing stage II osteonecrosis (*arrows*). The LHI was 23%. **b** Radiography after a 23° simple varus osteotomy fixed with an AO double-angle blade-plate. The postoperative LHI was 70%. **c** Radiography 16 years after osteotomy. Reduction in the size of necrotic lesions was found (*arrows*), and the clinical result was excellent

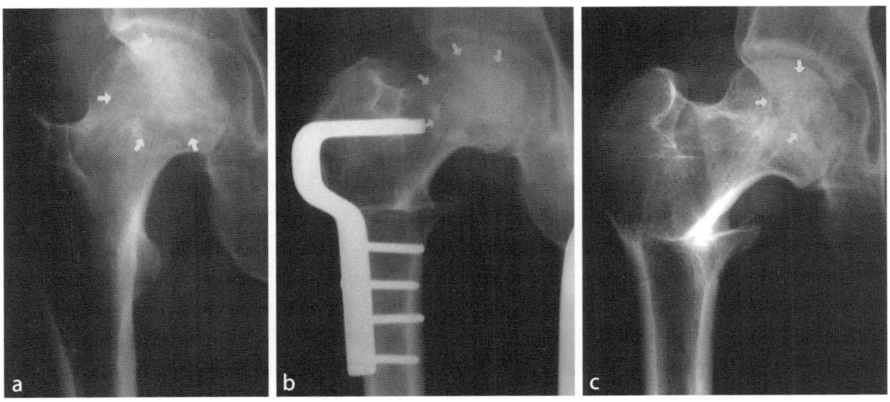

Fig. 4. Radiographic findings of a 27-year-old man with steroid-induced osteonecrosis of the left hip. **a** The LHI was 20% and the superolateral portion of the femoral head remained normal (*arrows*). **b** Radiography after 35° simple varus osteotomy fixed with a Wainwright–Hammond plate. Postoperative LHI was 37%. **c** Radiography 15 years after the osteotomy. The patient reported no hip pain; however, a limp due to limb shortening was observed

with placement of a bone graft that later showed radiographic union. One patient needed total hip arthroplasty. An average shortening of the leg length was 1.8 cm (range, 1.0–3.5 cm). In the group of 6 hips with varus correction greater than 25°, the rate of limping at the final outcome (4 of 6) was significantly higher than that of the remaining 34 hips with varus correction less than 25° (6 of 34) (Fisher's exact test, $P < 0.03$). There were no other significant complications such as deep infection or pulmonary embolism.

Discussion

Several studies have advocated varus intertrochanteric osteotomy in hips in which a lateral intact area of the femoral head can be placed into the acetabular weight-bearing portion by osteotomy [1,14,15,19–21]. Kerboul et al. [15] emphasized that the purpose of osteotomy was to remove the necrotic part of the femoral head from the zone of maximum pressure and to replace it with the normal posterolateral part. They reported that when the superolateral and posterior surfaces of the femoral head remained normal, good results were obtained. Our findings indicate that if necrotic lesions are limited medially and the lateral part of the femoral head remains intact, good long-term results can be obtained by simple varus osteotomy, which supports the results of Kerboul et al. [15].

Excessive varus correction is related to a high incidence of postoperative limp because of abductor muscle weakness and limb shortening. Jacobs et al. [14] reported that the results of intertrochanteric osteotomies were closely related to the size of the necrotic lesions and a relatively high incidence of limp in the varus osteotomy patients. Sakano et al. [21] reported good clinical results using Nishio's curved intertrochanteric varus osteotomy. Our results indicated that excessive varus correction should be avoided and that the correction angle should be planned up to 25°. In hips with correction angles within 25°, postoperative limp was sometimes found several months after the osteotomy, but this usually improved within 1 or 2 years.

Sugioka reported a technique of transtrochanteric anterior rotational osteotomy for osteonecrosis in 1978. Successful results by this technique were described by several other Japanese surgeons [10,18,23]. In the United States, however, successful results were not obtained with this technique [11,12,13]. Sugioka's osteotomy has sometimes been described as a technically demanding procedure [11–13,19]. Atsumi et al. [10] emphasized the importance of the postoperative varus position rather than the valgus position and described their technique of posterior rotational osteotomy and excellent results.

In the surgical technique of intertrochanteric osteotomy, it is often difficult to obtain precise correction angles as preoperatively planned. Kerboul et al. [15] reported that the angulation after osteotomy was exactly as planned in 45% of the operations, but only approximately so in the remaining cases. Varus-valgus angulation correction is relatively easy by measuring the angle of the guided Kirschner wires in relation to the femur shaft. Flexion-extension correction is sometimes difficult because the intra-operative lateral views of intertrochanteric regions are sometimes slightly oblique when the patient is in the operative lateral decubitus position, and corrective guides such as Kirschner wires on the true lateral view sometimes do not depict true flexion-extension correction angles. We therefore prefer simple varus osteotomy in which flexion-extension correction does not have to be considered.

In the radiographic follow-up, a demarcation line and sclerotic change in the necrotic area were found during the follow-up period in successfully treated hips. Demarcation lines and sclerotic changes in the necrotic lesions that gradually reduce in size represent the repair process of osteonecrosis. Sugioka et al. [24] reported that necrosis can heal when mechanical stress is withdrawn from the necrotic lesion. Varus intertrochanteric osteotomy may be indicated if the intact area occupies a larger area in the superolateral portion, an assertion that coincides with the findings of the present study.

In conclusion, hips with a small-to-medium necrotic lesion, a medial necrotic location, postoperative LHI greater than 25%, and a thick demarcation line seen on radiography with sclerotic change in the necrotic lesion are the best indications for osteotomy.

References

1. Merle d'Aubigné R, Postel M, Mazabraud A, et al (1965) Idiopathic necrosis of the femoral head in adults. J Bone Joint Surg 47B:612–633
2. Ohzono K, Saito M, Takaoka K, et al (1991) Natural history of nontraumatic avascular necrosis of the femoral head. J Bone Joint Surg 73B:68–72
3. Shimizu K, Moriya H, Akita T, et al (1994) Prediction of collapse with magnetic resonance imaging of avascular necrosis of the femoral head. J Bone Joint Surg 76A:215–223
4. Takatori Y, Kokubo T, Ninomiya S, et al (1993) Avascular necrosis of the femoral head: natural history and magnetic resonance imaging. J Bone Joint Surg 75B:217–221
5. Musso ES, Mitchell SN, Schink-Ascani M, et al (1986) Results of conservative management of osteonecrosis of the femoral head: a retrospective review. Clin Orthop 207:209–215
6. Cornell CN, Salvati EA, Pellicci PM (1985) Long-term follow-up of total hip replacement in patients with osteonecrosis. Orthop Clin N Am 16:757–769
7. Dorr LD, Takei GK, Conaty JP (1983) Total hip arthroplasties in patients less than forty-five years old. J Bone Joint Surg 65A:474–479
8. Mont MA, Hungerford DS (1995) Non-traumatic avascular necrosis of the femoral head. J Bone Joint Surg 77A:459–474.
9. Fairbank AC, Bhatia D, Jinnah RH, et al (1995) Long-term results of core decompression for ischaemic necrosis of the femoral head. J Bone Joint Surg 77B:42–49
10. Atsumi T, Kuroki Y (1997) Modified Sugioka's osteotomy: more than 130° posterior rotation for osteonecrosis of the femoral head with large lesion. Clin Orthop 334: 98–107
11. Dean MT, Cabanela ME (1993) Transtrochanteric anterior rotational osteotomy for avascular necrosis of the femoral head: long-term results. J Bone Joint Surg 75B: 597–601
12. Eyb R, Kotz R (1987) The transtrochanteric anterior rotational osteotomy of Sugioka. Early and late results in idiopathic aseptic femoral head necrosis. Arch Orthop Trauma Surg 106:161–167
13. Tooke SMT, Amstutz HC, Hedley AK (1987) Results of transtrochanteric rotational osteotomy for femoral head osteonecrosis. Clin Orthop 224:150–157
14. Jacobs MA, Hungerford DS, Krackow KA (1989) Intertrochanteric osteotomy for avascular necrosis of the femoral head. J Bone Joint Surg 71B:200–204
15. Kerboul M, Thomine J, Postel M, et al (1974) The conservative surgical treatment of idiopathic aseptic necrosis of the femoral head. J Bone Joint Surg 56B:291–296
16. Maistrelli G, Fusco U, Avai A, et al (1988) Osteonecrosis of the hip treated by intertrochanteric osteotomy: a four- to 15-year follow-up. J Bone Joint Surg 70B:761–766
17. Marti RK, Schüller HM, Raaymakers ELFB (1989) Intertrochanteric osteotomy for non-union of the femoral neck. J Bone Joint Surg 71B:782–787
18. Masuda T, Matsuno T, Hasegawa I, et al (1988) Results of transtrochanteric rotational osteotomy for nontraumatic osteonecrosis of the femoral head. Clin Orthop 228: 69–74

19. Mont MA, Fairbank AC, Krackow KA, et al (1996) Corrective osteotomy for osteonecrosis of the femoral head: the results of a long-term follow-up study. J Bone Joint Surg 78A:1032–1038
20. Saito S, Ohzono K, Ono K (1988) Joint-preserving operations for idiopathic avascular necrosis of the femoral head: results of core decompression, grafting, and osteotomy. J Bone Joint Surg 70B:78–84
21. Sakano S, Hasegawa Y, Torii Y, et al (2004) Curved intertrochanteric varus osteotomy for osteonecrosis of the femoral head. J Bone Joint Surg 86B:359–365
22. Scher MA, Jakim I (1993) Intertrochanteric osteotomy and autogenous bone-grafting for avascular necrosis of the femoral head. J Bone Joint Surg 75A:1119–1133
23. Sugano N, Takaoka K, Ohzono K, et al (1992) Rotational osteotomy for non-traumatic avascular necrosis of the femoral head. J Bone Joint Surg 74B:734–739
24. Sugioka Y, Hotokebuchi T, Tsutsui H (1992) Transtrochanteric anterior rotational osteotomy for idiopathic and steroid-induced necrosis of the femoral head: indications and long-term results. Clin Orthop 277:111–120
25. Sugioka Y, Katsuki I, Hotokebuchi T (1982) Transtrochanteric rotational osteotomy of the femoral head for the treatment of osteonecrosis: follow-up statistics. Clin Orthop 169:115–126
26. Wagner H, Zeiler G (1981) Segmental idiopathic necrosis of the femoral head. Springer-Verlag, Berlin, pp 87–116
27. Willert HG, Buchhorn G, Zichner L (1981) Segmental idiopathic necrosis of the femoral head. Springer-Verlag, Berlin, pp 63–80
28. Urbaniak JR, Coogan PG, Gunneson EB, et al (1995) Treatment of osteonecrosis of the femoral head with free vascularized fibular grafting: a long-term follow-up study of one hundred and three hips. J Bone Joint Surg 77A:681–694
29. Steinberg ME, Hayken GD, Steinberg DR (1995) A quantitative system for staging avascular necrosis. J Bone Joint Surg 77B:34–41

Transtrochanteric Rotational Osteotomy for Severe Slipped Capital Femoral Epiphysis

Satoshi Nagoya, Mitsunori Kaya, Mikito Sasaki,
Hiroki Kuwabara, Tomonori Iwasaki, and Toshihiko Yamashita

Summary. We performed transtrochanteric rotational osteotomy to treat severe slipped capital femoral epiphysis in four young patients. All four male patients, with an age range of 12–22 years, were followed for an average of 2 years and 10 months. The JOA score of 37 points preoperatively improved to an average of 90 points postoperatively. The posterior tilt angle (PTA) of 82° preoperatively improved to an average of 24° postoperatively. The flexion angle of the affected hip joint in neutral improved from 10°–25° to 70°–90°. Although one patient with acute on chronic type of SCFE developed osteonecrosis of the femoral head after the operation, the function of the hip joint was restored. Our results suggest that transtrochanteric rotational osteotomy is a valuable option for the treatment of severe slipped capital femoral epiphysis in young patients.

Key words. Transtrochanteric rotational osteotomy (TRO), Slipped capital femoral epiphysis, Posterior tilt angle

Introduction

The rationale of treatment for slipped capital femoral epiphysis (SCFE) is prevention of deterioration of slip angle and restoration of the range of motion in young patients. However, it is difficult to treat severe slipping greater than 70°. We have employed transtrochanteric rotational osteotomy (TRO) with varus angulation for such severe cases. The aim of this study is to report the clinical results and to clarify the usefulness of this procedure for severe SCFE.

Materials and Methods

Since 1996, 19 consecutive patients with SCFE were treated in our department. TRO with varus angulation was applied for patients with severe slipping greater than 70°. All patients were male; age at operation ranged from 12 to 22 years. A 22-year-old

Department of Orthopedic Surgery, Sapporo Medical University, South 1 West 16 Chuo-ku, Sapporo 060-8543, Japan

man developed SCFE secondary to hypopituitarism. Three patients were categorized to chronic type, and 1 patient was acute on chronic type. To evaluate the severity of posterior shifting of the femoral head, we used posterior tilt angle (PTA), which is an angle between the epiphyseal line and a line perpendicular to the femoral shaft axis (Fig. 1). PTA in the lateral view was 70°–89° preoperatively. Hip flexion angle was 10°–25°, and Drehmann sign was positive in all cases before surgery. All patients needed a relatively long time interval to obtain an adequate diagnosis from initial onset of the symptoms because of late consultation with an orthopedic surgeon.

The operative procedure is determined according to PTA. For a PTA less than 40°, we used in situ pinning with screws. Three-dimensional corrective femoral osteotomy, such as the Southwick osteotomy [1], is employed when the PTA is between 40° and 70°. When the PTA exceeds 70°, we need to lift up the slipped epiphysis to the weight-bearing rim by anterior rotation of the femoral head in TRO. Because anterior rotation results in valgus position of the femoral head, we need to apply varus angulation simultaneously.

The operation was performed according to Sugioka's femoral osteotomy [2] with anterior rotation of 60°–70° and varus angulation of 40° (Fig. 2A,B). After 2 days bed rest, wheelchair transfer was prescribed, and partial weight-bearing was allowed 8 weeks after operation; full-weight bearing was then permitted after 4 months. Bone scintigraphy was planned 1 week after the operation to confirm that the blood supply was preserved in the rotated femoral head.

The Japanese Orthopedic Association (JOA) score was used to evaluate the clinical results. Complications such as infection, deep venous thrombosis, pulmonary embolism, massive bleeding, and nerve palsy were investigated.

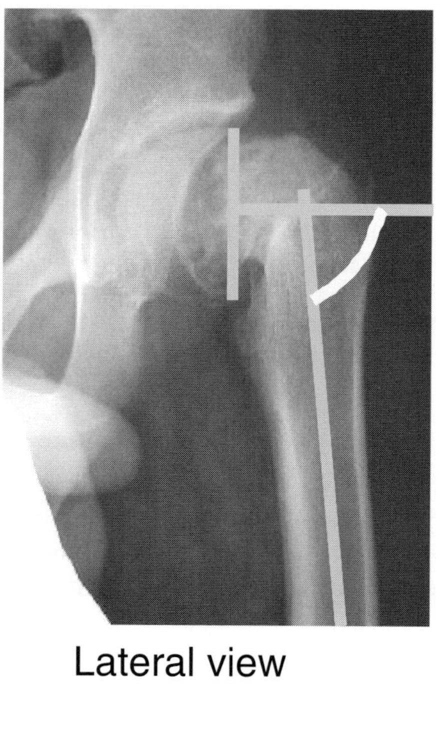

Fig. 1. Radiograph shows the posterior tilt angle (PTA), an angle between a line perpendicular to the epiphyseal line and the femoral shaft axis

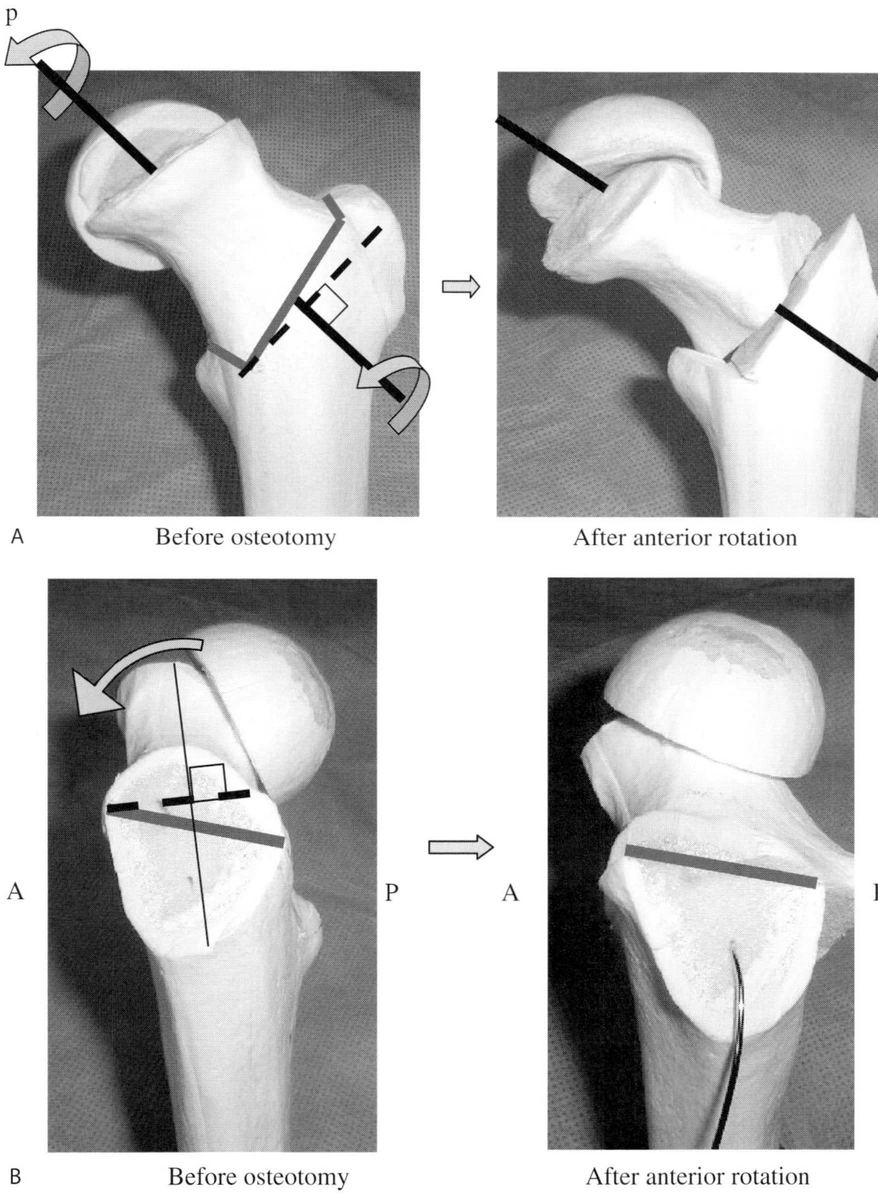

FIG. 2. **A** Anteroposterior (AP) view of left hip joint. *Solid line* indicates osteotomy line, which declined 20° varus to the line perpendicular to the femoral neck axis. **B** Lateral view of left hip joint. *Solid line* indicates osteotomy line, which declined 20° to the baseline perpendicular to the femoral neck axis. *Dashed line* indicates base line perpendicular to the femoral neck axis. *A*, anterior aspect; *P*, posterior aspect

Results

The JOA score of 37 points preoperatively improved to an average of 90 points postoperatively. The PTA of 82° preoperatively improved to an average of 24° postoperatively (Table 1). The flexion angle improved from 10°–25° to 70°–90° (Table 2). There was an average of leg discrepancy of 2–4 cm postoperatively. One patient had decreased blood supply of the femoral head detected in bone blood scintigraphy 1 week after operation, which resulted in partial osteonecrosis of the femoral head with segmental collapse (Fig. 3). There was no infection, deep venous thrombosis, pulmonary embolism, massive bleeding, or nerve palsy after the operations. Case 3 is a representative case (Fig. 4).

TABLE 1. Comparision of preoperative and postoperative posterior tiltangle (PTA)

Case	Preoperative (°)	Postoperative (°)
1	89	40
2	88	28
3	80	15
4	70	12
Average	82	24

TABLE 2. Restoration of range of motion (ROM) of the hip joint by the transtrachanteric rotational osteotomy (TRO)

Case number	Preoperative (°)	Postoperative (°)
1	10	70
2	15	80
3	30	80
4	45	100
Average	25	83

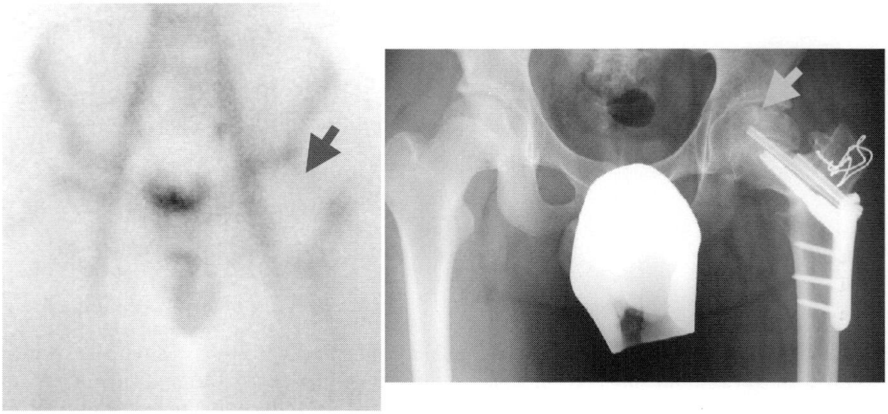

FIG. 3. Bone blood flow scintigraphy showing decreased blood supply in left femoral head of case 4 after TRO

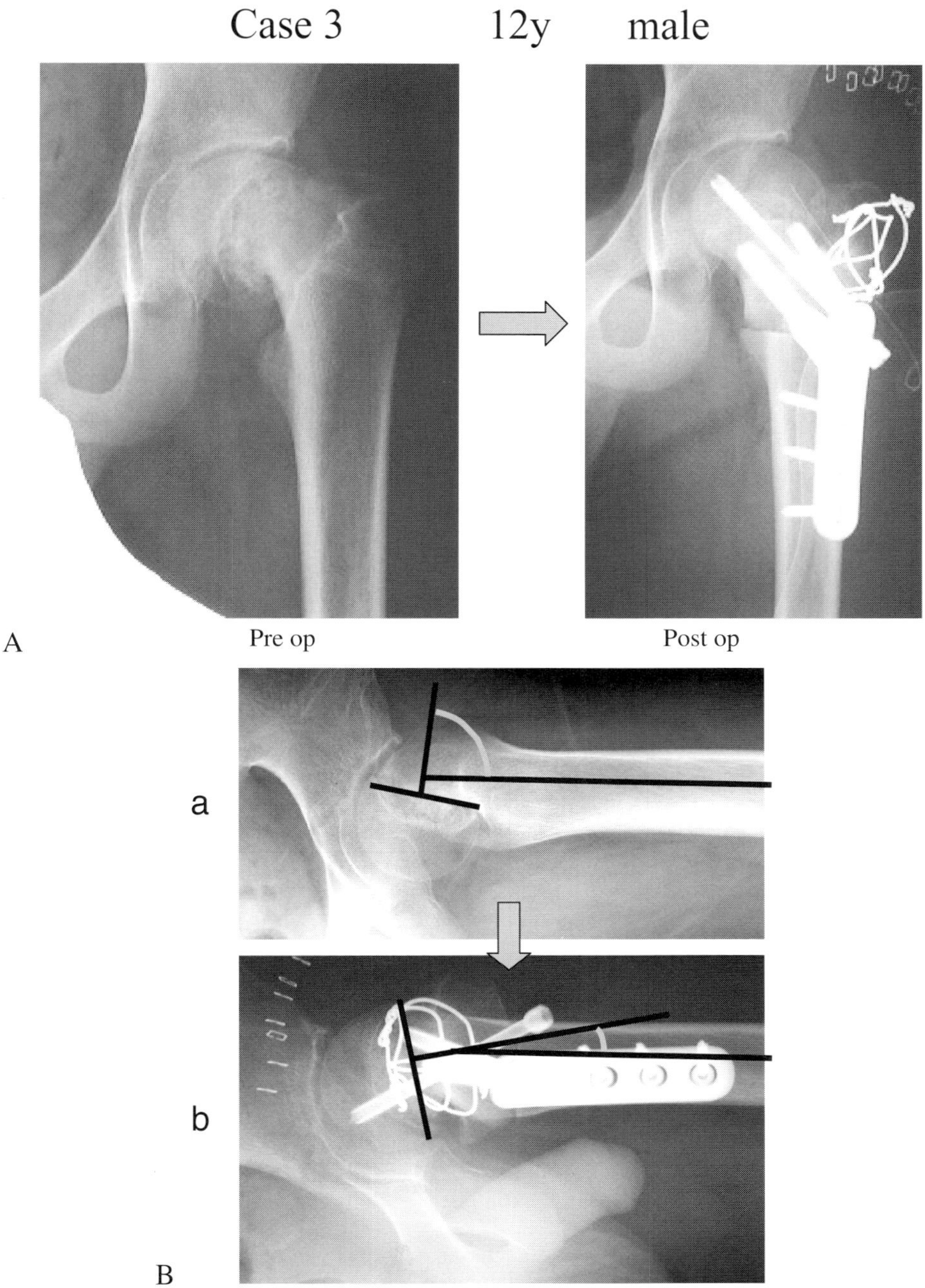

FIG. 4. **A** AP view of left hip joint before and after operation. **B** Radiograph shows severe slipped capital femoral epiphysis (SCFE) in case 3 with 80° of PTA (*a*). The configuration of the hip joint was successfully restored with 15° of PTA after the operation (*b*)

Discussion

In the natural history of untreated SCFE, more than one-third of severe cases develop end-stage degenerative arthritis of the hip joint [3]. An adequate surgical intervention might be required to prevent further joint destruction. The in situ pinning method is expected to prevent further slipping and restore the spherical shape of the femoral head in patients with PTA less than 30°. Three-dimensional corrective osteotomy [1] can be indicated for moderate cases with PTA less than 70°. However, because patients with severe slipping of femoral epiphysis have severe deformity of the femoral head and neck, sufficient correction is difficult to achieve. Several proximal osteotomies have been reported to be effective to correct slipped capital epiphysis [4,5]. TRO with varus angulation of the femoral head conferred restoration of configuration of the proximal femur and improvement of the range of flexion.

There are only a limited number of reports in which TRO was employed for the treatment of severe SCFE. Sugioka et al. [2] reported ten young patients with SCFE treated with TRO, and these patients had a good clinical course. In this series, five patients had severe SCFE with PTA greater than 70°. Masuda et al. [6] also reported that two of five cases treated with TRO had severe SCFE with PTA greater than 70°. Sugioka experienced one osteonecrosis of the femoral head, and Masuda et al. also had one case who developed osteonecrosis after the operation. We had one patient who developed osteonecrosis of the femoral head; bone scintigraphy indicated decreased blood supply to the bone 1 week after the operation. Because of the complicated technique of TRO, there may be a risk of some vascular problems of the femoral head. We, however, had confirmed that vascularity was preserved in the rotated femoral head during the operation. The other three patients without a necrotic event had the chronic type of SCFE. Because this patient with osteonecrosis had an acute on chronic type of SCFE, this may have led to osteonecrosis of the femoral head.

Although the treatment strategy for severe SCEF remains controversial, our results suggest that TRO is a valuable option for treating severe SCFE with little risk of osteonecrosis of the femoral head.

References

1. Southwick WO (1967) Osteotomy through the lesser trochanter for slipped capital femoral epiphysis. J Bone Joint Surg 49A:807–835
2. Sugioka Y (1984) Transtrochanteric rotational osteotomy in the treatment of idiopathic and steroid-induced femoral head necrosis, Perthes' disease, slipped capital femoral epiphysis, and osteoarthritis of the hip. Clin Orthop 184:12–23
3. Carney BT, Weinstein SL (1996) Natural history of untreated chronic slipped capital femoral epiphysis. Clin Orthop 322:43–47
4. Dunn DM (1978) Replacement of the femoral head by open operation in severe adolescent slipping of the upper femoral epiphysis. J Bone Joint Surg [Br] 60:394–403
5. Kramer WG, Craig WA, Noel S (1976) Compensating osteotomy at the base of the femoral neck for slipped capital femoral epiphysis. J Bone Joint Surg 58A:796–800
6. Masuda T, Matsuno T, Hasegawa I, et al (1986) Trochanteric anterior rotational osteotomy for slipped capital femoral epiphysis: a report of five cases. J Pediatr Orthop 6:18–23

Corrective Osteotomy with an Original Plate for Moderate Slipped Capital Femoral Epiphysis

Takahiko Kitakoji[1], Hiroshi Kitoh[2], Mitsuyasu Katoh[2], Tadashi Hattori[1], and Naoki Ishiguro[2]

Summary. We investigated, at skeletal maturity, the radiographic and clinical results of 20 patients with slipped capital femoral epiphysis (SCFE) who were treated by corrective osteotomy (CO). Mean age was 13.1 years at the time of operation and 19.8 years at the final examination. CO was performed by the intertrochanteric open-wedge method using an original plate without physeal fixation. The mean posterior tilt angle (PTA) was 47° before CO, 12° after CO, and 9° at the final examination, which indicated that 35° correction was obtained by CO and that this was maintained to skeletal maturity. Physeal closure was recognized in all cases without further slippage. Fifteen of the 20 patients had remodeling of the proximal femur according to the criteria of Jones et al. Six patients had very mild osteoarthritis (OA) changes according to the criteria of Boyer et al. at the final examination. Clinical results were also good with a low incidence of complications. We think that CO using the original plate is a useful method for moderate SCFE because its radiographic and clinical results are good with a simple technique. We emphasize the needlessness of physeal fixation at CO because natural physeal closure occurs without further slippage.

Key words. Slipped capital femoral epiphysis (SCFE), Corrective osteotomy (CO), Remodeling, Osteoarthritis (OA)

Introduction

There is still controversy about corrective osteotomy (CO) for slipped capital femoral epiphysis (SCFE). The location and method of osteotomy vary. Also, there is controversy about the necessity of physeal fixation for stabilization at the time of osteotomy. Of course, there is still also expansion of the indications for in situ pinning [1–5], and also the indications for pinning or osteotomy have not yet been clarified. In our institution, for moderate SCFE we have performed CO by the intertrochanteric open-wedge method using an original plate without physeal fixation. The purpose of this

[1] Department of Orthopaedic Surgery, Aichi Children's Health and Medical Center, 1-2 Osakada, Morioka-cho, Oobu, Aichi 474-8710, Japan
[2] Nagoya University School of Medicine, Nagoya, Japan

chapter is to investigate the radiographic and clinical results at skeletal maturity of SCFE patients treated by CO using the original plate.

Patients and Methods

From 1980 to 2000, 40 patients with SCFE were treated by CO using an original plate, and 20 of the 40 patients were followed up to bone maturity. The 20 patients were reviewed clinically and radiologically after an average follow-up of 6.7 years. The mean age was 13.1 years at the operation and 19.8 years at the final examination. There were 4 females and 16 males.

CO was performed by the intertrochanteric open-wedge method using the original plate without fixation of the capital femoral physis. The original plate, made from titanium, had 40° flexion and 15° inner rotation (Fig. 1). Accommodating to the original plate provided correction of posterior tilting deformity. Correction of varus deformity was possible by the blade insert angle; however, normally we produced slight valgus by inserting the blade into the axis of the femur vertically. There was of course a limitation of the correction angle because we corrected the deformity by accommodating to the plate. However, this technique was very simple, and certain correction was obtained (Fig. 2). For the opposite side, we performed prophylactic pinning; this was done when the case was diagnosed as preslippage on radiogram and the patient was obese or had an endocrine abnormality.

For the radiographic estimation, we measured the posterior tilt angle (PTA) before and after CO and at the final examination to clarify actual performance and maintenance of correction. Duration until union of osteotomy site and duration until physeal closure after surgery were also investigated. Remodeling after surgery was defined by Jones's classification [2]. In type A, the profile of the anterior head and neck was

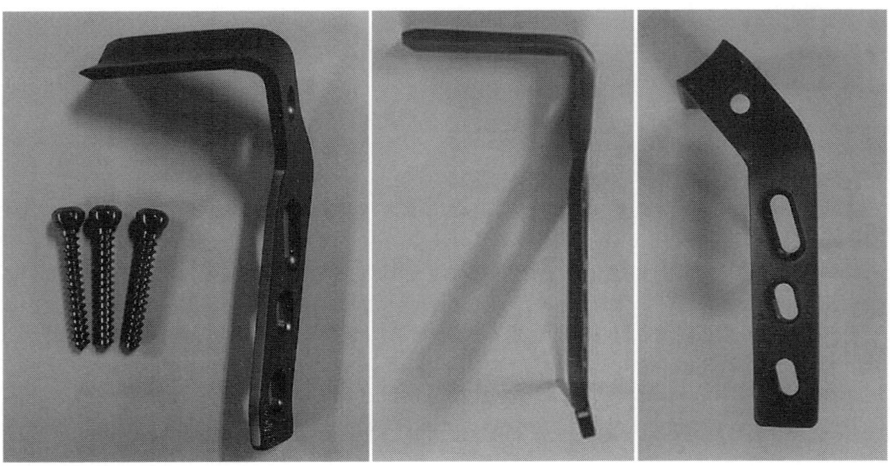

Fig. 1. An original plate for corrective osteotomy (CO) in the treatment of slipped capital femoral epiphysis (SCFE). The original plate is made from titanium and has 40° flexion and 15° internal rotation (Nagoya U. plate for SCFE, Mizuho, Tokyo, Japan)

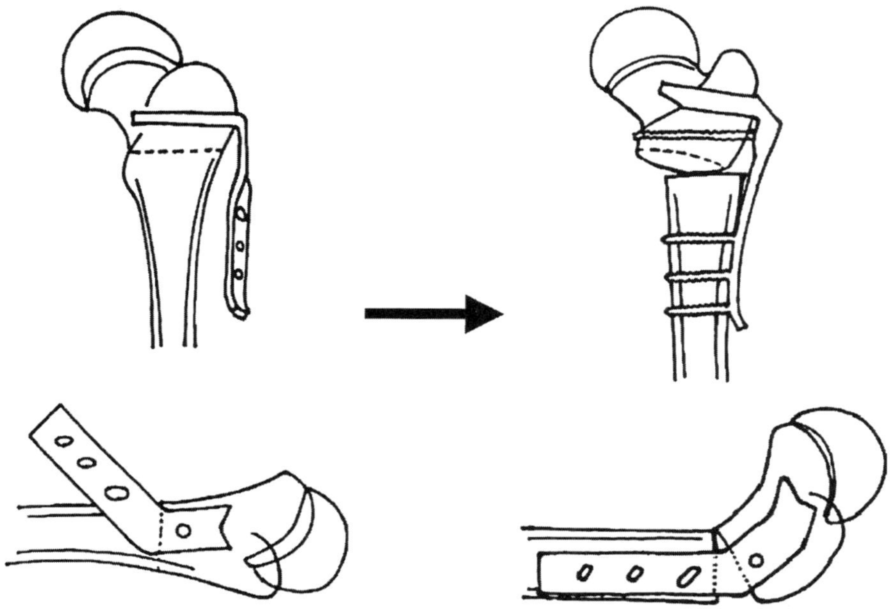

Fig. 2. Simple and certain correction with an original plate. Accommodating to the original plate provides correction of posterior tilting deformity. Varus deformity can be corrected by the blade insert angle; however, normally the blade is inserted into the axis of the femur vertically

normal with the convexity of the anterior margin of the femoral head running into a concavity, which was the anterior border of the neck; in type B, the anterior outline of the head and neck appeared as a straight line; and in type C, the profile was convex, the anterior margin of the femoral head being posterior to the anterior margin of the neck. Types A and B were defined as being remodeled and type C represented failure of remodeling. We also estimated changes in osteoarthritis from the radiogram at the time of final examination according to Boyer's classification: grade 0, no degenerative changes; grade I, no more than one subchondral cyst or one osteophyte, no bone sclerosis, and the joint space of normal width; grade II, one or a few subchondral cysts as well as osteophytes, minimum subchondral sclerosis, and slight joint space narrowing; and grade III, multiple subchondral cysts and osteophytes, with joint space narrowing [6].

As for the clinical results, we investigated pain, limping, range of hip motion, and leg length discrepancy (LLD) at the final examination. The presence of avascular necrosis and chondrolysis were also investigated as complications.

Results

Average PTA was 47° before the surgery, 12° after the surgery, and 9° at the final examination. A 35° correction was obtained on average by the surgery and was maintained after surgery to bone maturity. Average bone healing time is 5.6 months. Also, at the time of the osteotomy, we did not use physeal fixation; the physis was closed 16 months after surgery, on average, without having any further slippage.

According to Jones's classification, we classified 10 cases of type A, 5 cases of type B, and 5 cases of type C, and 15 of 20 cases were remodeled. Again, according to Boyer's classifications, we found 1 case of grade II with slight joint space narrowing, and this case had the complication of chondrolysis. We also found 5 cases of grade I with a few bone cysts or osteophytes. There was 1 case of chondrolysis; however, no case developed to avascular necrosis of the femoral head.

One case showed slight pain at the final examination, and five cases showed slight limping. Also, five cases showed limitation of internal rotation of more than 20°, and average LLD was 1.6 cm.

Case Presentation

A 12-year-old boy with hip pain on the right side presented to our hospital. Radiographic examination revealed slippage with 62° of PTA (Fig. 3a). Corrective osteotomy using the original plate without physeal fixation was performed, and PTA improved to 12°. Union of osteotomy site was achieved 4.5 months after the operation (Fig. 3b). Proximal femoral physeal closure on the right side was recognized without further slippage 18 months after the operation. At the age of 18, he had no limping,

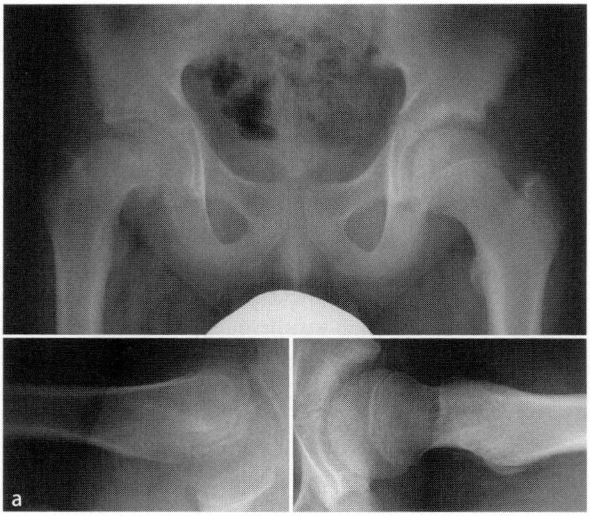

Fig. 3. A 12-year-old boy with SCFE on the right side treated by CO with an original plate. **a** Anteroposterior and lateral roentgenograms of both hips at presentation revealed slipping of the capital femoral epiphysis on the right side. Posterior tilt angle (PTA) was 62° on the right side. **b** Roentgenograms made 4.5 months after CO with an original plate showed union of the osteotomy site. PTA had improved to 12°. **c** Roentgenograms at the age of 18 showed the right hip joint was remodeled (type A according to Jones's classification), and it was classified as grade I osteoarthritis according to Boyer's classification

FIG. 3. *Continued*

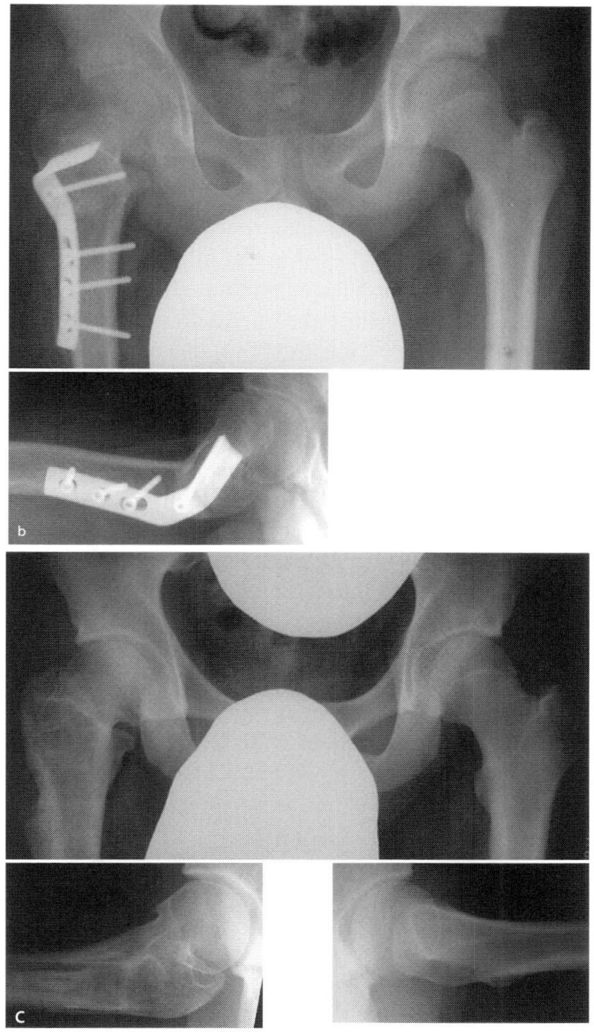

pain, or LLD. According to Jones's classification, his right hip was remodeled (type A), and according to Boyer's classification it was grouped into grade I with a few osteophytes (Fig. 3c).

Discussion

Location of proximal femoral osteotomies for SCFE was classified in three categories: subcapital, base of neck, and intertrochanteric [7]. The rate of complications such as chondrolysis or avascular necrosis is more or less directly related to the proximity of the osteotomy to the apex of the deformity, being highest for osteotomies at the apex (intracapsular in subcapital) and lowest for osteotomies performed extracapsularly in the intertrochanteric area. On the other hand, the greater the distance between the corrective osteotomy and the apex of deformity, the more severe the secondary compensating deformity will be, and the greater the difficulty of further reconstructive procedures, such as total joint arthroplasty. We always try to correct deformity at the intertrochanteric area because of lesser concern about complications.

Representative intertrochanteric osteotomies for SCFE are Southwick's and Imhaeuser's osteotomy [8,9]. We think these are good methods theoretically; however, the technique is complicated and not always easy to carry out. There is discrepancy between planning before the operation and radiograms after the operation in their procedures. So, we have done the simpler and more certain CO using an original plate. We think it is a useful method for moderate SCFE because the radiographic and clinical results at maturity are good, with a low incidence of complications. There is, of course, limitation of correction angle normally because we correct the deformity by accommodating to the plate; however, we believe perfect correction is not necessary. Fifteen of the 20 patients in this study had remodeling after the operation. We also emphasize the needlessness of the physeal fixation at CO as natural physeal closure occurs without further slippage. Physeal fusion is promoted by reorienting the plane of the capital physis into a more horizontal position [7].

There is still expansion of the indications for in situ pinning for SCFE [1–5], and also the indications for pinning or osteotomy for SCFE have not yet been made clear. Also, in our hospital, we expanded its indication in 1995, although it was PTA less than 30° until 1994. Jones et al. reported that no hip with PTA greater than 46° remodeled after in situ pinning for SCFE [2]. So, we presently select in situ pinning for SCFE with PTA 45° or less and CO for SCFE with PTA more than 45°.

References

1. O'Brien ET, Fahey JJ (1977) Remodeling of the femoral neck after in situ pinning for slipped capital femoral epiphysis. J Bone Joint Surg [Am] 59:62–68
2. Jones JR, Paterson DC, Hillier TM, et al (1990) Remodeling after pinning for slipped capital femoral epiphysis. J Bone Joint Surg [Br] 72:568–573
3. Rostoucher P, Bensahel H, Pennecot GF, et al (1996) Slipped capital femoral epiphysis: evaluation of different modes of treatment. J Pediatr Orthop B 5:96–101
4. Bellemans J, Fabry G, Molenaers G, et al (1996) Slipped capital femoral epiphysis: a long-term follow-up, with special emphasis on the capacities for remodeling. J Pediatr Orthop B 5:151–157
5. Boero S, Brunenghi GM, Carbone M, et al (2003) Pinning in slipped capital femoral epiphysis: long-term follow-up study. J Pediatr Orthop B 12:372–379
6. Boyer DW, Mickelson MR, Ponseti IV (1981) Slipped capital femoral epiphysis: long-term follow-up study of one hundred and twenty-one patients. J Bone Joint Surg [Am] 59:62–68
7. Herring JA (2002) Tachdjian's pediatric orthopaedics. Saunders, Philadelphia, pp 711–764
8. Southwick WO (1967) Osteotomy through the lesser trochanter for slipped capital femoral epiphysis. J Bone Joint Surg [Am] 49:807–835
9. Imhauser G (1977) Late results of Imhauser's osteotomy for slipped capital femoral epiphysis. Z Orthop 115:716–725

Follow-up Study After Corrective Imhäuser Intertrochanteric Osteotomy for Slipped Capital Femoral Epiphysis

Shigeru Mitani, Hirosuke Endo, Takayuki Kuroda, and Koji Asaumi

Summary. We investigated 28 hips in 26 patients with slipped capital femoral epiphysis who were treated by the Imhäuser intertrochanteric osteotomy, with subsequent removal of implants. The mean age at operation was 13 years, and the mean age at the time of the final follow-up was 19 years. The physeal stability was unstable for 15 hips and stable for 13. Posterior tilting angle (PTA) ranged from 33° to 72° before operation. PTA became restored to within the allowable range of up to 30° in all patients. The limitation of range of motion completely resolved in all patients, and none had necrosis of the femoral head postoperatively. There was a mean reduction in leg length by 0.7 cm. Four patients had a fracture due to bone fragility from long-term traction and bed rest. Chondrolysis developed in only 1 male classified as unstable. The Imhäuser treatment system for mild to severe cases may be said to be reasonable in that the physeal stability is rendered stable by traction and then the PTA is reduced to 30° or less by osteotomy to lessen the severity to mild. So, satisfactory results were obtained both clinically and roentgenographically in short- or midterm outcome.

Key words. Slipped capital femoral epiphysis, Intertrochanteric osteotomy, In situ pinning, Posterior tilting angle, Physeal stability

Introduction

Since 1977, we have been treating slipped capital femoral epiphysis at our hospital using the Imhäuser treatment system [1]. According to this system (Fig. 1), mild cases with a posterior tilting angle (PTA) of 30° or less are treated with the in situ pinning technique, whereas intertrochanteric osteotomy is indicated for moderate to severe cases. In patients incapable of walking or suffering from hip joint pain on exertion, traction is undertaken until irritant pain in the hip joint disappears. This treatment is not intended for reduction of slipped epiphysis but is aimed at attaining fibrous or osseous stabilization of the slippage site. Therefore, the Imhäuser treatment system may be characterized by these two surgical procedures used according to disease

---

Department of Orthopaedic Surgery, Okayama University Hospital, 2-5-1 Shikata-cho, Okayama 700-8558, Japan

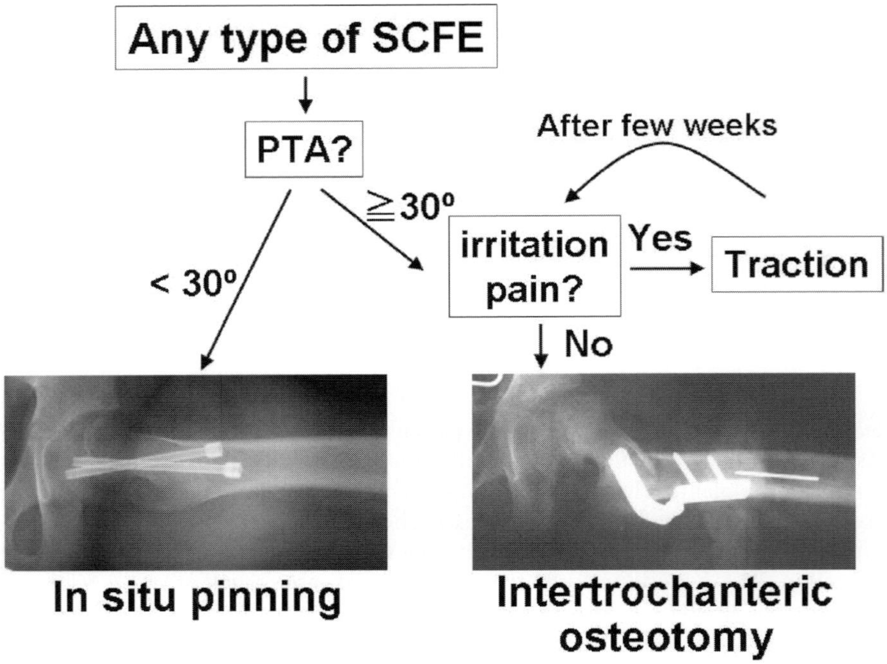

FIG. 1. Imhäuser's treatment system for slipped capital femoral epiphysis (*SCFE*). *PTA*, posterior tilt angle

severity and preoperative attainment of stabilization of the slippage site. Imhäuser [2] has documented that gratifying treatment results were obtained from a follow-up investigation in patients with slipped capital femoral epiphysis conducted over 11 to 22 years, showing that arthrotic changes had been seen in as few as 2 of 68 hip joints treated. To date, we also have had favorable results using this treatment system, as previously reported [3]. However, because several complications have been noted and because some other investigators [4] demonstrated, even in severe cases, that better treatment results were obtained with the in situ pinning technique than with osteotomy, we considered it necessary to reexamine this treatment system. The present study was performed to evaluate the treatment system for its usefulness and for any problems involved by reviewing retrospectively patients with slipped capital femoral epiphysis showing a PTA of 30° or greater that was treated by intertrochanteric osteotomy.

Patients

We investigated 28 hips in 26 patients, which were treated by the Imhäuser intertrochanteric osteotomy, with subsequent removal of implants. There were 24 male and 2 female patients. Of the 28 affected hip joints studied, 22 were unilateral in unilaterally affected cases, 2 were unilateral in bilaterally affected cases, and 4 were in 2 bilaterally affected cases. The age at onset of the disorder, estimated from the medical history taken at clinic interview, ranged from 8 years and 6 months to 22 years and 9 months (mean, 12 years and 4 months), and the age at which surgical treatment was performed was between 8 years and 10 months and 23 years and 2 months (mean, 13 years and 2 months). Age at the time of the final follow-up was between 13 years and 8 months and 28 years and 3 months (mean, 18 years and 9 months). The postoperative follow-up duration ranged from 2 to 11 years (mean, 5 years and 7 months). According to the classification defined by Campbell Operative Orthopaedics [5], the type of onset was chronic for 11 hips, acute on chronic for 15, and acute for 2. The physeal stability, as described by Loder et al. [6], was unstable for 15 hips and stable for 13. In situ pinning on unaffected hips for epiphyseodesis was performed on 20 hips.

Methods

Pertinent data were reviewed as to duration of preoperative traction and intraoperative correction angle by osteotomy and such clinical parameters as range of motion of the hip joint, any pain, and, in unilaterally affected cases, difference in leg length. Roentgenographically, the apparent neck–shaft angle was measured in the anteroposterior (AP) view and the pre- and postoperative PTA in the lateral view. Each patient was also assessed for complications.

Results

Duration of Traction

The duration of preoperative traction ranged from 2 to 114 days (mean, 45 days). According to the classification based on physeal stability, the range of this duration was 2 to 53 days (mean, 21 days) for stable cases and 36 to 114 days (mean, 58 days) for unstable cases.

Correction Angle

The intraoperative correction angle was 15° to 40° (mean, 31°) on flexion, 10° to 30° (mean, 24°) on valgus, and 25° to 50° (mean, 37°) on anterotation.

Clinical Results

For range of motion of the hip joint, flexion angle was 20° to 120° (mean, 67°) before operation and improved to 90° to 135° (mean, 118°) at the final follow-up (Fig. 2). Internal rotation angle also improved to 0° to 80° (mean, 34°) at the final follow-up from −30° to 35° (mean, −10°) before operation. External rotation angle, which was 10° to 90° (mean, 59°) before operation, was noted to have improved to 10° to 60° (mean, 40°) at the last follow-up (Fig. 3). None of the patients had a difference in range of motion by 20° or greater at the final checkup. In other words, external rotation contracture of the hip joint and Drehman's sign, which had been evident before operation, were noted to have disappeared in all patients. At the final follow-up, hip

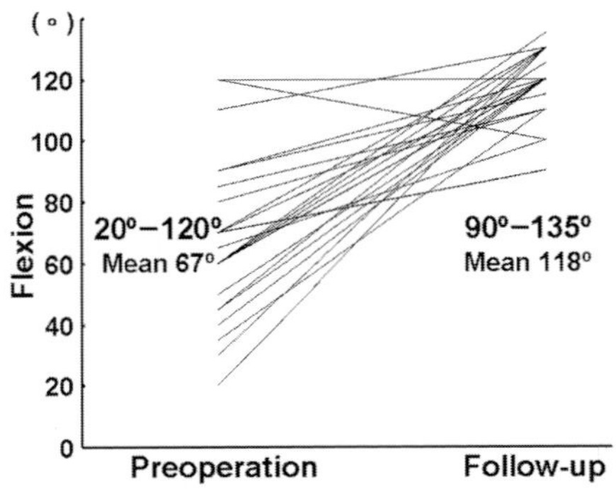

Fig. 2. Change of flexion angle of the hip joint

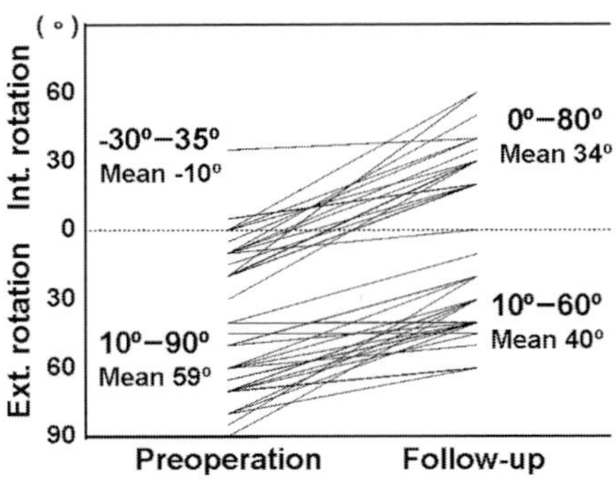

Fig. 3. Change of rotation angle of the hip joint

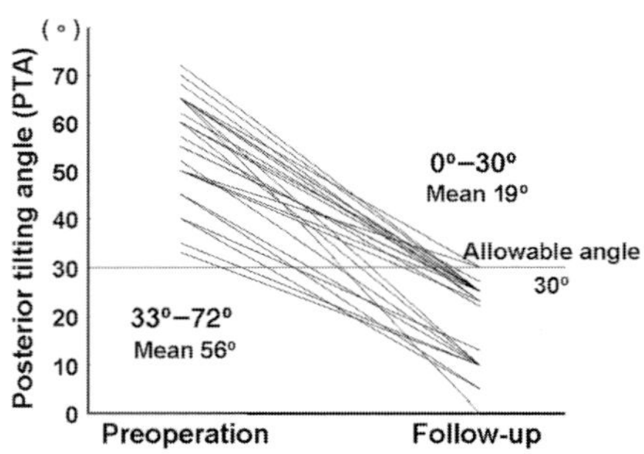

Fig. 4. Development of posterior tilting angle (PTA)

joint pain developed in 1 patient in whom there was narrowing of the joint space. There was a difference in leg length, ranging from 0.5 to 3.5 cm (mean, 0.7 cm), in 11 of the 22 unilaterally affected cases.

Roentgenographic Results

PTA ranged from 33° to 72° (mean, 56°) before operation. Postoperatively, it was between 0° and 30° (mean, 19°); the PTA became restored to within the allowable range of up to 30° in all patients (Fig. 4).

Apparent neck–shaft angle was between 120° and 155° (mean, 134°) on the first examination and from 140° to 170° (mean, 150°) at the last checkup, hence exhibiting a tendency to coxa valga (Fig. 5).

FIG. 5. Change of neck–shaft angle

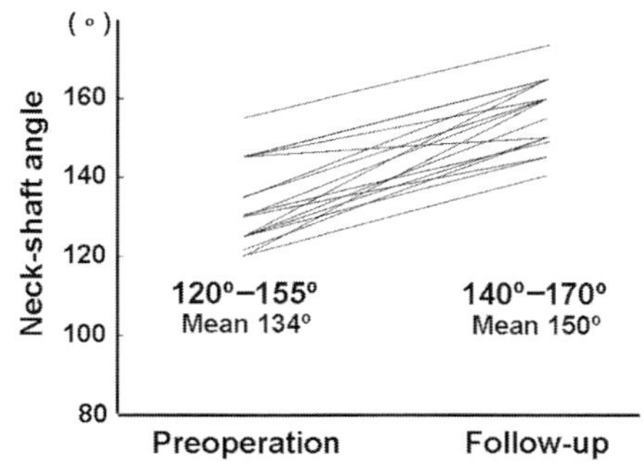

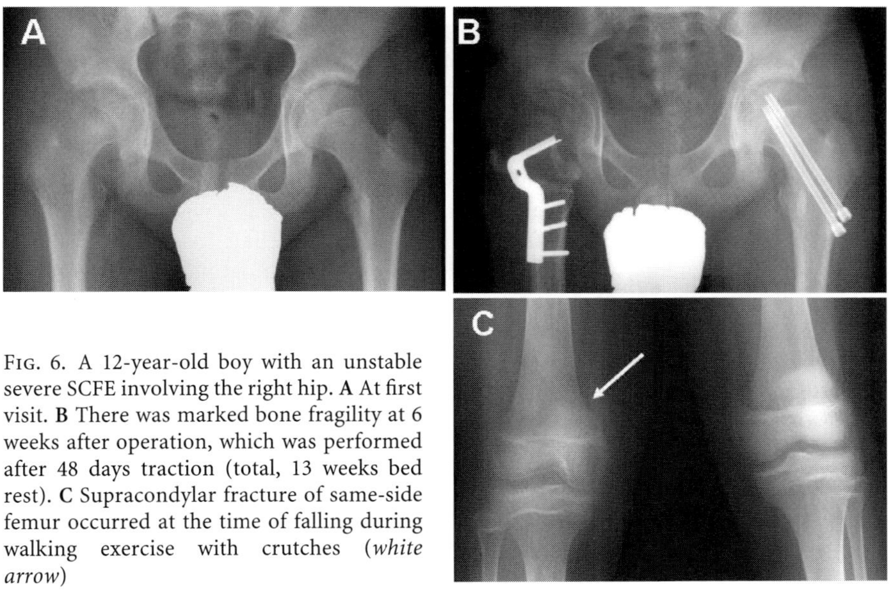

FIG. 6. A 12-year-old boy with an unstable severe SCFE involving the right hip. **A** At first visit. **B** There was marked bone fragility at 6 weeks after operation, which was performed after 48 days traction (total, 13 weeks bed rest). **C** Supracondylar fracture of same-side femur occurred at the time of falling during walking exercise with crutches (*white arrow*)

Complications

Avascular necrosis of the femoral head occurred in a male patient classified as an unstable (acute), with its onset at the age of 12 years and 1 month; this was considered to be not attributable to operative manipulation because a change in epiphyseal intensity had been noted on preoperative radiograms. The necrotic region was found to have been repaired with bone grafting following a 2-year relief of body weight by walking with crutches. Another male patient classified as an unstable (acute on chronic) with its onset at the age of 12 years and 3 months developed chondrolysis. Narrowing of the joint space became reversed following 2-year relief of body weight with a pogo-stick brace. A patient who complained of coxalgia was noted to have arthrotic changes. A reoperation was performed on a patient who incurred breakage of a plate postoperatively and two patients who had postoperative loosening and rotation of a plate because of bone fragility. Four patients suffered a fracture intra- or postoperatively (Fig. 6).

Discussion

The aim of treatment of slipped capital femoral epiphysis is to stabilize the slipping region, improve congruity of the hip joint, and maintain hip joint function through life without causing any complication. Treatment methods are classified as follows: in situ pinning aimed at stabilization of the slipped epiphysis without correction, various osteotomy procedures involving corrections at sites other than the deformed region, and open reduction, consisting of closed manipulation for correction at the slippage site and subcapital femoral neck osteotomy.

The in situ pinning method is performed to stabilize the slipped epiphysis, expecting postoperative remodeling to improve congruity of the hip joint. Various reduction procedures are designed to improve hip joint congruity by aiming for anatomical reduction, whereupon the slippage region becomes stabilized. The in situ pinning method has been described to be safest and noticeably effective even in severe cases, according to the American Academy of Orthopaedic Surgeons (AAOS) overview [6] of the varieties of treatment methods for slipped capital femoral epiphysis, but the overview includes fairly outdated reports and can hardly find categorical acceptance. Jones et al. [7] reported that there had been failure in attaining a spherical remodeling in cases with a PTA of 46° or more, whereas remodeling was obvious in more than 90% of mild cases. Thus, not all treated cases gain remodeling. Rab [8] conducted a study using three-dimensional models and showed that formation of articulation of the metaphysis with the acetabular shelf occurred in 1 of 6 of cases with a PTA of 30°, in 1 of 3 of cases with a PTA of 60°, and in 1 of 2 of cases with a PTA of 90°, and that this might cause arthrosis. Carney et al. [9] documented that long-term follow-up indicated that the more severe or more progressive the slipped capital femoral epiphysis, the greater the extent of aggravation with lapse of time. It follows that it is too risky to have improvement in hip joint congruity totally depend on remodeling.

Manual reduction is commonly used when the physeal stability is rated as unstable, and it reportedly entails a rather reduced risk of avascular necrosis of the femoral head if performed with tender care. Nevertheless, it cannot be ruled out that closed manipulations may possibly cause injury to nutrient arteries in the case where epiphyseal excursion is decreased; the incidence of avascular necrosis of the femoral head was reported to be 14% by Peterson et al. [10] and to be about 12% in Japan by Otani et al. [11]. While it has been described that, if physeal stability is stable, the risk of avascular necrosis of the femoral head can be reduced by concomitant application of subcapital femoral neck osteotomy in the open reduction of the epiphysis, the incidence of the necrosis is 4.5% as reported by Fish [12] and 14.8% by DeRosa et al. [13]. Open reduction involves complicated operative procedures and has the drawback of exposing the joint cartilage to air upon deployment of the articular capsule.

Intertrochanteric osteotomy entails problems such as development of deformity and reduction in leg length because the surgical correction is made at a site distant from the deformed area. However, its operative technique poses no problem in regard to avascular necrosis of the femoral head and has the advantage of providing an early closure of the growth plate and of no deployment of the articular capsule [14].

Factors that affect long-term results in cases of slipped capital femoral epiphysis include type of disorder, severity, any complications, and treatment methods. Loder et al. [6] have described how results of treatment depend on stability of the epiphysis, in that the results were gratifying in 96% of cases with stable physeal stability and in only 47% of cases with unstable physeal stability. They also reported that none developed avascular necrosis of the femoral head among the "stable" cases while it occurred in 47% of "unstable" cases. Without needing mention, the above-cited reports of Jones et al. [7] and Carney et al. [9] indicated results of treatment are more favorable in milder cases. That is, to achieve the best therapeutic results, it is necessary to perform treatment without causing complications in stable, mild cases.

It may be said to stand to reason that the Imhäuser treatment system ensures a stable physeal stability of the affected hip joint by pinning in mild cases, whereas in more severe cases the physeal stability of the joint is rendered stable by traction and then the PTA is reduced to 30° or less by osteotomy to lessen the severity to mild. In the present study, limitation of range of motion completely resolved in all patients following treatment, and none had necrosis of the femoral head postoperatively. Consistent with the reports of Imhäuser [2] and Kartenbender et al. [15], rather gratifying results were obtained both clinically and roentgenographically in short- or mid-term outcomes. As shown in Fig. 7, most cases had good congruity of the hip joint as a result of both the correction osteotomy and remodeling after operation. However, the apparent neck–shaft angle was 150° on average at the time of this investigation, thus indicating a tendency toward coxa valga (Fig. 7). There was a mean reduction in leg length by 0.7 cm, so there is a possible influence of an altered functional axis on the knee joint. Further investigation is necessary, therefore, to investigate osteotomy angle, especially with respect to anterotation and valgus. Four patients

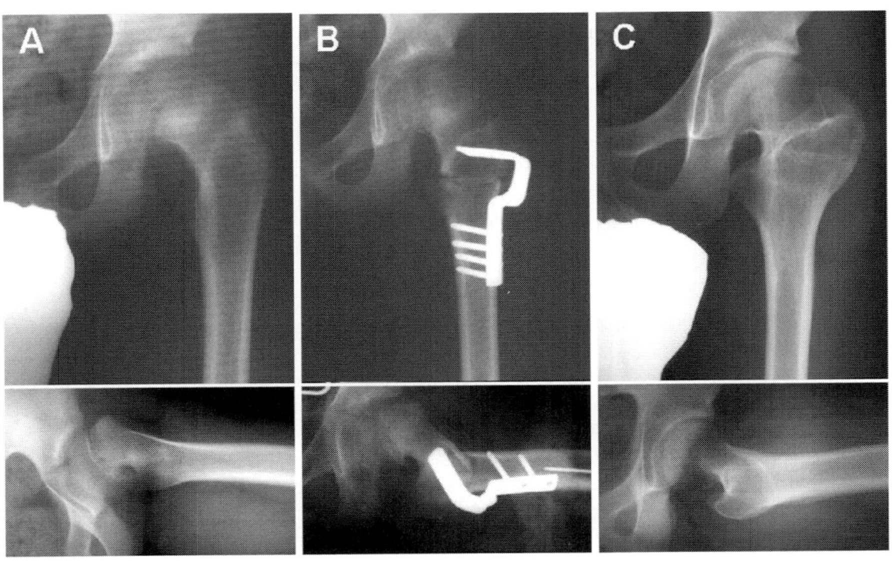

Fig. 7. A 12-year-old boy with a stable SCFE involving the left hip. **A** PTA was 65° at first visit (12 years and 5 months old). **B** PTA was 20° immediately after operation (12 years and 6 months old). **C** Good congruity of the hip joint was obtained at the final visit (18 years and 11 months old), and neck–shaft angle was 155°

had a fracture as a result of bone fragility from long-term traction and bed rest. The treatment scheme is under reconsideration with regard to preoperative duration of traction, based also on the recent medical care situation.

Intertrochanteric osteotomy in the Imhäuser treatment system is considered a useful procedure because it is relatively simple in technique and involves no development of avascular necrosis of the femoral head. As Schai et al. [16] reported that results of treatment with the Imhäuser method were superior to those by other procedures but entailed development of arthrosis in 45% of cases, it seems that matters relating to treatment of this disorder are yet to be resolved. Indeed, there are problems peculiar to this treatment method that remain to be solved, as has been disclosed by the present study; further long-term follow-up for treated joints is needed.

References

1. Imhäuser G (1986) Spontane Epipyhsendislokation am koxalen Femurende. Orthopäde in Praxis und Klinik, vol VII. Thieme, Stuttgart, pp 115–148
2. Imhäuser G (1977) Spätergebnisse der sog. Imhäuser-Osteotomie bei der Epiphysenlösung. Z Orthop 115:716–725
3. Oda K, Mitani S (1998) Slipped capital femoral epiphysis (in Japanese). Orthop Surg Traumatol 41:439–448
4. Loder RT, Aronsson DD, Dobbs MB, et al (2001) Slipped capital femoral epiphysis. Instr Course Lect 50:555–570
5. Canal ST (2003) Fractures and dislocations in children. Slipped capital femoral epi physis. In: Campbell's operative orthopaedics, 10th edn. Mosby, Philadelphia, pp 1481–1483
6. Loder RT, Richards ABS, Shapiro PS, et al (1993) Acute slipped capital femoral epiphysis: the importance of physeal stability. J Bone Joint Surg 75A:1134–1140
7. Jones JR, Paterson DC, Hillier TM, et al (1990) Remodelling after pinning for slipped capital femoral epiphysis. J Bone Joint Surg 72B:568–573
8. Rab GT (1999) The geometry of slipped capital femoral epiphysis: implications for movement, impingement, and corrective osteotomy. J Pediatr Orthop 19:419–424
9. Carney BT, Weinstein SL, Noble J (1991) Long-term follow-up of slipped capital femoral epiphysis. J Bone Joint Surg 73A:667–674
10. Peterson MD, Weiner DS, Green NF, et al (1997) Acute slipped capital femoral epiphysis: the value and safety of urgent manipulative reduction. J Pediatr Orthop 17:648–654
11. Otani T, Saito M, Kawaguchi Y, et al (2004) Short-term clinical results of manipulative reduction for acute-unstable slipped capital femoral epiphysis (in Japanese). Hip Joint 30:223–225
12. Fish JB (1994) Cuneiform osteotomy of the femoral neck in the treatment of slipped capital femoral epiphysis. A follow-up note. J Bone Joint Surg 76A:46–59
13. DeRosa GP, Mullins RC, Kling TF Jr (1996) Cuneiform osteotomy of the femoral neck in severe slipped capital femoral epiphysis. Clin Orthop 322:48–60
14. Crawford AH (1996) Role of osteotomy in the treatment of slipped capital femoral epiphysis. J Pediatr Orthop 5B:102–109
15. Kartenbender K, Cordier W, Katthagen BD (2000) Long-term follow-up study after corrective Imhäuser osteotomy for severe slipped capital femoral epiphysis. J Pediatr Orthop 20:749–756
16. Schai PA, Exner GU, Hänsch O (1996) Prevention of secondary coxarthrosis in slipped capital femoral epiphysis: a long-term follow-up study after corrective intertrochanteric osteotomy. J Pediatr Orthop 5-B: 135–143

Slipping of the Femoral Capital Epiphysis: Long-Term Follow-up Results of Cases Treated with Imhaeuser's Therapeutic Principle

MUROTO SOFUE[1] and NAOTO ENDO[2]

Summary. Slipping of the femoral capital epiphysis is a common problem in growing children. For the treatment of this disease, it is of the utmost importance to prevent complications that would adversely affect normal development of the hip joint. Therefore, it is absolutely necessary to choose a treatment that will allow the hip joint to develop normally and which will prevent osteoarthritic changes in the future. The long-term results of cases treated with Imhaeuser's method [1,2] are reported here. The results were very satisfying, and this treatment should be continued in the future.

Key words. Slipping of the femoral capital epiphysis, Aseptic necrosis of the femoral head, In situ pinning, Imhaeuser's osteotomy [1,2], Three-dimensional osteotomy

Introduction

Slipping of the femoral capital epiphysis (SFCE) has recently become more commonplace in Japan. Figure 1 shows a patient with SFCE who was treated in the 1960s in Niigata University Hospital. At that time, manual reduction followed by pinning was common in Japan. However, by the age of 31, a severe arthritic change occurred in this patient.

Authors [3,4,5] reviewed the cases in the hospitals associated with Niigata University and found that of five cases that underwent manual reduction, unfortunately four of them had femoral head necrosis, which resulted in osteoarthritic change at an early age. Therefore, forceful reduction is contraindicated.

The aim of the treatment for SFCE is first to improve joint incongruity and correct the range of motion (ROM) without complications. This procedure will prevent the development of osteoarthritis in the hip joint. With these points in mind, we chose Imhaeuser's method and treated the patients according to his principles. This chapter is the report of the treatment of those patients along with their long-term follow-up.

[1] Department of Orthopaedic Surgery, Nakajo Central Hospital, 12-1 Nishihoncho, Tainai, 959-2656 Niigata, Japan

[2] Division of Orthopedic Surgery, Niigata University Graduate School of Medical and Dental Sciences, 1-757 Asahimachi-dori, Niigata 951-8510, Japan

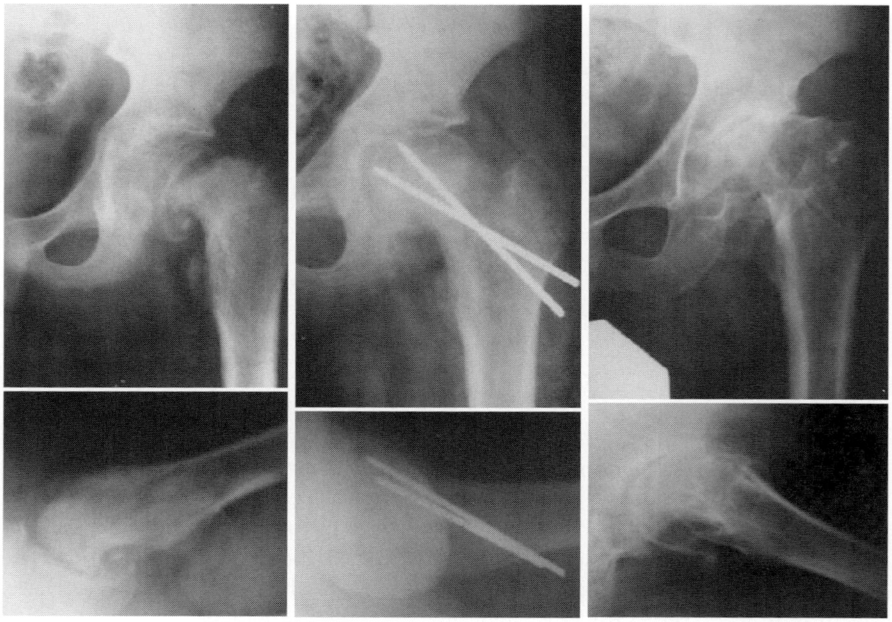

A B C

FIG. 1. **A** A 14-year-old boy, posterior tilt 65°. **B** Manual reduction and pinning. **C** Osteoarthritic change after femoral head necrosis at the age of 31 years old

Materials and Methods

In accordance with Imhaeuser's principles [1,2], we have treated 76 cases, 79 joints of SFCE, from 1976 to 2003.

In this study, the cases that were treated up to 1993 and followed over a period of longer than 10 years are investigated. The 47 cases in all included 42 males and 5 females, ranging in age from 9 to 14 years old at the time of surgery, except for 1 patient treated at 20 years of age with endocrinopathy. Two cases were bilateral and 45 cases were unilateral. In the unilateral cases, 20 joints were right side and 25 were left side. The type of slip was acute on chronic in 3 joints and chronic in 46 joints. The direction of slip was posteroinferior in 48 cases, and 1 was posterosuperior (Table 1).

The course of treatment is shown in Table 2. Forty-five hips of the normal side received prophylactic pinning, and 23 hips with less than 30° of slipping and 3 hips with more than 30° of slipping, which were gently reduced to less than 30° by supracondylar skeletal traction, have been treated with in situ pinning. In total, 71 hips have been pinned. Twenty-three hips with more than 30° of slipping, which were not reduced to less than 30° in spite of direct traction, were treated by Imhaeuser's osteotomy. In all, 94 hips comprising 47 cases were clinically analyzed.

TABLE 1. Cases treated with Imhaeuser's method [1,2], 1976–1993

Total cases: 47 (42 boys, 5 girls)
Follow-up: 10 years or more
Age: 9–14 years (except for 1 case of a 20-year-old)
Slip side: 2 bilateral, 45 unilateral (20 right, 25 left)
Slip type: 3 acute on chronic, 46 chronic
Slip direction: 1 posterosuperior, 48 posteroinferior

TABLE 2. Course of treatment

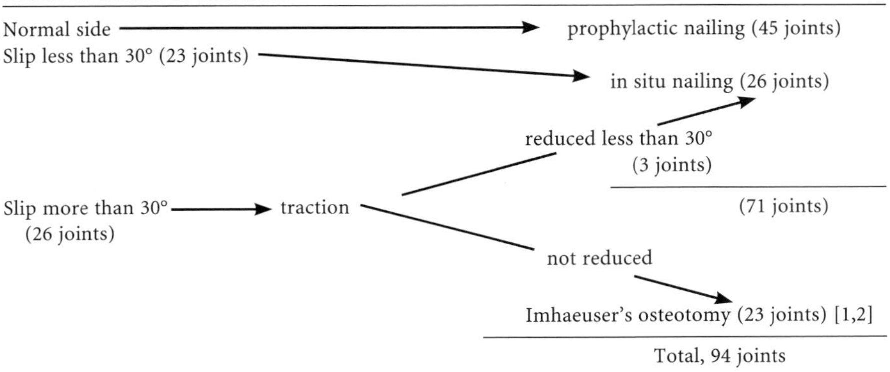

Case Reports

Pinning Cases

Case 1: An 11-year-old boy with mild slipping of 20° on the right side (Fig. 2) was treated with in situ pinning on the right side and prophylactic pinning on the left side (Fig. 3). Sixteen years later, when he was 27 years old, a slight shortening of the femoral neck with good joint congruency can be seen (Fig. 4). Clinically, he has no problems and even plays soccer on a club team.

Case 2: A 14-year-old boy with bilateral slipping of 25° on the right and 20° on the left (Fig. 5) was treated with in situ pinning on both sides (Fig. 6). Seventeen years later, at 28 years old, there is some tendency of coxa vara in the X-ray findings, but joint congruency is very good (Fig. 7). Clinically, he has no problems and enjoys early-morning baseball with his club team.

Case 3: A 13-year-old boy with acute on chronic slipping of 65° on the left side (Fig. 8). After applying supracondylar skeletal traction for 3 weeks, good reduction of the epiphysis was achieved (Fig. 9B), and in situ pinning was performed (Fig. 9C). At the 25-year postoperative follow-up examination, when he was 37 years old, very good joint congruency can be seen (Fig. 10). He works as a long-distance driver and does not have any complaints about his hip joints.

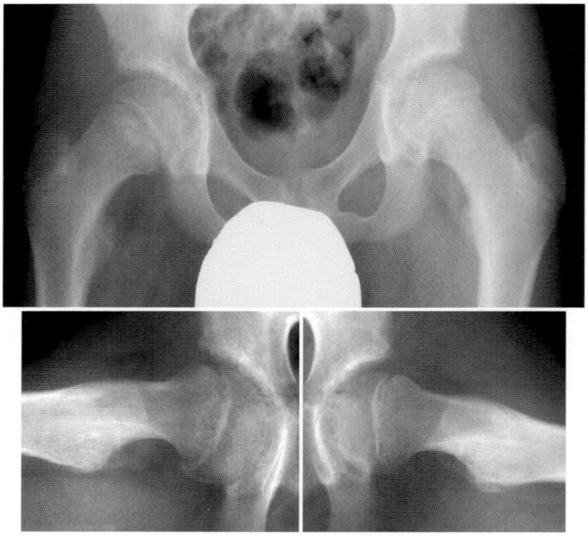

Fig. 2. An 11-year-old boy, right chronic slip, posterior tilt 20°

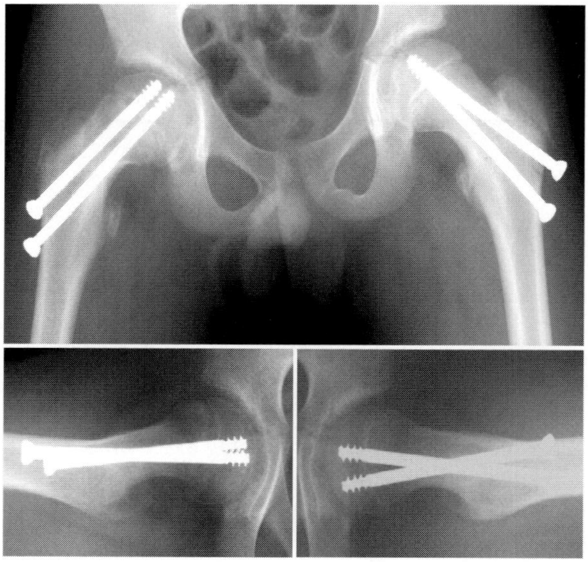

Fig. 3. An 11-year-old boy. *Right*, in situ pinning; *left*, prophylactic pinning

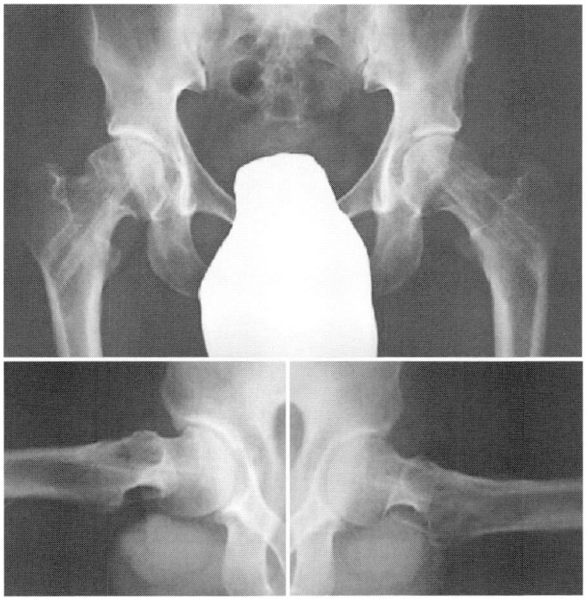

FIG. 4. A 27-year-old man, 16 years after surgery, with good joint congruity

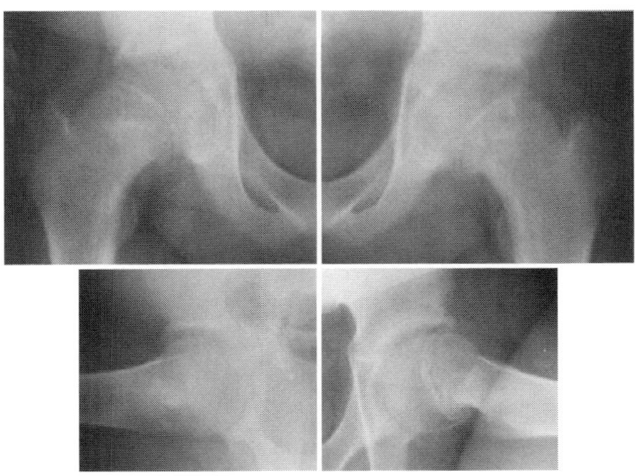

FIG. 5. A 14-year-old boy, bilateral chronic slip, posterior tilt: right, 25°, left, 20°

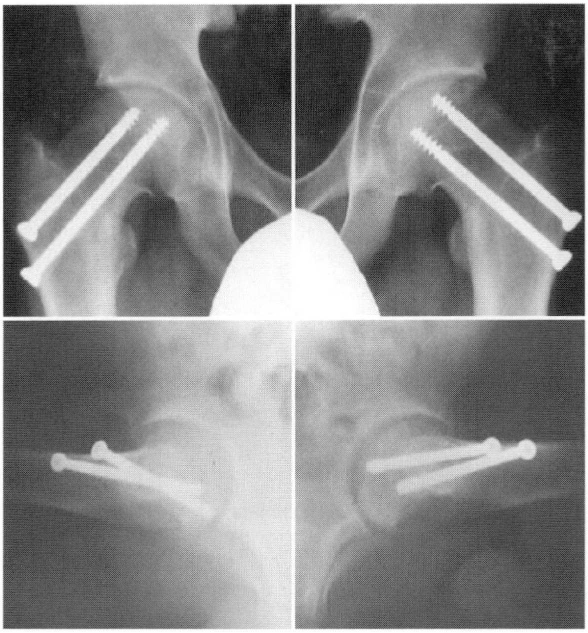

FIG. 6. A 15-year-old boy, bilateral in situ pinning, 1 year after surgery

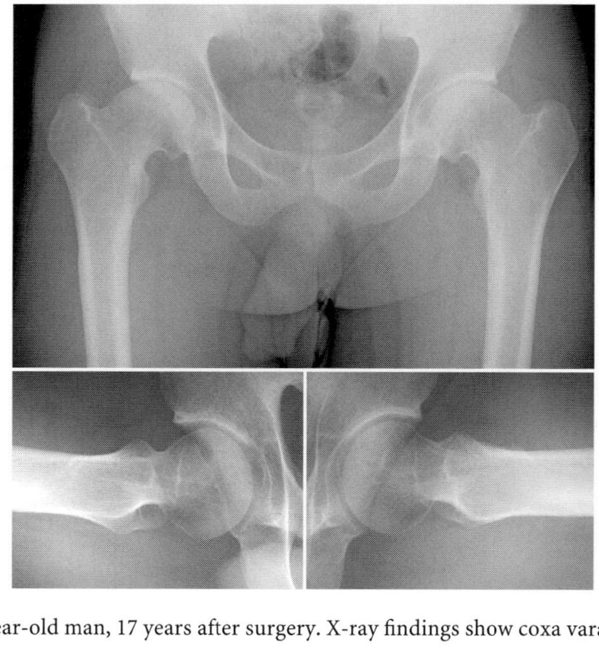

FIG. 7. A 28-year-old man, 17 years after surgery. X-ray findings show coxa vara but good joint congruity

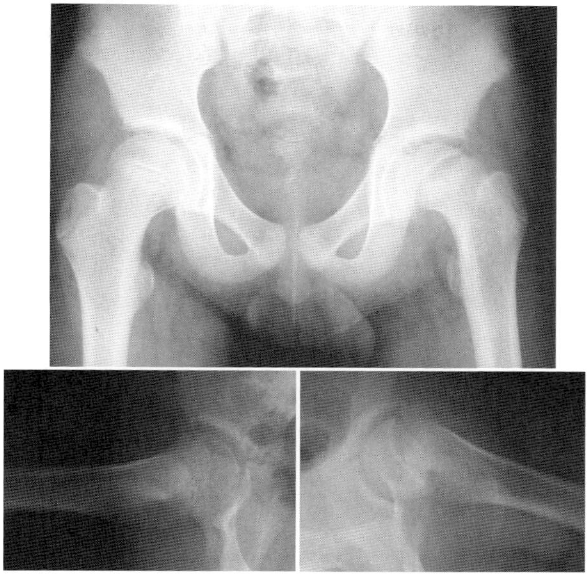

FIG. 8. A 13-year-old boy, left acute on chronic slip, posterior tilt 65°

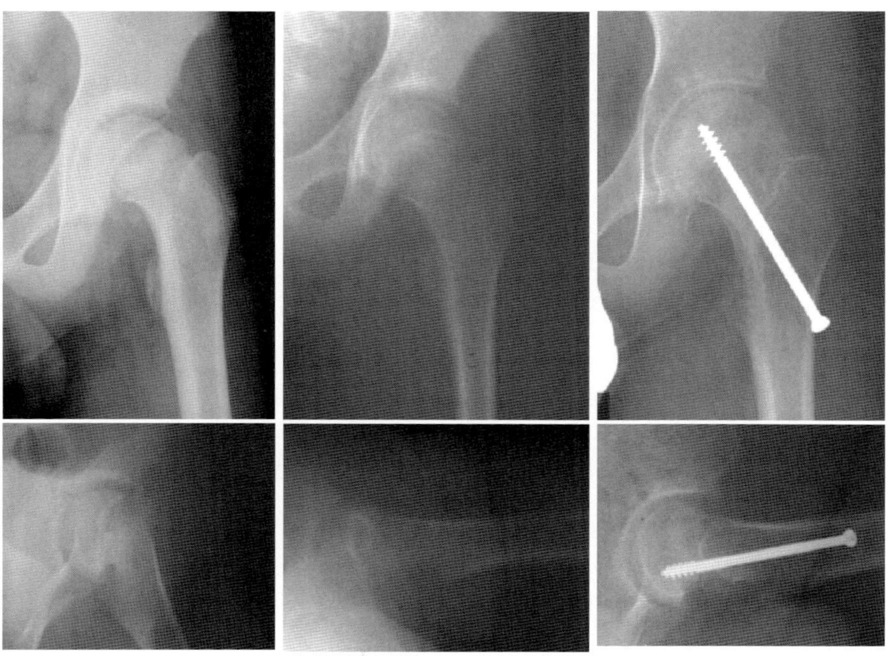

A B C

FIG. 9. Progression of treatment. **A** Slipping with posterior tilt 65°. **B** After 3 weeks of skeletal traction, slipped epiphysis was gently reduced. **C** In situ pinning

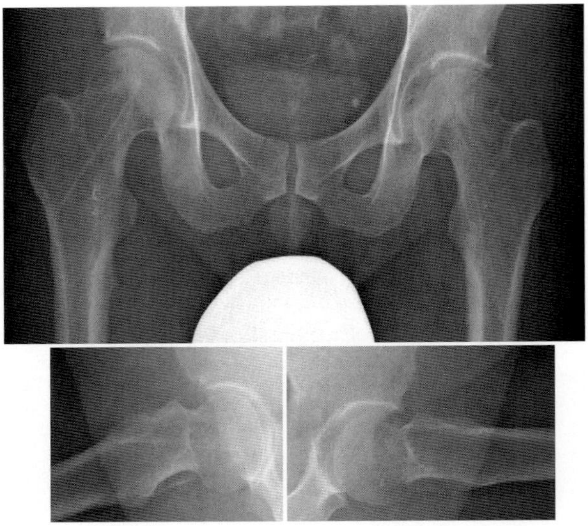

Fig. 10. A 37-year-old man, 25 years after surgery. Bilateral hips show good joint congruity

Table 3. The elements of Imhaeuser's osteotomy [1,2]

1. Internal rotation to correct the external rotated midpoint
2. Valgisation of 20° to 30°
3. Flexion to correct the posterior tilting of epiphysis to maximum permissible angle of 30°

Three-Dimensional Osteotomy (Imhaeuser's Osteotomy) Cases

Imhaeuser's osteotomy [1,2] consists of the following elements (Table 3):

1. Internal rotation to correct the external rotated midpoint.
2. Valgisation of 20° to 30°.
3. Flexion to correct the posterior tilting angle to a maximum permissible angle of 30°.

The valgus element (2) is necessary, because this osteotomy is performed at the intertrochanteric region of the femur, which has a neck-shaft angle of about 140°. Figure 11 shows an example case with external rotation from 10° to 70° (midpoint, 40°).

Case 4: A 13-year-old girl with right hip slipping of 60° (Fig. 12). In spite of direct traction, the slip could not reduced. Imhaeuser's osteotomy was performed. Figure 13 shows the patient's postoperative findings with good progression. Twenty-one years later, she is 34 years of age. The X-ray findings show good joint congruency

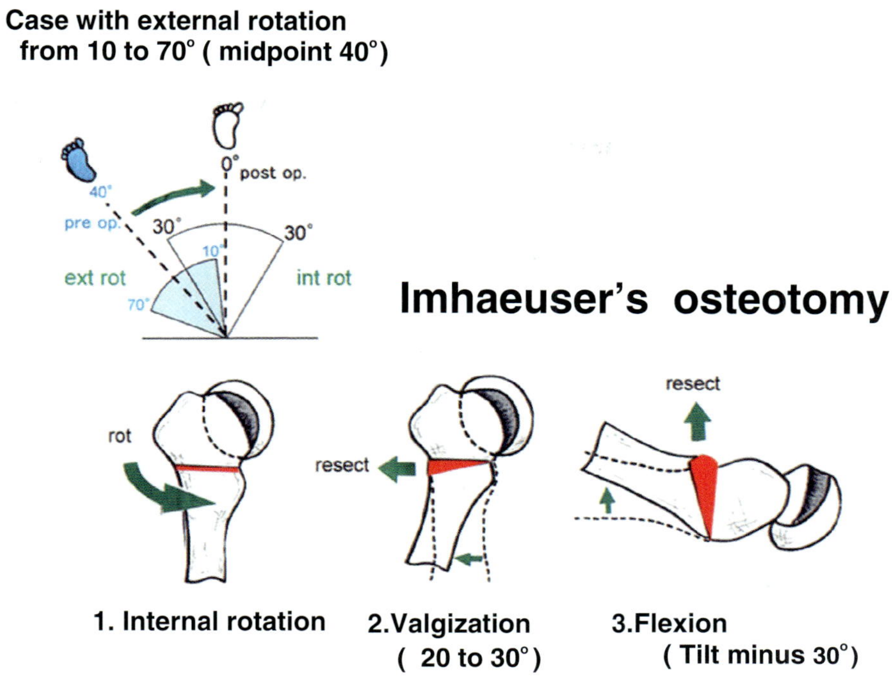

FIG. 11. Scheme of Imhauser's osteotomy [1,2] shown by an example case with external midpoint of 40° (from 10° to 70° external rotation)

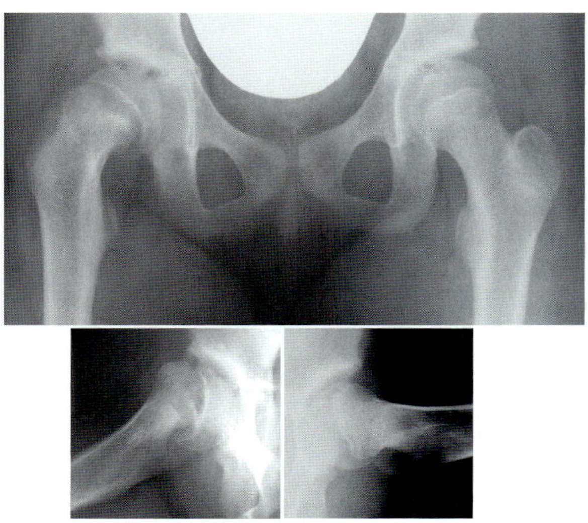

FIG. 12. A 13-year-old girl, right chronic slip, posterior tilt 60°

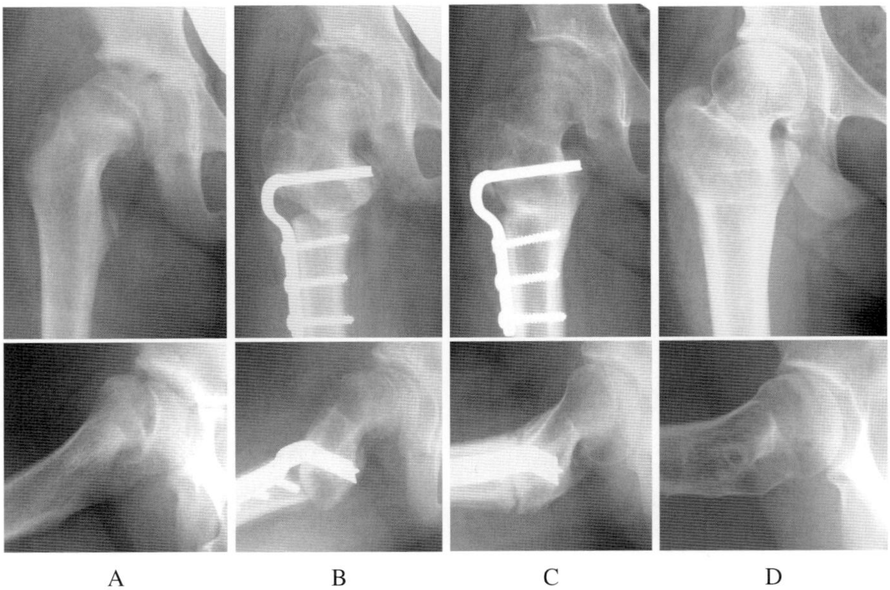

FIG. 13. Progression after Imhauser's osteotomy. **A** Preoperative. **B** Operative. **C** Postoperative, 1 year. **D** Postoperative, 8 years

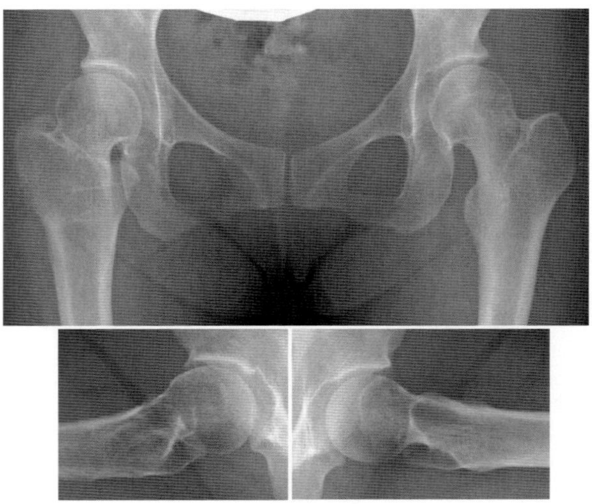

FIG. 14. A 34-year-old woman, 21 years after the osteotomy. X-ray shows good joint congruity

(Fig. 14). She has two children, has no clinical complaints, and lives an active life as a housewife.

Case 5: A 13-year-old boy with slipping of 45° on the left hip (Fig. 15). Imhaeuser's osteotomy [1,2] was performed on the left hip and a prophylactic pinning was done on the right hip (Fig. 16). Fifteen years later, he is 28 years of age. X-ray findings show good joint congruity (Fig. 17), and the range of motion is free. He works in a restaurant as a cook and does not have any complaints about either leg.

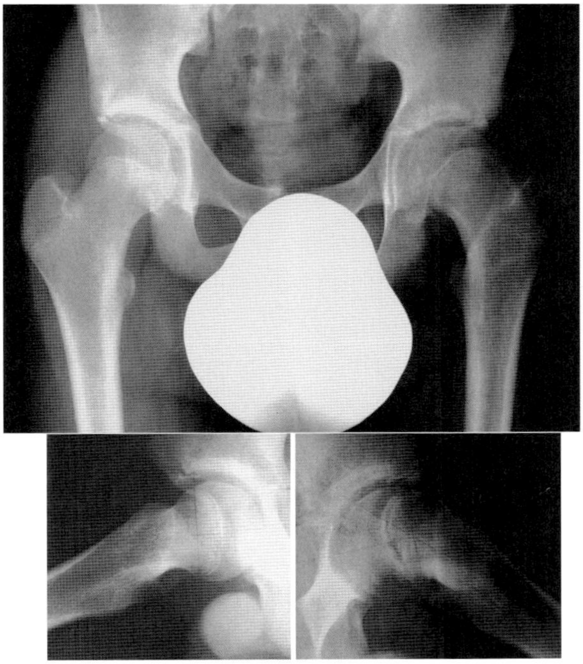

FIG. 15. A 13-year-old boy, left chronic slip, posterior tilt 45°

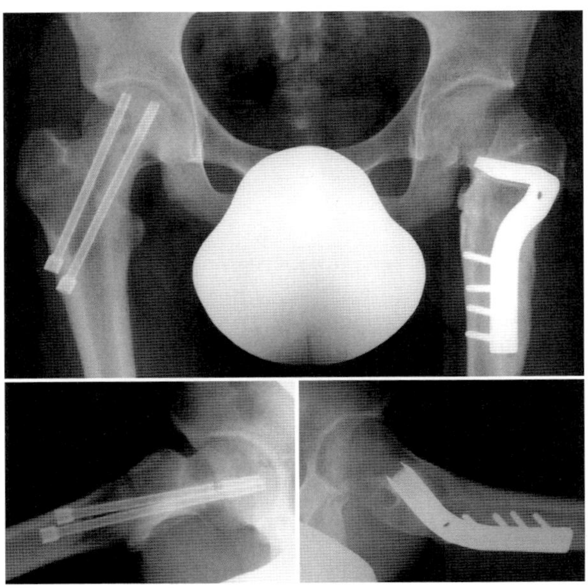

FIG. 16. A 14-year-old boy. *Right*, prophylactic pinning; *left*, Imhaeuser's osteotomy [1,2], 1 year postoperative

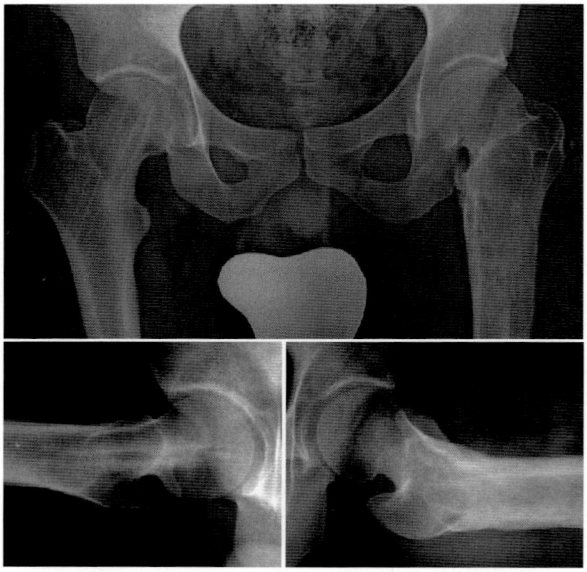

Fig. 17. A 28-year-old man, 15 years postoperative. X-ray shows good joint congruity

Table 4. Pinning results

Number of joints:	71
JOA hip score:	100 points for all joints
Complications (AVN, chondrolysis, etc.):	None
Epiphyseal line:	closed on all 71 joints
Bilateral pinning cases:	24 cases
Leg length discrepancy	
No discrepancy:	20 cases
Discrepancy ≦1 cm:	4
Discrepancy >1 cm:	0

JOA, Japanese Orthopaedic Association; AVN, avascular necrosis

Results

The results of the 71 joints that received pinning were investigated (Table 4). In all cases the Japanese Orthopaedic Association (JOA) hip score was 100 points of a possible 100 points. Complications such as avascular necrosis (AVN) of the femoral head or chondrolysis were not observed. In all 71 joints, the epiphyseal lines were closed. Leg length was examined in 24 cases that were pinned on both hips; 20 cases had no discrepancy and 4 cases had some leg length discrepancy less than or equal to 1 cm. There were no leg length discrepancies of more than 1 cm.

TABLE 5. Imhaeuser's osteotomy results

Number of cases (joints):	22 (23)
JOA score:	>90 points
Complication (AVN, chondrolysis, etc.):	none
Drehmann's sign [6]:	none
Tilt angle:	
Before surgery:	average 52°
After surgery:	average 22° (all cases less than 30°)
Leg length discrepancy:	
<1 cm:	20 cases
≧2 cm and <3 cm:	2
OA change:	
(—):	15 joints
Coxa valga:	7 joints
Advanced stage:	1 joint

OA, osteoarthritis

The results of Imhaeuser's osteotomy [1,2], which was done in 22 cases on 23 joints, were also investigated (Table 5). The postoperative JOA hip score was more than 90 points of a possible 100 points. Early complications, including femoral head necrosis or chondrolysis, were not observed. There was no persisting Drehmann's sign [6] in any of the cases. The preoperative tilt angle of epiphysis, on average 52°, was reduced to less than 30° with an average of 22° after surgery.

As for leg length, 20 cases had a discrepancy of less than 1 cm, whereas the remaining 2 cases had a discrepancy less than 3 cm. Except for 1 hip with an advanced stage of osteoarthritic (OA) change, 15 hips developed normally. Although 7 hips showed coxa valga, there was good joint congruity and no findings of OA change.

Conclusion

Long-term follow-up of SFCE, treated in accordance with Imhaeuser's principle, showed satisfying results. This treatment should be continued in the future.

References

1. Imhaeuser G (1962) Ueber Dislokation der proximalen Femurepiphyse durch Schaedigung der Wachstumzone (Dislokation der Hueftkopfepiphyse nach vorn-unten). Z Orthop 96:265–276
2. Imhaeuser G (1977) Spaetergebnisse der sog. Imhaeuser Osteotomie bei der Epiphysenloesung. Z Orthop 115:716–725
3. Sofue M, Endo N (1993) Slipping of the femoral capital epiphysis (in Japanese). In: Yamamuro T, Inoue S (eds) Comprehensive textbook of orthopaedic operations, vol 11. Kanahara, Tokyo, pp 145–175
4. Sofue M, Endo N (1997) The results of epiphyseal slipping of femoral head treated with Imhaeuser's method (in Japanese). Cent Jpn J Orthop Traum 40:821–822

5. Sofue M, Hatakeyama S, Endo N, et al (2005) Imhaeuser's three dimensional osteotomy for slipped femoral capital epiphysis (in Japanese). J Joint Surg 24:82–88
6. Drehmann F (1979) Das Drehmannsche Zeichen. Eine klinische Untersuchungsmethode bei Epiphyseolysis capitis femoris. Zeichenbeschreibungen, aetiopathogenetische Gedanken, klinische Erfahrungen. Z Orthop 117:333–344

In Situ Pinning for Slipped Capital Femoral Epiphysis

Satoshi Iida and Yoshiyuki Shinada

Summary. We reviewed retrospectively 28 hips of 25 patients (22 boys and 3 girls) after in situ pinning for slipped capital femoral epiphysis. The mean follow-up period was 5 years (range, 1.5–17). The mean age at surgery was 12.1 years (range, 10–14). Twenty-four hips were stable slips and 4 hips were unstable. Fourteen hips were mild slips (lateral head–shaft angle less than 30°), 10 hips were moderate (30°–59°), and 4 hips were severe (60° or greater). All patients had no hip pain at the latest follow-up; however, the range of internal rotation was mildly limited in 11 hips. Osteonecrosis and chondrolysis were not detected radiographically. Remodeling occurred in 21 of 23 hips (91%) and was not dependent on the degree of slip. The mean period from surgery to physeal closure was 16.1 months (range, 3–57). Progressive slippage occurred in 1 patient after pinning with a single screw. The patient (an 11-year-old boy with a mild chronic slip) started to do hard activities before the physeal closure, and an additional surgery was performed 29 months after the initial pinning. Moderate and severe slips can be treated by in situ pinning; however, careful postoperative management will be required.

Key words. Slipped capital femoral epiphysis, In situ pinning, Lateral head–shaft angle, Progressive slippage, Remodeling

Introduction

Pinning in situ for slipped capital femoral epiphysis (SCFE) is generally considered to produce satisfactory results in cases of mild slip. Recently, the use of fluoroscopic imaging and improved cannulated screw technique makes percutaneous screw fixation the treatment of choice for most cases of SCFE. On the other hand, progressive slippage has been reported in the literature [1,2]. The best method of treatment for moderate and severe slip remains controversial.

Remodeling after in situ pinning has been reported in the literature. Jones et al. advocated a new classification of remodeling and demonstrated the frequency and what factors would influence it [3].

Department of Orthopaedic Surgery, Matsudo City Hospital, Kamihongou 4005, Matsudo, Chiba, 271-0064, Japan

We have assessed the radiographic and clinical results after in situ pinning for SCFE and evaluated the extent of remodeling at follow-up.

Materials and Methods

Between July 1983 and July 2003, 40 hips of 35 patients were treated at Matsudo City Hospital for SCFE. Of these, 12 hips of 12 patients were treated with gently manipulative reduction and pinning [4]. One hip with an unstable and severe slip demonstrated osteonecrosis after the manipulative reduction and pinning. Thereafter, we have not performed manipulative reduction intentionally and also have not done primary osteotomy [5].

Twenty-eight hips of 25 patients that were treated with in situ pinning attended this review. There were 22 boys and 3 girls. The mean age at surgery was 12 years (range, 10–14). The mean follow-up period was 5 years (range, 1.6–17.1 years). One hip was an acute slip (onset within 3 weeks), 8 hips were acute on chronic slips and 19 hips were chronic slips. The distinction between a stable and an unstable slip was the ability to bear weight according to the classification of Loder et al. [6]. Five patients had bilateral slips. Of these, 2 had manipulative reduction in the contralateral hips, and they were free of complications. Another patient received manipulative reduction on the contralateral hip at a previous hospital and had already demonstrated osteonecrosis at the initial visit to our hospital.

All patients were treated with pinning on a fracture table under general anesthesia. Intraoperative fluoroscopy was used. No attempts at manipulative reduction intraoperatively were performed. Several K-wires or Knowles pins were used in 6 hips before 1992 and one or two SCFE screws (Depuy Orthopaedics, Warsaw, IN, USA) in 22 hips after 1992.

Clinical and radiographic examinations were undertaken in all patients. Clinically, we reviewed the pain and the range of motion (ROM) in the involved hips. The clinical results were classified according to the criteria of Heyman and Herndon [7]. For an excellent result, the patient had to have a normal ROM, no hip pain, and no limp; for a good result, slight limitation of internal rotation, no pain, and no limp; for a fair result, limitation of abduction and internal rotation but no pain and no limp; for a poor result, mild limp, slight pain after strenuous exercise, and slight limitation of abduction, internal rotation, and flexion; and for a failed result, pain with activity, limp, and marked limitation of motion that would lead to a subsequent reconstructive procedure.

The lateral head–shaft angle was measured on the frog-leg lateral radiograph of the hips on preoperative, postoperative, and follow-up studies. This angle served as a comparison for the severity of the slip and a measurement of the presence or absence of slip progression. Severity of the slip was grouped as mild, 0° to 29°; moderate, 30° to 59°; and severe, 60° or greater. Serial follow-up radiographs were evaluated for physeal closure, and the time from the surgery to fusion was documented. Proximal capital femoral physeal fusion was determined to have occurred when 50% or more of the physis had undergone linear closure. Remodeling was assessed on lateral radiographs according to the classification of Jones et al. [3], as follows. Type A has a normal configuration with the convexity of the anterior margin of the femoral head.

In type B, the anterior outline of the head and neck appears as a straight line and the anterior margin of the femoral head and neck are the same line. In type C, the profile is convex, the anterior margin of the femoral head is posterior to the anterior margin of the neck, and there is a prominence in the midregion of the neck. Types A and B were defined as remodeled, and type C represented failure of remodeling. We assessed osteonecrosis, chondrolysis, and the difference of articulotrochanteric distance from the contralateral normal hip in the patients whose hip was involved unilaterally.

Postoperatively, the patients with mild slip were advised to walk with partial weight-bearing on crutches for 3 months. Patients who had moderate and severe slips were advised to use long-leg non-weight-bearing apparatus until physeal closure was completed radiographically.

For statistical analysis, Fisher's exact test was performed using StatView version 4.0 software (Abacus, Berkley, CA, USA).

Results

Fifteen hips were mild slips, 8 hips moderate slips, and 5 hips severe slips. Twenty-four hips were classified as a stable slip and 4 hips as an unstable slip. All patients had no hip pain at the latest follow-up. Seventeen hips had an excellent result with the criteria of Heyman and Herndon, and 11 hips had a good result. These patients with good results showed mild limitations of internal rotation; however, no patients revealed Drehman's sign or walking disturbance associated with external rotation contracture.

Radiographically, no evidence of osteonecrosis or chondrolysis was seen during the course of this study. Two hips with unstable slip showed an improvement of the slip intraoperatively in positioning on a fracture table, and one hip had been treated in direct traction with improvement of the slip. These patients were free of complications. The mean period from surgery to physeal closure was 16.1 months (range, 3–57 months). All patients, except 1, showed physeal closure without slip progression. The patient with slip progression was an 11-year-old boy who demonstrated a stable slip in the left hip at presentation. Five months before the onset of pain in the left hip, he suffered from a moderate slip in the right hip. In situ pinning with a single screw was performed in the right hip, and in the left hip a similar procedure was done. We advised him not to engage in any sports activities; however, despite our admonition he discarded the crutch and began to play basketball before physeal closure. The head–shaft angle of the left hip changed from 20° immediately after surgery to 45° at 29 months after the primary pinning. The radiograph showed a radiolucency around the screw in the anterolateral metaphysis and maintenance of screw position in the femoral head. We performed an additional surgery with two cannulated screws. Ultimately, in this patient it took 4 years to demonstrate physeal closure from the time of initial pinning (Fig. 1). In 18 patients with unilateral involvement, the mean difference of articulotrochanteric distance was 8.8 mm (range, 3–15 mm). Remodeling occurred in 21 hips (91%) of 23 hips in which the frog-leg lateral radiograph was available. According to Jones's classification, 16 hips were grouped in type A, 5 hips in type B, and 2 hips in type C (Fig. 2). In 13 hips with moderate and severe slips, 12 hips showed remodeling and 9 hips showed remodeling in

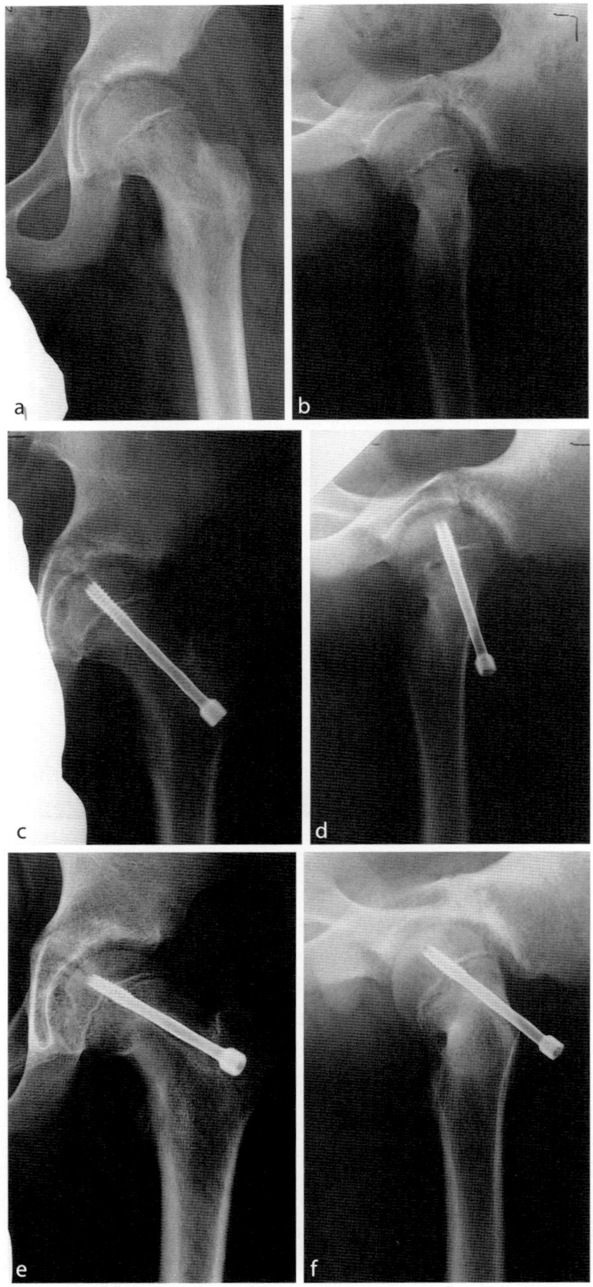

Fig. 1. An 11-year-old boy. **a,b** Stable slip with 20° head–shaft angle at presentation. **c,d** Pinning with single cannulated screw in good position. **e,f** Progressive slippage 2 years and 5 months after the surgery. **g,h** Additional surgery with two cannulated screws. **i,j** Physeal closure 4 years and 4 months after the initial surgery. (From [5], with permission)

FIG. 1. *Continued*

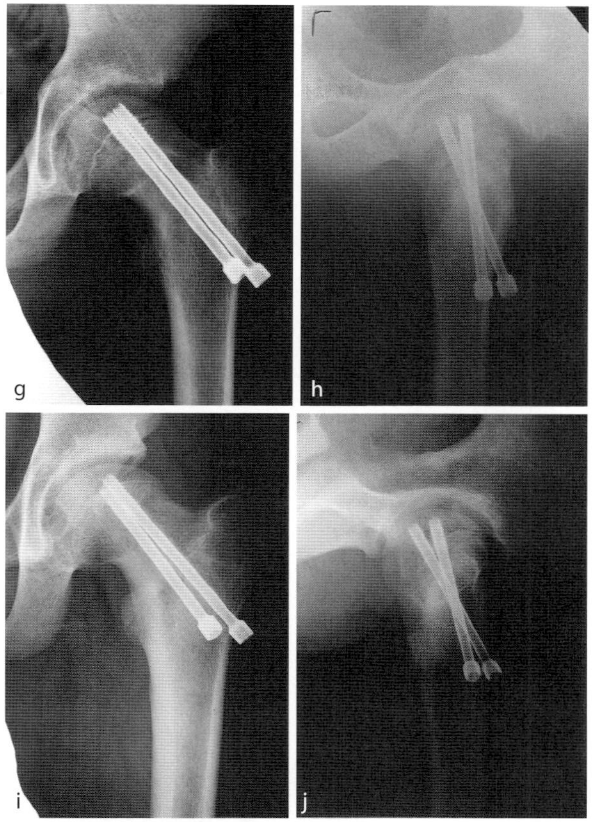

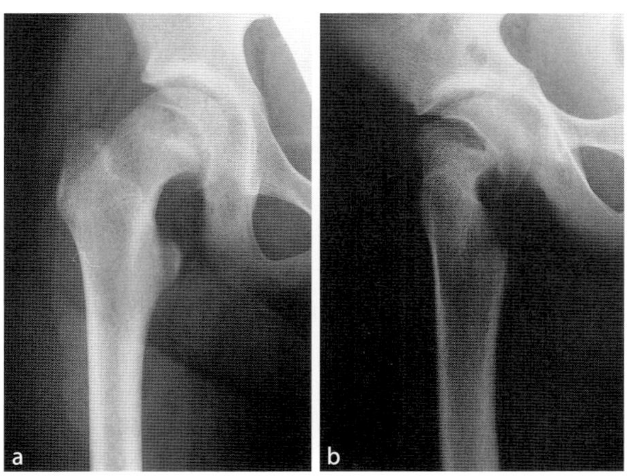

FIG. 2. An 11-year-old girl. **a,b** Stable slip with 60° head–shaft angle at presentation. **c,d** Immediately after in situ pinning with single cannulated screw. **e,f** At 4 years and 2 months after the surgery. Clinical result was excellent, and the radiograph showed type A remodeling. (From [5], with permission)

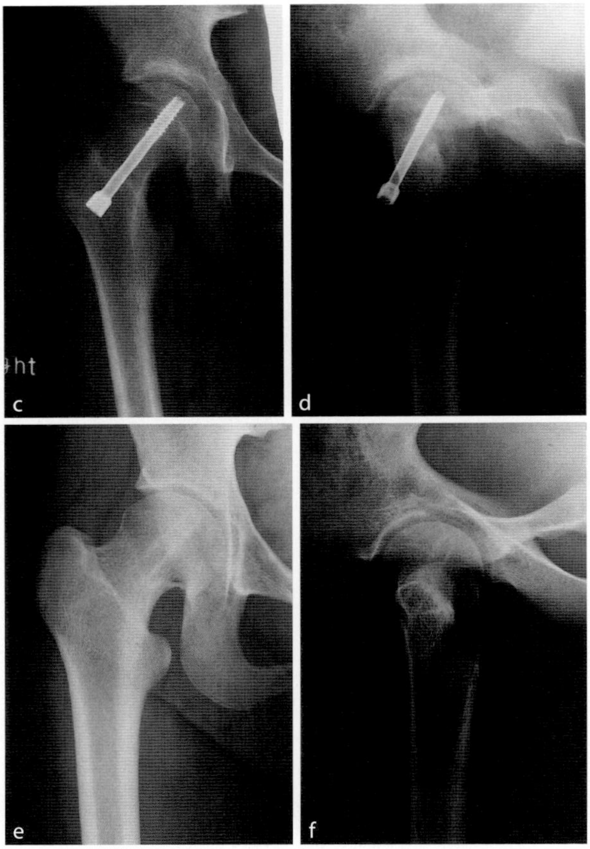

FIG. 2. *Continued*

TABLE 1. Remodeling and degree of slip

Head–shaft angle	Remodeled		Not remodeled
	Type A	Type B	Type C
0°–29°	9	0	1
30° or more	7	5	1

Between remodeled and not remodeled, Fisher's exact probability = 0.69; Between type A and type B, Fisher's exact probability = 0.039

10 hips with mild slips. Remodeling was not dependent on the degree of slip (Table 1). Excluding two hips that showed no remodeling (type C), mild slips demonstrated significantly better remodeling than moderate or severe slips. There was no significant correlation between triradiate cartilage status and remodeling (Table 2).

TABLE 2. Remodeling and triradiate cartilage

Triradiate cartilage	Remodeled		Not remodeled
	Type A	Type B	Type C
Open	10	3	1
Fusion	6	2	1

Between remodeled and not remodeled, Fisher's exact probability = 0.64

Discussion

The indication of in situ pinning for SCFE remains controversial. O'Brien and Fahey reported that in situ pinning might give satisfactory results even when the difference between the two lateral head–shaft angles approached 55° to 60°, and they advocated that if two or three pins could be inserted into the femoral epiphysis from the lateral aspect of the femoral shaft, then in situ pinning would be indicated [8]. Recently, the use of cannulated screws and pinning from the anterolateral aspect of the proximal femur makes in situ pinning an acceptable alternative in some patients who have rather advanced slipping. Aronson and Carlson [9] and Ward et al. [10] described satisfactory results that were obtained with in situ pinning for slips greater than 70°.

Several authors have reported that satisfactory results were obtained after intertrochanteric osteotomy for moderate and severe slips. Intertrochanteric osteotomy was regarded as a safe and effective procedure. Osteonecrosis and chondrolysis, however, were described to occur after intertrochanteric osteotomy [11].

Treatment for SCFE must be aimed at minimizing osteonecrosis and chondrolysis, which are the two main complications. To perform the safest procedure for SCFE, in situ pinning has been selected for most slips. In these series, in situ pinning gave satisfactory results for SCFE with a head–shaft angle less than 60°. Moreover, remodeling after slipping of the epiphysis has been reported, and the inherent capacity of remodeling makes in situ pinning the treatment of choice for more-advanced slips. O'Brien and Jones reported that remodeling occurred frequently after in situ pinning for SCFE [3,8]. Jones et al. reported that remodeling was dependent on the degree of the slip and that no hip with a head–shaft angle greater than 46° showed remodeling [3]. In this series, 6 hips remodeled among 7 hips with a head–shaft angle greater than 40°. Jones et al. also reported that remodeling was significantly more likely to occur if the triradiate cartilage was open at presentation [3]. However, we did not find a significant correlation between remodeling and triradiate status. It is necessary to evaluate what factors would influence the remodeling after in situ pinning.

In situ pinning is considered to be a less-invasive procedure. On the other hand, careful postoperative management is necessary, especially for moderate and severe slips. Carney et al. and Saunders et al. reported that in several cases slippage have progressed after in situ pinning [1,2]. We also experienced one patient with progressive slippage. The patient showed a stable and mild slip at presentation and pinning was performed in good position, but he started to play basketball without medical permission. In this patient, time to physeal closure from the initial pinning was prolonged (4 years and 4 months). It should be considered that slip progression may occur after in situ pinning until the accomplishment of physeal closure because the epiphysis continues to slip and shear stress may act on the proximal physis. Therefore, we recommend a long-leg non-weight-bearing apparatus for the patients with head–shaft angle greater than 30°. Moreover it is expected that reducing the mechanical stress on the physis may promote better remodeling. It should be evaluated if careful postoperative management with limitation of weight-bearing can influence remodeling.

In situ pinning in our institute for slip with head–shaft angle less than 60° showed satisfactory clinical results and revealed good remodeling radiographically for short- and midterm periods. Taking into account that all the patients are adolescent, a longer follow-up is needed.

References

1. Carney BT, Birnbaum P, Minter C (2003) Slip progression after *in situ* single screw fixation for stable slipped capital femoral epiphysis. J Pediatr Orthop 23(5):584–589
2. Saunders JO, Smith WJ, Stanley EA, et al (2002) Progressive slippage after pinning for slipped capital femoral epiphysis. J Pediatr Orthop 22:239–243
3. Jones JR, Paterson DC, Hillier TM, et al (1990) Remodelling after pinning for slipped capital femoral epiphysis J Bone Joint Surg 72B:568–573
4. Iida S, Shinohara H, Fujitsuka M, et al (1992) Manual reduction for slipped capital femoral epiphysis (in Japanese). Rinsho Seikei Geka 27:771–777
5. Iida S, Shinada Y (2005) The indication and the limitation of in situ pinning for slipped capital femoral epiphysis (in Japanese). J Joint Surg 24:76–81
6. Loder RT, Richards AABS, Shapiro PS, et al (1993) Acute slipped capital femoral epiphysis: the importance of physeal stability. J Bone Joint Surg 75A:1134–1140
7. Heyman CH, Herndon CH (1954) Epiphyseodesis for early slipping of the upper femoral epiphysis. J Bone Joint Surg 36A:539–554
8. O'Brien CE, Fahey JJ (1977) Remodeling of the femoral neck after *in situ* pinning for slipped capital femoral epiphysis. J Bone Joint Surg 59A:62–69
9. Aronson DD, Carlson WE (1992) Slipped capital femoral epiphysis. A prospective study of fixation with a single screw. J Bone Joint Surg 74A:810–819
10. Ward WT, Stefko J, Wood KB, et al (1992) Fixation with a single screw for slipped capital femoral epiphysis. J Bone Joint Surg 74A:799–809
11. Jerre R, Hansson G, Wallin J, et al (1996) Long-term results after realignment operations for slipped capital femoral epiphysis. J Bone Joint Surg 78B:745–750

Retrospective Evaluation of Slipped Capital Femoral Epiphysis

Meishuu Ko[1], Kouji Ito[1], Keiji Sano[1], Naoki Miyagawa[1], Kengo Yamamoto[2], and Youichi Katori[2]

Summary. We treated 16 patients (16 hips) with slipped capital femoral epiphysis (12 boys and 4 girls) encountered during the previous 16-year period. Their age ranged from 8 to 15 years (mean, 11.1 years), and the observation period ranged from 18 to 82 months (mean, 37 months). The evaluation items were chief complaint, mechanism of injury, initial diagnosis, disease type, radiographic findings, physique and endocrinological abnormalities, treatment methods, and complications. The disease type was acute slip in 2 patients, chronic slip in 8, and acute on chronic slip in 6. Mild slip was observed in 10 patients, moderate slip in 5, and severe slip in 1. Only 31.3% of the patients were diagnosed as having slipped capital femoral epiphysis. The mean interval from the first visit to diagnosis was 30 days. Surgery was performed in all patients; Southwick intertrochanteric osteotomy was performed in 5 patients and in situ pinning in 11. Concerning surgical complications, methicillin-resistant *Staphylococcus aureus* infection developed in 1 patient and k-wire breakage in 1. Most patients had satisfactory results. No avascular necrosis occurred. Limitation of motion remained in 6 hips, but no hip pain, and normal gait was attained.

Key words. Slipped capital femoral epiphysis, Retrospective evaluation, Osteotomy, In situ pinning, Early diagnosis

Introduction

The report in 2004 by the Multicenter Study Committee of the Japanese Pediatric Orthopaedic Association showed a definite increase in patients with slipped capital femoral epiphysis during the previous 25-year period in Japan [1]. However, physicians other than pediatric surgeons are infrequently aware of slipped capital femoral epiphysis and do not include this entity in diseases for differential diagnosis; therefore, its diagnosis rate is low. In addition, there are no treatment methods with established evidence at present. We encountered 16 patients with slipped capital

[1] Department of Orthopedic Surgery, Tokyo Medical University Hachioji Medical Center, 1163 Tatemachi, Hachioji, Tokyo 193-0944, Japan
[2] Department of Orthopedic Surgery, Tokyo Medical University, Tokyo, Japan

femoral epiphysis during the previous 16-year period and clinically evaluated this disease.

Subjects and Methods

The subjects were 16 patients (12 boys and 4 girls) encountered during the previous 16-year period. Their age ranged from 8 to 15 years (mean, 11.1 years), and the observation period ranged from 18 to 82 months (mean, 37 months). The evaluation items were chief complaint, mechanism of injury, initial diagnosis, disease type, radiographic findings such as the slipping angle, physique and endocrinological abnormalities, treatment methods, and complications.

For radiographic evaluation, the head–shaft angle on frontal images and the posterior tilting angle in the frog-leg position were measured, and the right–left difference was regarded as the slipping angle. The severity of the disease was evaluated mainly based on the posterior tilting angle.

Results

The chief complaint was hip joint pain in 11 patients, pain from the hip joint to the knee in 3, pain from the hip joint to the thigh in 1, femoral pain in 1, and lower limb pain in 1. The mechanism of injury was sports in 8 patients, falling during running in 1, falling on the stairs in 1, long-distance walking in 1, and unknown in 3: most patients had relatively mild injuries. The mean interval between the onset of symptoms to the initial visit to the hospital was 69 days and that from the initial visit to diagnosis was 30 days. The duration until diagnosis was relatively short in patients with acute slip but considerably longer in some patients with chronic or acute on chronic slip.

The coefficient of the correlation between the onset of symptoms and diagnosis was 0.632, and the correlation was marked in patients with a long course.

The initial treatment was performed by an orthopedic surgeon in 11 patients, a surgeon in 3, a pediatrician in 2, and a bonesetter in 1. The initial diagnosis was slipped capital femoral epiphysis in 5 patients, absence of abnormalities in 3, Perthes disease in 2, unknown in 2, and growing pain, transient synovitis of the hip, and femoral neck fracture in 1 each. Only 31.3% of the patients were diagnosed as having slipped capital femoral epiphysis, and this correct diagnosis was made only by orthopedic surgeons. At the time of the visit to our hospital, a correct diagnosis was soon made in all patients.

The disease type was acute slip in 2 patients, chronic slip in 8, and acute on chronic slip in 6. The head–shaft angle at the first visit was 2°–42° (mean, 17.9°), and the posterior tilting angle was 7°–78° (mean, 29.6°). Mild slip (between 0° and 30°) was observed in 10 patients, moderate slip (between 30° and 60°) in 5, and severe slip (>60°) in 1 (Fig. 1).

The mean interval between the onset of symptoms and the initial visit to the hospital was 69 days and that from the first visit to diagnosis was 30 days.

The physique (height, weight) of the patients was compared with its distribution according to age reported by the School Health Statistic Survey in 2005. Compared

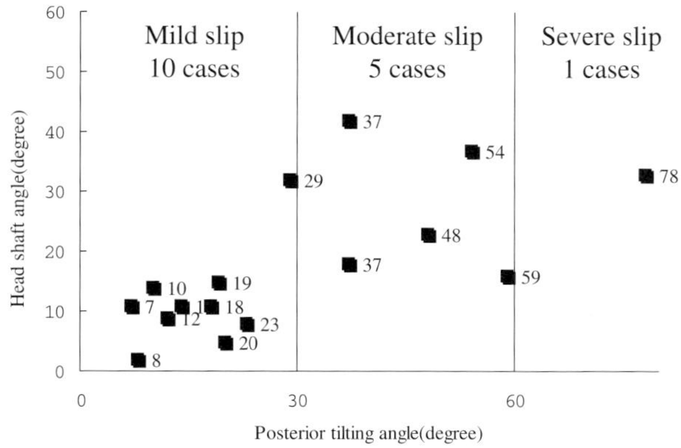

FIG. 1. Relation between head-shaft angle and posterior tilting angle

with the mean statistical values, the height of the patients was −10.1 to +19.9 cm (mean, +6.0 cm), and height below the mean was observed in only 2 patients. Compared with the mean statistical values, the weight of the patients was −10.4 to +39.7 kg (mean, +17.6 kg), and weight below the mean was observed in only 1 patient. Body mass index was 14.2–33.4 (mean, 24.6) and ≥25 in 8 patients (50%). The underweight patient with a body mass index of 14.2 was a 12-year-old girl who was 3 cm taller than the mean height.

Endocrinological examination showed a low testosterone level in one patient. However, abnormalities could not be confirmed in any patient because they were in the growth stage.

Surgery was performed in all patients; Southwick intertrochanteric osteotomy [2] was performed in 5 patients and in situ pinning in 11. Contralateral preventive bone epiphyseal fixation was performed in all except 1 patient.

The implant used for in situ pinning was the Knewles pin in 2 patients, Kirschner wire (k-wire) with thread in 3, and ACE(R) SCFE screw in 6. For contralateral preventive pinning, the Knewles pin was used in 2 patients, k-wire with thread in 3, ACE SCFE screw in 9, and Hannson pin in 1. For fixation after Southwick intertrochanteric osteotomy, the AO double angle plate (MIZUHO, Tokyo, Japan) was used. In all patients, epiphyseal fixation was added, and the implants used were the same materials as those used in preventive pinning. The flexion osteotomy angle was frequently 20°–30°, although it was 50° in 1 patient. Changes in the slipping angle after osteotomy are shown in Fig. 2. Good reductions in both the posterior tilting angle and head–shaft angle were observed.

Concerning surgical complications, methicillin-resistant *Staphylococcus aureus* infection associated with Southwick intertrochanteric osteotomy developed in one patient and k-wire breakage associated with in situ pinning in one. Leg length discrepancy after Southwick intertrochanteric osteotomy until the final observation was observed in three of five patients (0.5, 0.8, and 1.0 cm, respectively), but this presented no clinical problems. Limitation in range of motion was present in six patients; only

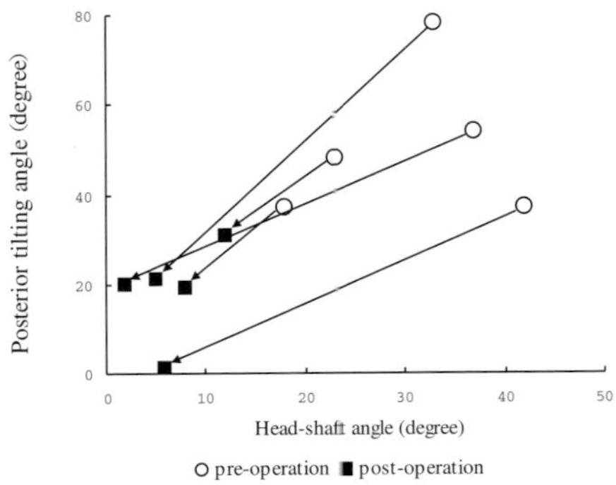

Fig. 2. Changes of head-shaft angle and posterior tilting angle after osteotomy

limitation in flexion was observed in two, only that in internal rotation in two, and that in both flexion and internal rotation and both flexion and internal/external rotation in one each.

Concerning sequelae, one patient showed narrowing of the joint space at the initial consultation, and although postoperative changes were negligible, the course has been observed. No avascular necrosis of the femoral head occurred, no pain of hip, and the patient has acquired a normal gait.

Case Presentations

Patient 1: 10-Year-Old Boy

He noticed right hip joint pain in February 2002. On March 30 of the same year, he fell on the stairs, sustained injury, and was transported to a local hospital by ambulance. A diagnosis of femoral neck fracture was made by a surgeon at the first consultation, and he was referred to our hospital (Fig. 3A). A diagnosis of unstable slipped capital femoral epiphysis was made, and direct wire traction was performed for about 2 weeks from immediately after admission. Because the slipping angle as the posterior tilting angle was reduced from 59° to 17° by traction, in situ pinning was performed (Fig. 3B). Five years and 4 months after operation, he has no pain or limitation in the range of motion, showing a good course (Fig. 3C).

Patient 2: 12-Year-Old Girl

She noticed hip joint pain about 1 year earlier, visited a local hospital, but was told that there was no abnormality. After an athletic meeting, her hip joint pain increased, and she visited our hospital, was diagnosed as having slipped capital femoral epiphysis, and admitted (Fig. 4A). Even after direct traction, adequate reduction could not be achieved, and Southwick intertrochanteric osteotomy was performed. The osteotomy angle was 35° in flexion and 20° in abduction. The internal rotation collection was 20° (Fig. 4B). Three years and 8 months after operation, remodeling of the femoral head was good, but limitation in the range of motion in flexion (5°) remained (Fig. 4C).

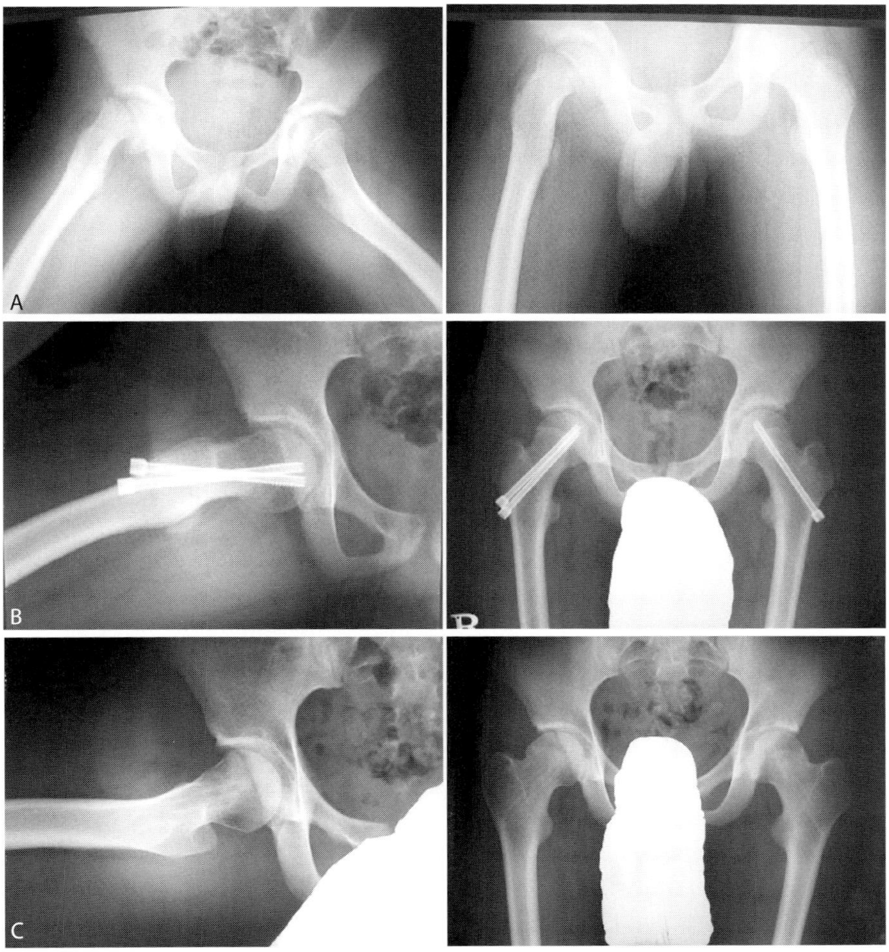

FIG. 3. Case 1 10-year-old boy. **A** Pre-operative roentgenogram of the hip. **B** Postoperative roentgenogram of the hip. **C** Roentgenogram of the hip 64 months postoperation

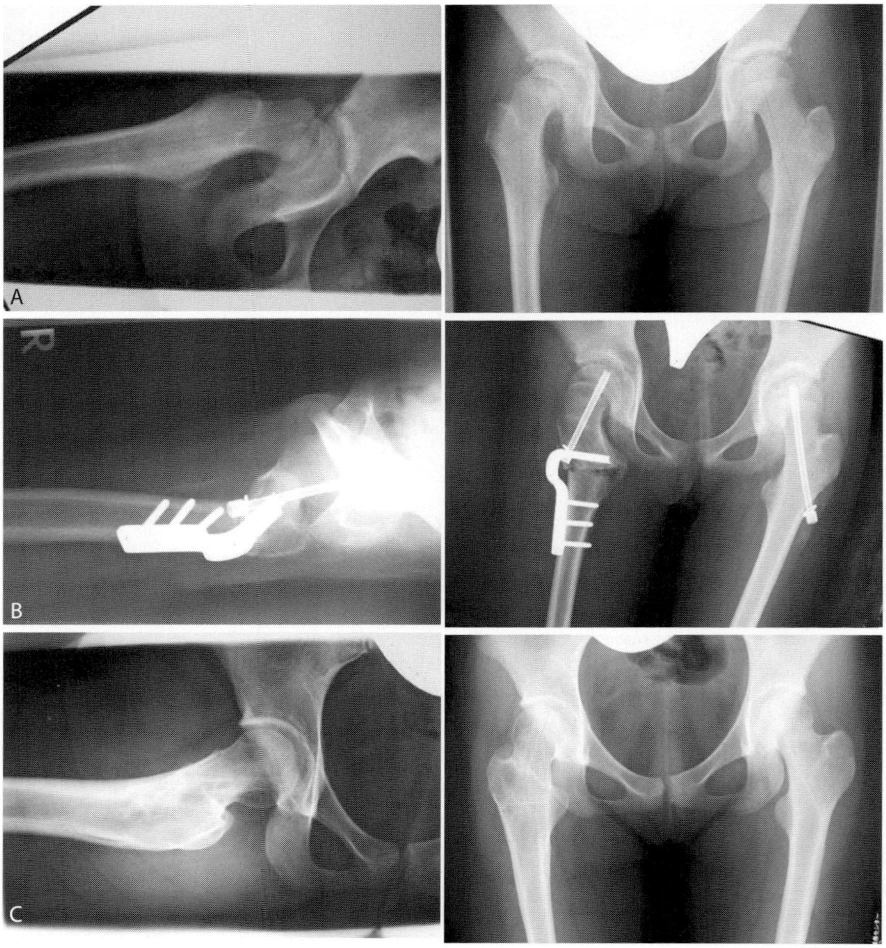

FIG. 4. Case 2 12-year-old girl. **A** Pre-operative roentgenogram of the hip. **B** Postoperative roentgenogram of the hip. **C** Roentgenogram of the hip 44 months postoperation

Discussion

In our patients, the correct initial diagnosis rate was only 31.3%, and some patients with an incorrect diagnosis showed a change to acute on chronic slip.

The coefficient of the correlation between the duration until diagnosis and the slipping angle was 0.632 (see Table 1). Saisu et al. [3] and Kocher et al. [4] reported a significant association between duration until diagnosis and slipping angle. Some patients in this study required a considerably long time for diagnosis, increasing the slipping angle, and thus we confirmed the importance of early diagnosis.

Our treatment principles are as follows (Fig. 5). In patients in whom instability is suspected at the first visit and reduction can be expected, direct wire traction is performed, and the severity of the disease is evaluated based on the posterior tilting angle. In situ pinning is performed when the angle is less than 30° and Southwick intertrochanteric osteotomy when the angle is ≥30°. Because no manual reduction is performed either before or during operation, there is no method of confirming instability. Therefore, we perform direct wire traction in patients with a posterior tilting angle of ≥30° on the affected side and prophylactic pinning on the contralateral side in principle. Castro et al. [5] stated that "close follow-up and not prophylactic pinning was most supported by the literature." In contrast, Schultz et al. [6] reported "a benefit in the long-term outcome for patients who had prophylactic of the contralateral hip." A review of the literature shows arguments both for and against prophylactic pinning but no studies with a large body of evidence. We perform prophylactic pinning because we have previously encountered children with contralateral slip and fully realized that children at this age when this disease frequently develops do not often follow instructions to rest.

We perform in situ pinning in patients with a posterior tilting angle of <30°. However, some studies have shown good results after in situ pinning in patients with an angle of ≥30°. In patients with this disease not complicated by femoral head necrosis or acute cartilage necrosis, short-term results are good. Even if short- or middle-term results are good, however, because osteoarthrosis of the hip develops at middle age or later, the expansion of the indications of this method should be carefully evaluated.

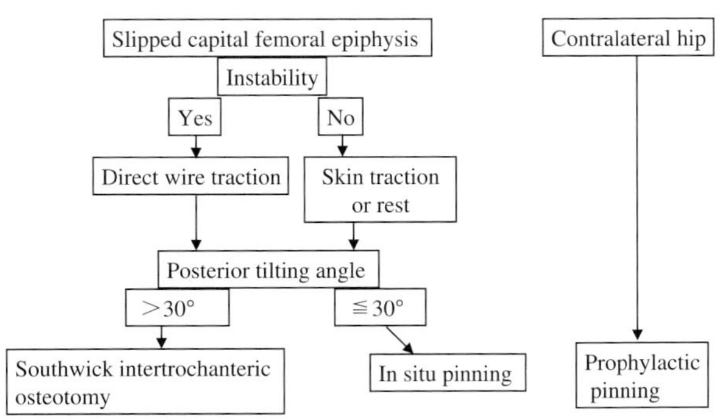

Fig. 5. Algorithm of treatment for slipped capital femoral epiphysis

Various osteotomy methods have also been reported. We use Southwick intertrochanteric osteotomy because operation-associated femoral head necrosis rarely occurs, no high-level technique is necessary, and stable results can be expected.

References

1. Noguchi Y, Sakamaki T(2004) Epidemiology and demographics of slipped capital femoral epiphysis in Japan. J Jpn Pediatr Orthop Assoc 13(2):235–243
2. Southwick WO (1967) Osteotomy through the lesser trochanter for slipped capital femoral epiphysis. J Bone Joint Surg [Am] 49(5):807–835
3. Saisu T, Kamegaya M, Ochiai N, et al (2003) Importance of early diagnosis for treatment of slipped capital femoral epiphysis. J Jpn Pediatr Orthop Assoc 12(1–2):61–64
4. Kocher MS, Bishop JA, Weed B (2004) Delay in diagnosis of slipped capital femoral epiphysis. Pediatrics 113(4):322–325
5. Castro FP Jr, Benett JT, Doulens K (2004) Epidemiological perspective on prophylactic pinning in patients with unilateral slipped capital femoral epiphysis. J Pediatr Orthop 20(6):745–738
6. Schultz WR, Weinstein JN, Weinstein SL (2002) Prophylactic pinning of the contralateral hip in slipped capital femoral epiphysis: evaluation of long-term outcome for the contralateral hip with use of decision analysis. J Bone Joint Surg [Am] 84A(8): 1305–1314

Part II
Avascular Necrosis of the Femoral Head

Osteotomy for Osteonecrosis of the Femoral Head: Knowledge from Our Long-Term Treatment Experience at Kyushu University

Seiya Jingushi

Summary. Many young patients suffer from osteonecrosis of the femoral head (ONFH). For this reason, osteotomy is considered to be an important treatment option, and their survival after osteotomy of the hip is expected to be of long duration. Cases that survived more than 25 years after osteotomy were investigated to reconfirm the principles or the indication based upon our previous experience about osteotomy treatment for ONFH. Fifteen cases were divided into two groups with or without advanced osteoarthritis at the last follow-up and were compared. The mean follow-up periods were 28 and 27 years, respectively. All the cases with advanced osteoarthritis (OA) had collapse progression. All the cases in which the preoperative stage was advanced were included in those with advanced OA at the last follow-up. In contrast, collapse progression was not observed in the cases without advanced OA at the last follow-up. All these cases had minimum collapse before operation. According to these data, we reconfirmed that collapse progression is the main cause for poor outcome after osteotomy, and that cases operated on at an early stage are apt to experience a good prognosis. When the indication and the operation are appropriate, osteotomy could prevent disease deterioration even more than 25 years after the operation.

Key words. Osteonecrosis of the femoral head, Osteotomy, Transtrochanteric anterior rotational osteotomy, Collapse, Clinical outcome

Introduction

Once collapse occurs at the necrosis area of the femoral head, it usually progresses. Collapse causes incongruity and instability of the hip joint, and the progression of collapse causes incongruity and instability to increase and finally results in secondary osteoarthritis (Fig. 1). The purpose of osteotomy for osteonecrosis of the femoral head (ONFH) is to prevent the progression of collapse and secondary osteoarthritis. A principle of osteotomy is to support weight-bearing with intact or live bone instead

Department of Orthopaedic Surgery, Graduate School of Medical Sciences, Kyushu University, 3-1-1 Maidashi, Higashi-ku, Fukuoka 812-8582, Japan

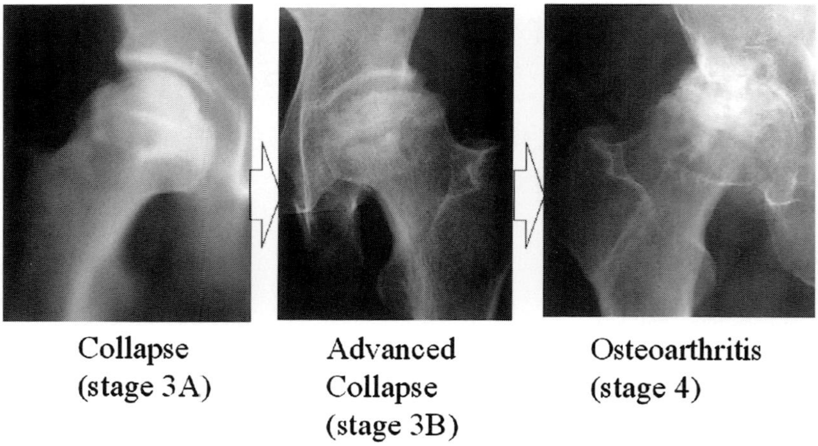

FIG. 1. Natural course of osteonecrosis of the femoral head (ONFH)

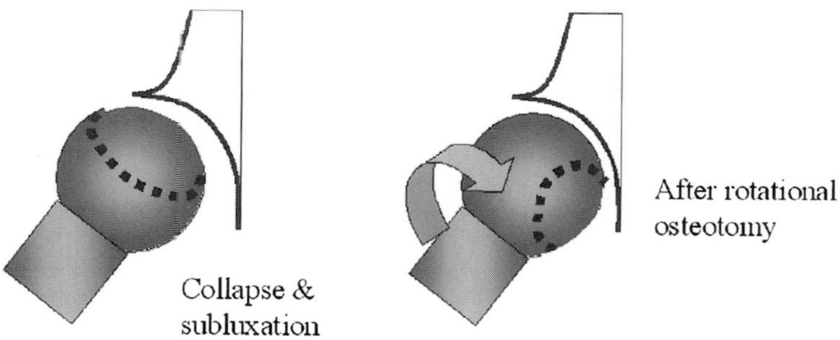

FIG. 2. A principle of anterior rotational osteotomy for ONFH. The *dashed line* shows the osteonecrosis area of the femoral head from the anterior view

of the necrotic bone and to restore the subluxated femoral head (Fig. 2). In other words, osteotomy is on-site vascularized bone grafting with articular cartilage and with good congruency. Options of osteotomy for ONFH are transtrochanteric anterior or posterior rotational osteotomy (ARO or PRO) developed by Sugioka et al. [1,2], and intertrochanteric curved varus osteotomy developed by Nishio and Sugioka [3]. The treatment option is chosen depending on the lesion of osteonecrosis or on where and how wide is the osteonecrosis area in the femoral head. Stage and age at the operation are also considered in this choice.

Many young patients suffer from the disease. Especially for young patients, osteotomy is an important treatment option to be considered, and they are expected to survive for a long time after their hip osteotomy. Osteotomy in Kyushu University Hospital started in 1972. Sugioka developed transtrochanteric rotational osteotomy

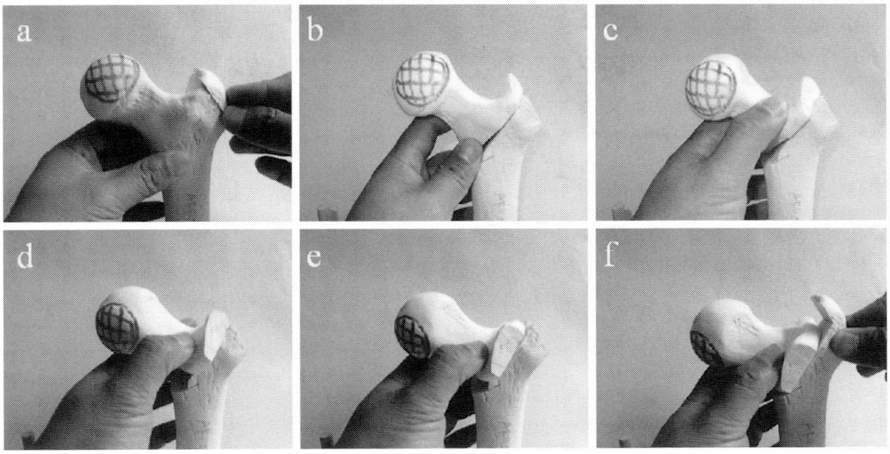

FIG. 3. Sequential photographs of anterior rotation of the femoral head show a model of anterior rotational osteotomy (ARO) with 20° varus position and indicate how ARO results in weight-bearing with the living posterior surface of the femoral head (**a–f**). *Hatched area* indicates necrotic area. All the photographs show the anterior view. According to anterior rotation, the osteotomy line is 10° inclination away from the perpendicular to the neck (**a**) and 10° retroversion. The result is 20° varus position after anterior rotation of the femoral head (**f**)

of the femoral head, so-called "rotational osteotomy" or "Sugioka's osteotomy" [1]. Anterior rotation of the femoral head with vascularity results in weight-bearing with the live posterior surface of the femoral head (Fig. 3).

Experience of Osteotomy in Kyushu University Between 1972 and 1979

The cases that survived more than 25 years after the operation were investigated to reconfirm the principles or the indication based upon our previous experience with osteotomy treatment for ONFH [1,2,4].

Patients and Methods

Between 1972 and 1979, 128 patients with idiopathic ONFH underwent osteotomy in our department. Fifteen hips of 9 patients, who had been visiting our outpatient office and had their living hip joints more than 25 years after operation, were examined. The hips were separated into two groups (Table 1). One group includes the hips that had advanced or terminal osteoarthritis (OA) at the last follow-up. Another group includes those that had no OA or early OA. Age at operation and period after operation were similar in both the groups. Clinical scores were assessed according to the hip scoring system by the Japanese Orthopaedic Association.

TABLE 1. Characterization of the hips in two groups

	With advanced OA	Without advanced OA
Number of examined hips	9	6
Age at operation (years)	31 (19–52)	31 (24–38)
Involved in the contralateral side	6 (67%)	3 (50%)
Period after operation (years)	28 (25–30)	27 (26–29)
Stage	3A: 5 (56%); 3B: 4 (44%)	3A: 6 (100%)
Collapse progression	9 (100%)	0 (0%)
JOA score[a] at the last follow-up	55 (34–82)	86 (54–100)

OA, osteoarthritis

[a] In the clinical scoring system for hip joints developed by the Japanese Orthopaedic Association, the maximum score is 100 points

Results

All hips that had no or early OA at the last follow-up were at stage 3A at operation and had no collapse progression after osteotomy (see Table 1). The average of their clinical scores was promising. In contrast, approximately half of the hips that had advanced or terminal OA at the last follow-up were at stage 3B at operation. Furthermore, all of them had collapse progression and had poor clinical scores at the last follow-up.

Representative Cases

Case 1

The patient was male and had bilateral ARO at 38 years old (Fig. 4a). Preoperative stage of the right and left hip was 3A or 3B, respectively. Twenty-eight years after operation, collapse had progressed in the left hip, and that hip showed terminal OA at the last follow-up (Fig. 4b). The clinical score was 34 points. The right hip had early OA at the last follow-up, and the clinical score was 54 points, although collapse did not progress after the operation.

Case 2

This patient was male and underwent ARO and varus osteotomy, respectively, in the right and left hips at 33 years of age (Fig. 5a). Preoperative stage was 3A in both hips. Twenty-seven years after the operation, collapse of the femoral head had not progressed, and OA changes were not observed (Fig. 5b). The clinical scores were 92 and 82 points, respectively. Note that good bone regeneration was observed in the osteonecrosis area of the bilateral femoral head.

Case 3

This patient was male and had ARO bilaterally at 24 years old at the time of operation (Fig. 6a). Preoperative stage was 3A in both hips. Twenty-six years after the operation, collapse of the femoral head had not progressed, and OA changes were not observed (Fig. 6b). The clinical score was 100 points in both the joints.

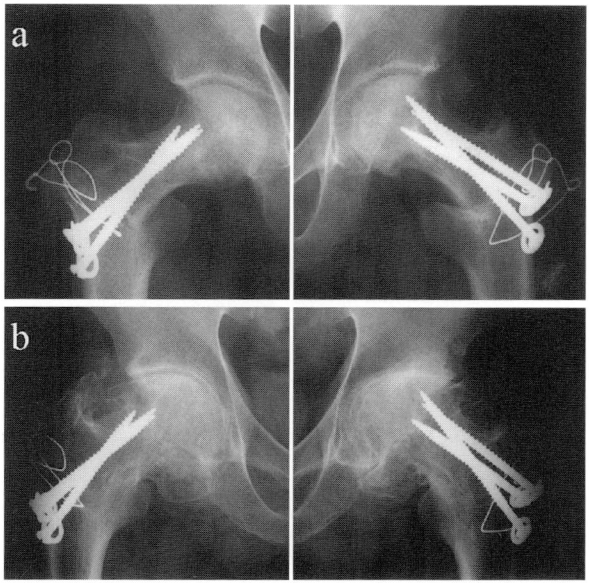

FIG. 4. A representative case (case 1) that had advanced osteoarthritis (OA) 28 years after operation. **a** Just after osteotomy; **b** 28 years after osteotomy

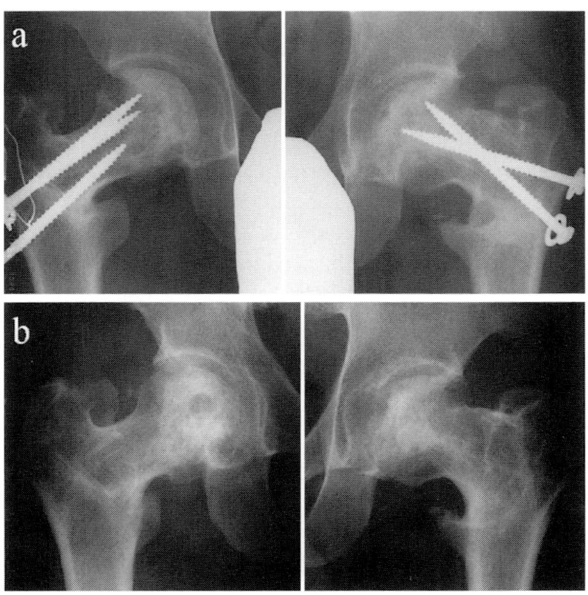

FIG. 5. A representative case (case 2) that had no OA changes 27 years after operation. **a** Just after osteotomy; **b** 27 years after osteotomy

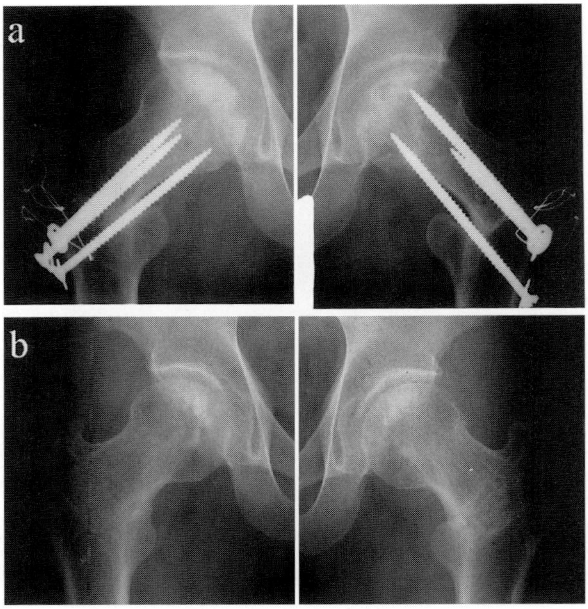

Fig. 6. A representative case (case 3) that had no OA changes 26 years after operation. **a** Just after osteotomy; **b** 26 years after osteotomy

Discussion

Based on the data, we reconfirmed that progression of collapse was the main cause of poor results after osteotomy, as previously described [1,2,4]. Cases operated on at an early stage are apt to experience good prognosis. Stage at operation is another important factor to influence the clinical outcome. When osteotomy is carried out at an early stage and prevents progression of collapse, this could prevent disease deterioration or maintain hip function without clinical symptoms even more than 25 years after operation.

Experience of Osteotomy in Kyushu University Between 1980 and 1988

Previously, we examined 125 cases that had undergone operations between 1980 and 1988 [5]. Twenty-eight hips had collapse progression more than 10 years after operation. We found that the postoperative intact ratio in the nonprogression group was significantly larger than that in the progression group. A minimum postoperative intact ratio to prevent collapse progression over a 10-year period was 34% (Fig. 7). According to that study, the aim of osteotomy is to achieve more than 34% of the

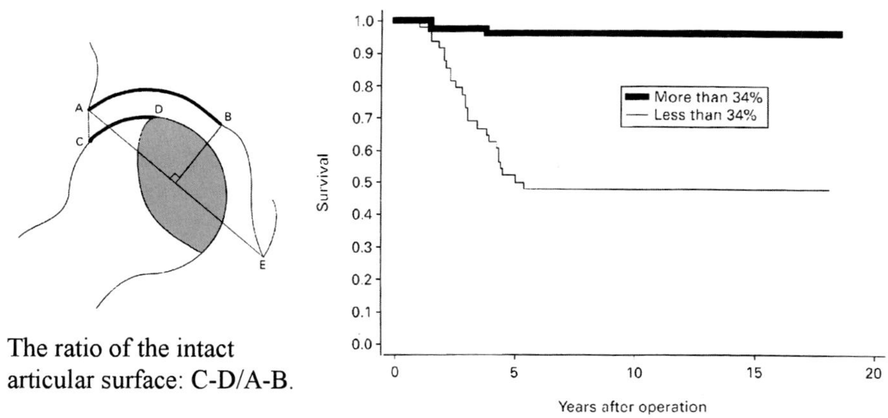

FIG. 7. Kaplan–Meier survival curve of groups with a postoperative intact ratio of more than 34% and with a ratio less than 34%. The occurrence of progressive collapse is used as an endpoint. (From [5], with permission.) The figure on the *left* shows how to calculate the intact ratio

ratio of the intact area postoperatively. We try to ensure this every time during preoperative planning.

A Current Representative Case

Sugioka has reported good clinical outcome of osteotomy for ONFH. However, there are many reports that show poor clinical outcome, especially as concerns rotational osteotomy [6–8]. The most important issue about osteotomy treatment may be whether osteotomy could be carried out successfully by others than Sugioka.

In our department, osteotomy treatment has been carried out according to the principles based on our long experience. A current representative case is shown, a 33-year-old woman who had bilateral steroid-induced osteonecrosis. Radiographs and magnetic resonance imaging (MRI) show a wide osteonecrosis area, and the intact area was limited to the posterior surface of the femoral head (Fig. 8). According to the preoperative planning, ARO with 20° varus position was expected to result in more than 34% of the ratio of the intact articular in both the joints. The osteotomy was carried out in the right hip joint, and then in the left hip 2 months after the first operation. Four years after operations, collapse has not progressed in either of the hip joints, and no OA changes are observed in the postoperative radiographs (Fig. 9). She has no problems in walking, squatting, and going up and down the stairs (Fig. 10) at 5 years after osteotomy. Clinical scores of both hip joints are 100 points, and she has returned to work.

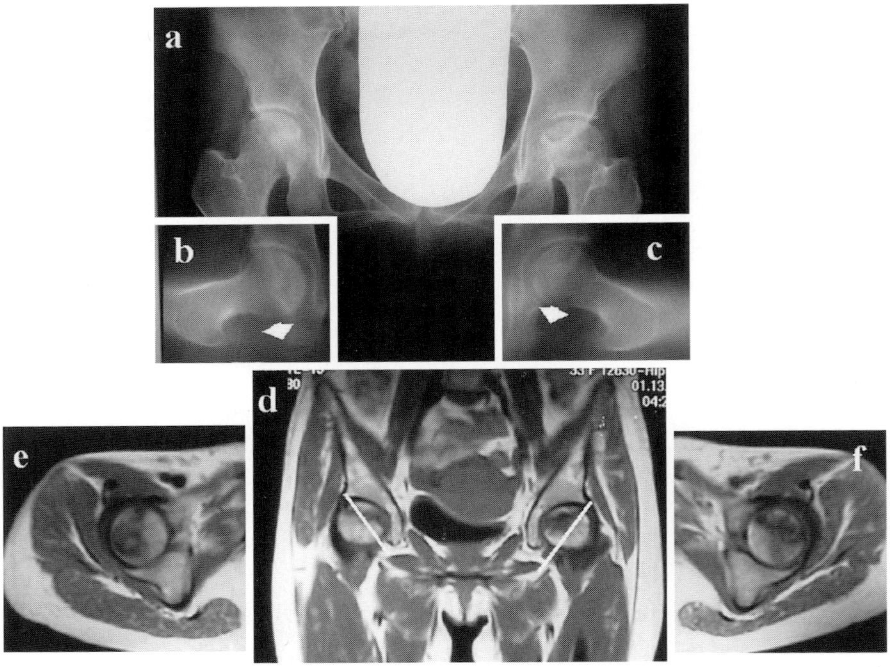

FIG. 8. Preoperative radiographs and magnetic resonance (MR) images of a current representative case. **a** Anteroposterior view radiograph of bilateral ONFH. **b, c** Tomography of the bilateral joints in a Lauenstein position. **d** Frontal section of T_1-weighted MRI of the bilateral hip joints. **e, f** View of vertical section to the femoral neck axis in right and left femoral head, respectively. Location of the section is indicated in **d**

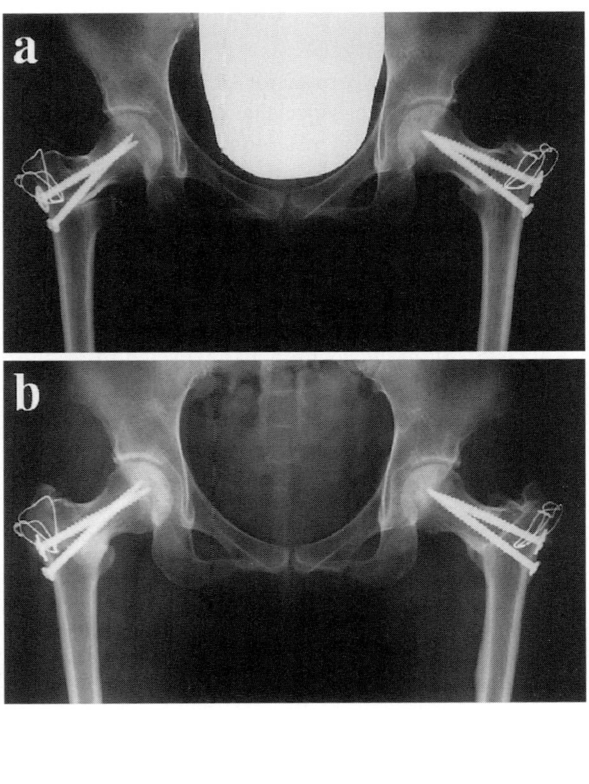

FIG. 9. Radiographs of bilateral hip joints just after osteotomy (**a**) or 4 years after osteotomy (**b**)

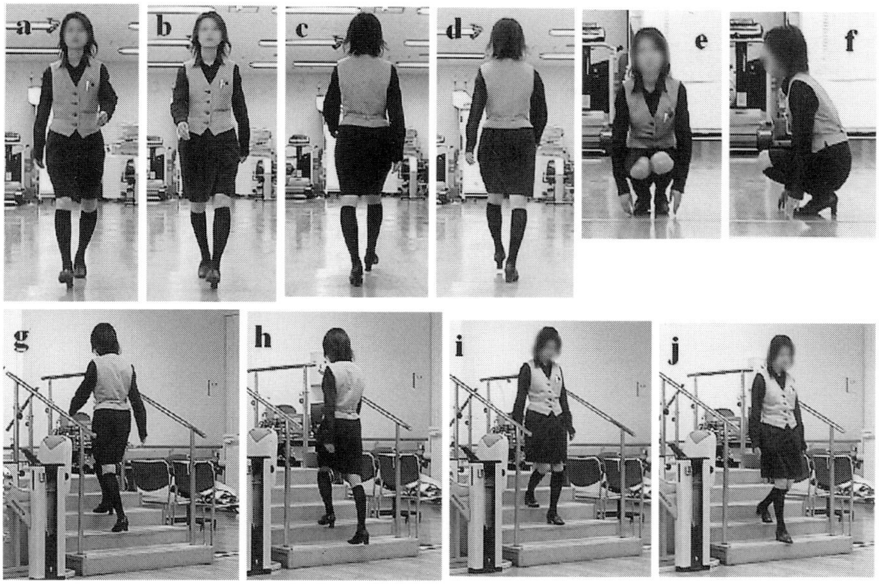

FIG. 10. Activities of daily life of the representative case. **a–d** Walking; **e, f** squatting; **g, h** going up stairs; **i, j** going down stairs

Conclusions

Osteotomy could maintain prevention of disease deterioration of ONFH even more than 25 years after the operation. Osteotomy is a promising treatment option for ONFH, especially for young patients. We believe that experienced hip surgeons can perform osteotomy, including ARO, successfully once they understand the indications and techniques.

References

1. Sugioka Y (1978) Transtrochanteric anterior rotational osteotomy of the femoral head in the treatment of osteonecrosis affecting the hip. A new osteotomy operation. Clin Orthop 130:191–201
2. Sugioka Y, Hotokebuchi T, Tsutsui H (1992) Transtrochanteric anterior rotational osteotomy for idiopathic and steroid-induced necrosis of the femoral head. Clin Orthop 277:111–120
3. Nishio A, Sugioka Y (1971) A new technique of the varus osteotomy at the upper end of the femur. Orthop Traumatol 20:381–386
4. Hosokawa A, Mohtai M, Hotokebuchi T, et al (1997) Transtrochanteric rotational osteotomy for idiopathic and steroid-induced osteonecrosis of the femoral head: indications and long-term follow-up. In: Urbaniak JR, Jones JP Jr (eds) Osteonecrosis, etiology, diagnosis and treatment. The American Orthopaedic Association, Rosemont, IL, pp 309–314

5. Miyanishi K, Noguchi Y, Yamamoto T, et al (2000) Prediction of the outcome of transtrochanteric rotational osteotomy for osteonecrosis of the femoral head. J Bone Joint Surg 82B:512–516
6. Belal MA, Reichelt A (1996) Clinical results of rotational osteotomy for treatment of avascular necrosis of the femoral head. Arch Orthop Trauma Surg 115(2):80–84
7. Dean MT, Cabanela ME (1993) Transtrochanteric anterior rotational osteotomy for avascular necrosis of the femoral head. Long-term results. J Bone Joint Surg [Br] 75(4):597–601
8. Tooke SM, Amstutz HC, Hedley AK (1987) Results of transtrochanteric rotational osteotomy for femoral head osteonecrosis. Clin Orthop 224:150–157

Joint Preservation of Severe Osteonecrosis of the Femoral Head Treated by Posterior Rotational Osteotomy in Young Patients: More Than 3 Years of Follow-up and Its Remodeling

Takashi Atsumi, Yasunari Hiranuma, Satoshi Tamaoki, Kentaro Nakamura, Yasuhiro Asakura, Ryosuke Nakanishi, Eiji Katoh, Minoru Watanabe, and Toshihisa Kajiwara

Summary. Posterior rotational osteotomy in 48 hips of 40 young patients with femoral head osteonecrosis with extensive and apparent collapsed lesions were reviewed with a mean of 9.2 years of follow-up. No viable area was seen on the articular surface of the femoral head of the loaded portion on preoperative anteroposterior radiographs in all femoral heads. All hips had greater than 3 mm collapse; 40 hips showed no apparent joint narrowing, and 8 hips revealed joint narrowing. Posterior viable area of joint surface before surgery ranged from 6% to 29%, with a mean of 19%, on lateral radiographs. Anterior viable area ranged from 6% to 42% with a mean of 21%. The mean age of the patients was 29 years, with 13 women and 27 men. Thirty-five hips were nontraumatic, and 13 were traumatic. Mean postoperative viable area below the acetabular roof was 59% on anteroposterior radiographs and 54% on 45° flexed radiographs. Recollapse was prevented in 44 hips (92%), with adequate viable area on the loaded portion on final follow-up radiographs. Progressive joint narrowing was found in 9 hips. Resphericity of the postoperative transferred medial collapsed area of the femoral head was observed on 34 of 35 hips on final anteroposterior radiographs. The joint space was increased in 6 of 8 hips. Posterior rotational osteotomy appeared to be effective in delaying the progression of degeneration in young patients with extensive collapsed osteonecrotic lesions.

Key words. Osteonecrosis, Osteonecrosis of the femoral head, Joint preservation, Posterior rotational osteotomy, Transtrochanteric rotational osteotomy

Introduction

Nontraumatic and posttraumatic osteonecrosis involving the femoral head frequently occurs in young patients. Preservation of the joint of the femoral head necrosis in young patients to avoid joint replacement procedures is widely accepted for

---

Department of Orthopaedic Surgery, Fujigaoka Hospital, Showa University School of Medicine, 1-30 Fujigaoka Aobaku, Yokohama 227-8501, Japan

orthopedic surgeons. However, in cases of extensive lesion and apparent collapse, some kinds of osteotomies [1,2], with vascularized fibular grafts [3], are usually not effective. Sugioka has reported transtrochanteric anterior rotational osteotomies for osteonecrosis of the femoral head and described excellent follow-up results [4–6]. The absolute indications for this operation were that the necrotic area is located on less than the posterior one-third of the entire femoral head on correct lateral radiographs [4]. Sugioka also mentioned indications for posterior rotational osteotomies, but he did not report the details of this procedure [5]. We have reported on the use of posterior rotational osteotomies including our modified approach, "high degree posterior rotation" [7,8], for femoral head osteonecrosis with extensive lesions. The advantages of posterior rotational osteotomies are as follows. (1) The posterior column artery branched off from the femoral medial circumflex artery is shifted medially and is not under tension without vascular damage by posterior rotation. We confirmed this condition by our angiographic studies [9]. (2) The necrotic area is transferred to the posteromedial non-weight-bearing portion. Postoperative uncollapsed anterior viable areas are moved to the loaded portion below the acetabular roof in flexed positions. After posterior rotation, congruency can be expected in a flexed position of daily life. The purpose of this study is to investigate the effectiveness of joint preservation by posterior rotational osteotomy for the treatment of severe femoral head osteonecrosis with extensive collapsed lesions in patients less than 50 years old.

Materials and Methods

Between 1985 and 2002, 60 hips with apparent collapse and extensive lesions of the femoral head in young patients (less than 50 years of age) were treated by posterior rotational osteotomies including high-degree posterior rotation. Of these hips, 48 hips of 40 patients with a minimum of 3 years follow-up were subjected in this study (follow-up range, 3–20 years; mean, 9.2 years). If the patients were converted to a prosthetic replacement, follow-up ended. The age of the patients at the time of surgery ranged from 15 to 49 years with a mean of 29 years; 13 patients were women and 27 were men. Of the hips, 23 had a history of corticosteroid administration, 9 had a history of alcohol abuse, 10 had a history of femoral neck fracture, and 3 had a history traumatic dislocation; the remaining 3 hips had no apparent risk factor. We excluded 12 of 60 hips from the study because 7 hips were lost to follow-up, 4 hips were conversion surgery of a prosthetic replacement less than 3 years after posterior rotational osteotomy because of early recollapse after trauma, and 1 patient died of underlying disease.

All 48 hips had extensive lesions from medial to lateral and from anterior to the posterior portion of the femoral head. No viable area was seen on the articular surface of the loaded portion of the femoral head facing the acetabular roof on preoperative anteroposterior radiographs (type C2 of criteria of Japanese Investigations Committee) [10] in all 48 hips. On correct lateral radiographs [4], the posterior viable area of joint surface of these hips before surgery ranged from 6% to 29% with a mean of 19%. The anterior viable area ranged from 6% to 42% with a mean of 21%. No hips were indicated for a traditional anterior rotational osteotomy. All 48 hips had apparent collapse (greater than 3 mm). In these hips, 40 hips showed no apparent joint space narrowing (stage 3B of criteria of Japanese Investigations Committee) [10]. The remaining 8 hips revealed apparent joint space narrowing (stage 4). Twenty-five cases were involved by osteonecrosis bilaterally on radiographs or magnetic resonance imaging. Of these hips, 11 were treated by bilateral posterior rotational osteotomy. Different procedures were elected for the contralateral hips of the other 14 cases: 2 anterior rotational osteotomies and 1 total hip arthroplasty. The remaining 4 cases were not treated because of small-size lesion without symptoms. These hips were not included in this study. All collapsed femoral heads were rotated in the posterior direction. Degrees of rotation ranged from 70° to 160° posteriorly (mean, 126°). Additional intentional varus positioning was done from 10° to 30° (mean, 19°) in all 48 hips to obtain an extensive noncollapsed viable articular surface of the femoral head in the loaded portion postoperatively. A summary of the patient population is shown in Table 1.

The rotational angle and intentional varus angle necessary for this procedure were determined by preoperative assessment, mainly on radiographic findings. Correct lateral radiographs (Fig. 1B) and anteroposterior radiographs in a flexed position were taken in all hips to observe the location and extent of necrotic region. Radiographs taken under these conditions can show the location and extent of the noncollapsed viable articular surface of the femoral head after posterior rotation. Magnetic resonance imaging and computed tomography can be available if the demarcation area between living and necrotic bone is not clearly visualized on radiographs.

A modified Southern approach [7,8] was applied in 47 hips. The modified Ollier approach as reported by Sugioka [4] was employed in 1 remaining operation. For the fixation of osteotomy plane after femoral head rotation, we used large screws (Sugioka) in 4 hips, an AO screw in 2, and an AO plate in 2. However, these fixation devices were not strong enough to allow for early motion. Thereafter, the authors made and used a customized device developed by Atsumi [7,8] in 40 hips.

Table 1. Patient population

Forty-eight hips, of 40 young patients
Age, 15–49 years old (mean, 29 years)
Sex: 13 women, 27 men
Etiological factor:
Steroid administration, 23 hips
Alcohol abuse, 9; traumatic, 13
No apparent factor, 3
Type C2: 48 hips (no viable area on articular surface of the femoral head of loaded portion on preoperative anteroposterior radiographs)
Stage 3B, 40 hips; 4, 8 hips (all 48 showed >3 mm collapse)
Anterior or posterior viable area on correct lateral radiographs
Anterior, 6%–42% (mean, 21); posterior, 6%–29% (mean, 19)
Posterior rotational angle: 70°–160° (mean: 126°)
Additional varus position 10°–25° (mean, 19°)
Follow-up, 3–20 years (mean, 9.2 years)
Excluded cases: lost to follow-up, 7; early revised surgery, 4; died, 1

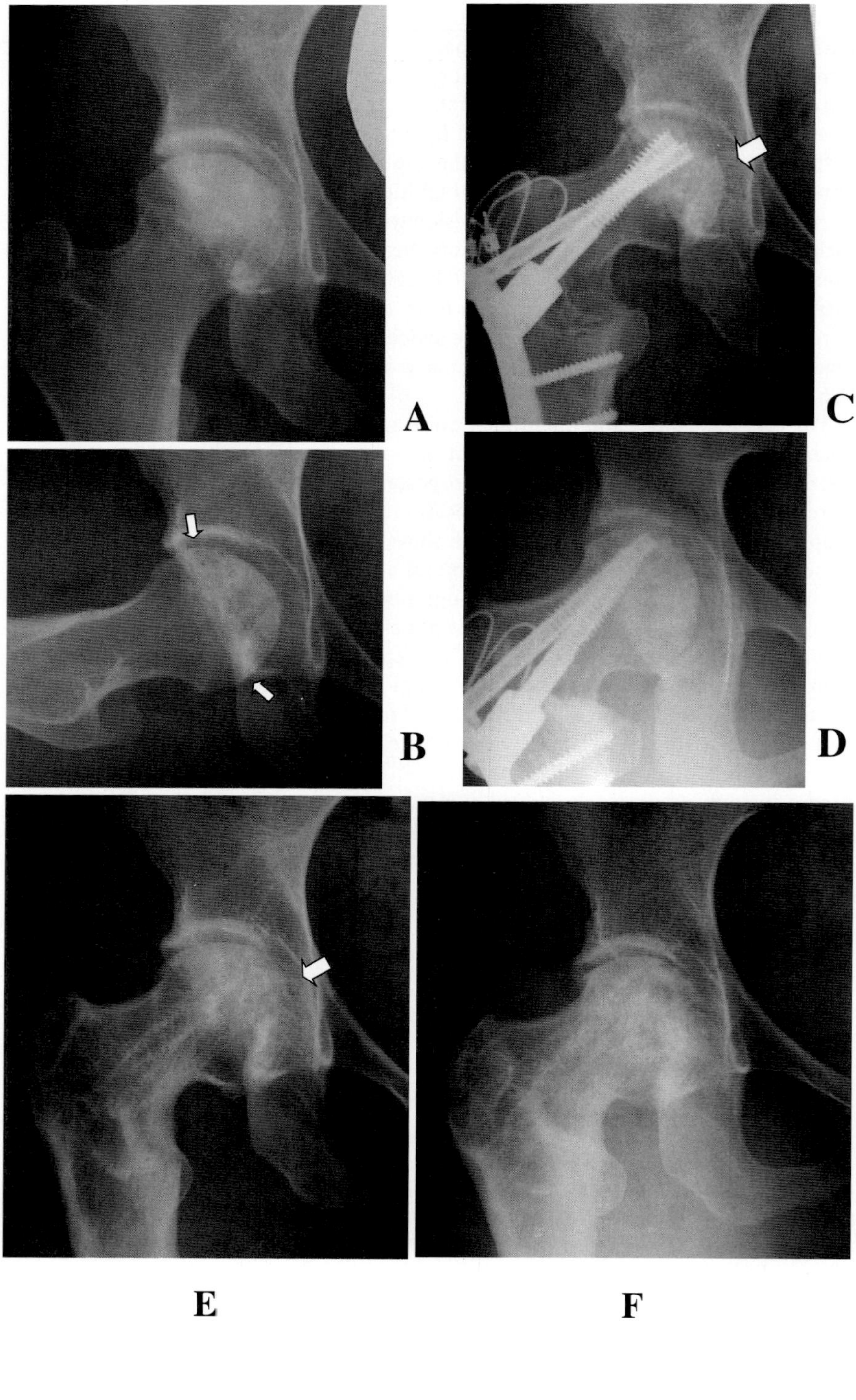
A
C
B
D
E
F

TABLE 2. Extent of viable area of femoral head on postoperative AP and 45° flexion AP radiographs

	Group A	Group B	Group C
	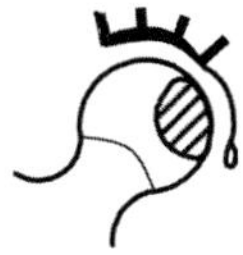 ≧2/3	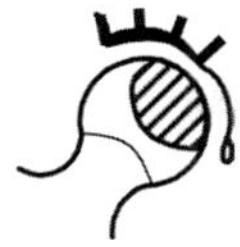 ≧1/3, 2/3	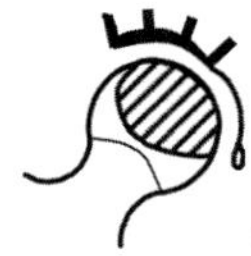 <1/3
Conventional AP ($n = 48$)	15 (31%)	27 (56%)	6 (13%)
45° Flexion AP ($n = 48$)	10 (21%)	33 (69%)	5 (10%)

AP, anteroposterior

For postoperative management, partial weight-bearing was permitted 5 to 6 weeks after operation using two crutches. Gait with one crutch was essential for 6 months to 1 year depending on the extent of lesion.

Radiographic outcome was influenced by the extent of the lateral noncollapsed living area of the femoral head corresponding to the acetabular roof on postoperative conventional anteroposterior radiographs. Extent of the noncollapsed viable area of the loaded portion of the femoral head was measured by angle [7], and the rate of extent was divided into three groups as follows: group A, less than the medial one-third of the weight-bearing area is involved; group B, more than one-third but less than two-thirds is involved; and group C, more than two-thirds is involved (Table 2). Anteroposterior radiographs were also taken in 45° of hip flexion [(7,8)] to observe the anterior viable portion of the femoral head. The extent of the viable area of the anterior femoral head was also divided into three groups as well on conventional anteroposterior radiographs. Prevention and progression of recollapse and progressive joint space narrowing were observed on the follow-up radiographs, and the relationship with the extent of viable articular surface of the femoral head was also studied. Of the remodeling after surgery, respherical contour on the collapsed area that moved medially and improvement of degenerative joint narrowing were investigated. The necrotic focus was moved to the medial portion of the femoral head on postoperative anteroposterior radiographs in all 48 hips. In 35 of 48 hips, collapsed

◄

FIG. 1. A 30-year-old woman receiving high doses of corticosteroids for treatment of multiple sclerosis. **A** Preoperative anteroposterior radiograph of her right hip showed extensive collapsed lesion without viable area on loaded portion below the acetabular roof. **B** Correct lateral radiograph showed extensively involved area. *Arrows* show anterior and posterior demarcation area between necrotic and noncollapsed viable portion. Anterior viable area is 13%, posterior viable area is 15%. **C** A 150° posterior rotational osteotomy with 15° varus position was performed. Anteroposterior (AP) radiograph taken 3 months after operation revealed adequate viable joint surface of the femoral head below the acetabular roof. Note the necrotic lesion is moved to the medial area (*arrow*). Extent of viable femoral head was 60%. **D** Viable area was 82% on 45° flexion AP radiograph taken at the same time. **E** AP radiograph taken 11 years after operation disclosed spherical contour of the medial femoral head (*arrow*). Joint space was well maintained, and the patient was free from pain. Flexion was 80°, abduction was 30°, and Japanese Orthopaedic Association (JOA) hip score was 96 points. **F** A 45° flexion AP radiograph taken 11 years after operation showed sphericity of the femoral head

areas were clearly observed at the medial portion of the femoral head on postoperative anteroposterior radiographs during less than 6 months after surgery. Respherical contour on the medial collapsed area on final anteroposterior radiographs of 35 hips was studied. Of the improvement of degenerative joint on 8 hips with joint space narrowing preoperatively, observation was made for changes of acetabular subchondral roof on anteroposterior radiographs at 6 months, 2 years, and final follow-up. Clinical evaluation was assessed on JOA hip score [11].

Results

On postoperative anteroposterior radiographs taken in the short period after surgery (less than 1 year), the lateral noncollapsed viable area of joint surface facing the acetabular roof was 21% to 100% (mean, 58) in all 48 hips. In these hips, 15 hips were group A, 27 were group B (Fig. 1C), and 6 were group C. On postoperative 45° flexion anteroposterior radiographs, the lateral noncollapsed viable area was 11% to 100% (mean, 54); 10 hips showed group A (Fig. 1D), 33 were group B, and 5 were group C (Table 2); and 4 hips (8%) resulted in recollapse at final follow-up. These 4 hips were in group C. Recollapse did not occur in 44 hips of groups A and B. Progressive joint space narrowing was found in 9 hips. Of the extent of viable area on anteroposterior radiographs, 3 hips were in group A, 2 were in group B, and 4 were in group A (Table 3). In 40 hips of stage 3B, recollapse was found in 3 hips and joint narrowing was noted on 7 hips. Recollapse occurred on 1 hip and joint narrowing was seen on 2 of 8 hips with stage 4 (Table 4).

Resphericity of the medial collapsed area of the femoral head was observed in 34 of 35 hips (97%) on the final anteroposterior radiographs (Fig. 1E). Of changes of the acetabular subchondral roof for the 8 hips with joint space narrowing before operation, atrophic changes of the acetabular subchondral roof were noted 6 months after operation in all hips. The shape of the acetabular roof was improved and reformed by 2 years after the procedure. The joint space was increased when comparing it to before the surgery and was maintained at final follow-up anteroposterior radiographs.

TABLE 3. Relationship between extent of viable area of femoral head after operation corresponding with acetabular roof, recollapse, and progressive joint space narrowing

Conventional AP radiographs (n = 48)	Total	Group A	Group B	Group C
Recollapse	4 (8%)	0	0	4
Progressive joint space narrowing	9 (19%)	3	2	4

TABLE 4. Relationship between stages, recollapse, and progressive joint space narrowing

Stage	Recollapse	Progressive joint space narrowing
3B	3/40 hips (8%)	7/40 hips (18%)
4	1/8 hips (12%)	2/8 hips (25%)

With regard to the range of motion, in hips without recollapse or joint space narrowing, the flexion angle was 60° to 130° (mean, 100°), and abduction angle was 15° to 40° (mean, 22°). Hips with either recollapse or joint space narrowing evidenced flexion from 40° to 100° (mean, 96°) and abduction from 5° to 25° (mean, 19°). Clinical evaluation according to the Japanese Orthopaedic Association hip score system was 84 to 100 points (mean, 91) in hips without recollapse or 50 to 83 points (mean, 67) in those without joint space narrowing. Two hips were revised with a total hip arthroplasty around 15 years after surgery. Four hips were waiting a total hip arthroplasty due to poor results. Causes of the unsuccessful results including early failure were postoperative inadequate viable area under the weight-bearing portion below the acetabular roof in 3 hips, vascular impairment by operation in 2, and living bone that fractured after a high level of activities in 2, degenerative change in 2, and challenging procedure in 1 because of the young age of the patient.

Discussion

Several kinds of procedures for joint preservation of femoral head osteonecrosis appear to be effective in early-stage and small or mid-sized necrosis [1–3,12]. Joint preservation of femoral head osteonecrosis with extensive and collapsed lesions in young patients may be an important challenge for orthopedic surgeons. The principal concept of femoral osteotomies for joint preservation in the treatment of femoral head osteonecrosis is that necrotic focus is moved away from the major weight-bearing portion on the acetabulum [2,4,7]. In this situation. weight-bearing forces are received by the transferred viable area. Reports of anterior rotational osteotomy described by Sugioka et al. showed good results if posterior noncollapsed viable bone remained in more than one-third of the entire femoral head and adequate viable area could be transferred to the loaded portion opposite the acetabular roof [4–6]. However, many young patients have extensive lesions that do not indicate anterior rotational osteotomy is suitable.

Our previous reports of posterior rotational osteotomies including "high degree posterior rotation" [7,8] for femoral head osteonecrosis with extensive lesions showed good results even if patients have extensive lesions and apparent collapse. In the present study, recollapse was prevented in cases with adequate viable area corresponding to the acetabular subchondral roof on conventional anteroposterior radiographs and 45° flexion on anteroposterior views. In these cases, the anterior viable area can be moved to the loaded portion by the use of the posterior rotational osteotomy, including the "high degree posterior rotation osteotomy" as described. The extent of the viable area corresponding to the weight-bearing portion below the acetabular roof on conventional anteroposterior radiographs was almost equivalent to the extent on the 45° flexion anteroposterior radiographs. Containment and congruency between the femoral head and the acetabulum was improved not only in the neutral position but also in flexion of daily activities after this posterior rotational osteotomy.

Extended joint space and remodeling of the acetabular subchondral shape were noted in hips with degenerative changes preoperatively. A regaining of the spherical contour of the collapsed femoral head was also found. It was believed that the reason for remodeling after operation was the containment and congruency of the joint as a result of the anterolateral adequate viable area of the femoral head. The authors assumed that the main causes of failure with recollapse were inadequate viable area under the weight-bearing portion below the acetabular roof, fracture of the viable bone with mechanical weakness after a high level of activities too soon after the operation, or vascular damage caused by the operation. In conclusion, posterior rotational osteotomy including the high degree posterior rotation appears effective for the treatment of nontraumatic and posttraumatic osteonecrosis of the femoral head with collapse and extensive involvement in young patients. The authors believe that this operation may delay the progression of degeneration if adequate viable area can be placed below the loaded portion of the acetabulum. Remodeling of the collapsed lesion and the degenerative acetabular subchondral roof might be one of the important factors for preserving the joints.

References

1. Kerboul M, Thomine J, Postel M (1974) The conservative surgical treatment of idiopathic aseptic necrosis of the femoral head. J Bone Joint Surg [Br] 56:291–296
2. Mont MA, Fairbank AC, Krackow KA et al (1996) Corrective osteotomy for osteonecrosis of the femoral head. J Bone Joint Surg [Am] 78:1032–1038
3. Urbaniak JR, Coogan PG, Gunneson, EB, et al (1995) Treatment of osteonecrosis of the femoral head with free vascularized fibular grafting. A long-term follow-up study of one hundred and three hips. J Bone Joint Surg [Am] 77:681–694.
4. Sugioka Y (1978) Transtrochanteric anterior rotational osteotomy of the femoral head in the treatment of osteonecrosis affecting the hip. A new osteotomy operation. Clin Orthop Relat Res 130:191–201
5. Sugioka Y (1980) Transtrochanteric rotational osteotomy of the femoral head. In: Riley LH Jr (ed) The hip. Proceedings of the eighth open scientific meeting of the Hip Society. Mosby, St. Louis, pp 3–23
6. Sugioka Y, Hotokebuti T, Tsutsui H (1992) Transtrochanteric anterior rotational osteotomy for idiopathic and steroid-induced necrosis of the femoral head. Indications and long-term results. Clin Orthop Relat Res 227:111–120
7. Atsumi T, Kuroki Y (1997) Modified Sugioka's osteotomy. More than 130° posterior rotation for osteonecrosis of the femoral head with large lesion. Clin Orthop Relat Res 334:98–107
8. Atsumi T, Muraki M, Yoshihara S, et al (1999) Posterior rotational osteotomy for the treatment of femoral head osteonecrosis. Arch Orthop Trauma Surg 119:388–393
9. Atsumi T, Yamano K (1997) Superselective angiography in osteonecrosis of the femoral head In: Urbaniak JR, Jones JP (eds) Osteonecrosis: etiology, diagnosis, and treatment. American Academy of Orthopaedic Surgeons, Rosemont, IL, pp 247–252
10. Sugano N, Atsumi T, Ohzono K et al (2002) The 2001 revised criteria for diagnosis, classification, and staging of idiopathic osteonecrosis of the femoral head. J Orthop Sci 7:801–805
11. Imura S, et al (1995) Japanese Orthopaedic Association hip score system. J Jpn Orthop Assoc 69:860–867
12. Fairbank AC, Bhatia D, Jinnah RH, et al (1995) Long-term results of core decompression for ischemic necrosis of the femoral head. J Bone Joint Surg [Br] 77:42–49

Limitations of Joint-Preserving Treatment for Osteonecrosis of the Femoral Head: Limitation of Free Vascularized Fibular Grafting

KENJI KAWATE[1], TETSUJI OHMURA[1], NOBUYUKI HIYOSHI[1], TOMOHIRO TERANISHI[2], HIROYUKI KATAOKA[3], KATSUYA TAMAI[1], TOMOYUKI UEHA[1], and YOSHINORI TAKAKURA[1]

Summary. Fifty-six hips of 46 patients undergoing free vascularized fibular grafting for the treatment of osteonecrosis of the femoral head were investigated. The average age at surgery was 39 years, and the average follow-up period was 6 years. Associated etiological factors included a history of high-dose steroids for 27 hips, consumption of alcohol for 25, and idiopathy for 4 hips. The radiographic appearance, determined according to the staging system of the Japanese Investigation Committee, was stage 1 for 2 hips, stage 2 for 28, stage 3A for 15, stage 3B for 10, and stage 4 for 1 hip. The radiographic type of necrosis, determined according to the radiographic classification of the Japanese Investigation Committee, was type B for 4 hips, type C-1 for 20, and type C-2 for 32 hips. The clinical results of steroid-induced osteonecrosis were poorest among the etiologies. Twenty-four hips collapsed or progressed radiographically. There was a significant relationship between preoperative stage and radiographic progression. There was also a significant relationship between preoperative type and radiographic progression. Eleven hips were converted to total hip arthroplasty. In conclusion, the current results show that vascularised fibular grafting is a good procedure for the precollapse stages and a valuable alternative for patients with stage 3A.

Key words. Osteonecrosis of the femoral head, Free vascularized fibular grafting, Indication, Etiology, Collapse

Introduction

Various procedures for salvaging the femoral head affected by osteonecrosis, such as core decompression, osteotomy, and curettage of the lesion followed by bone grafting, have been reported, especially in young patients, because total hip arthroplasty (THA) in young patients is associated with a high rate of revision surgeries [1–3]. However, the results reported for these methods are inconsistent. The results for core

[1] Department of Orthopaedic Surgery, Nara Medical University, 840 Shijo-cho, Kashihara, Nara 634-8522, Japan
[2] Department of Orthopaedic Surgery, Nara Prefectural Rehabilitation Center, Tawaramoto, Japan
[3] Department of Orthopaedic Surgery, Nara Prefectural Gojo Hospital, Gojo, Japan

decompression indicated that it is not effective for hips that have already collapsed [4]. Varus osteotomy is indicated only for patients with hips with a small area of necrosis [5]. Sugioka's rotational osteotomy is effective for hips that have already collapsed but is not suitable for hips with a large area of necrosis [6]. Curettage of the lesion followed by bone grafting is thought to be insufficient for revascularization [7]. Although the vessel transplantation procedure reported by Hori et al. is epoch making as a biological approach, it does not yield sufficient biomechanical support [8].

Yoo et al. reported excellent outcomes of free vascularized fibular grafting in 1992 [9]. Therefore, free vascularized fibular grafting, which is expected to provide both biological function and biomechanical support, has been used in our institution since 1992. The present study focused on the limitations of free vascularized fibular grafting.

Materials and Methods

Fifty-six hips of 46 patients undergoing free vascularized fibular grafting for treatment of osteonecrosis of the femoral head were investigated in the present study. There were 38 male and 8 female patients, whose mean age at surgery was 39 years (range, 22–60 years). The average follow-up period was 6 years (range, 3–12 years). The indications for surgery were age less than 60 years and pain at the time of preoperative evaluation.

Asymptomatic patients were not considered candidates for the procedure. Associated etiological factors included a history of high-dose steroids for 27 hips, consumption of alcohol for 25 hips, and idiopathic for 4 hips. The radiographic appearance, determined according to the staging system of the Japanese Investigation Committee, was stage 1 for 2 hips, stage 2 for 28 hips, stage 3A for 15, stage 3B for 10, and stage 4 for 1 hip [10] (Table 1). The radiographic type of necrosis, determined according to the radiographic classification of the Japanese Investigation Committee, was type B for 4 hips, type C-1 for 20, and type C-2 for 32 hips [10] (Table 2).

The Japanese Orthopaedics Association Hip Score (JOA score) was used for clinical evaluation in the present study [11]. Follow-up examination consisted of radiography and clinical evaluation using the JOA score every half-year. The radiographs were evaluated to determine disease progression. Clinical assessment was made using four classes: excellent, no hip pain, and a hip rating more than 90 points; good, a hip rating of 80 to 89 points; fair, a hip rating of 70 to 79 points; and poor, a hip rating less than 69 points.

TABLE 1. Preoperative stage determined according to the staging system of the Japanese Investigation Committee [10]

Stage	1	2	3A	3B	4
Steroid-induced ON	1	13	7	5	1
Alcohol-related ON	1	13	6	5	0
Idiopathic ON	0	2	2	0	0
Total	2	28	15	10	1

Data are number of cases

ON, osteonecrosis

TABLE 2. Preoperative type determined according to the staging system of the Japanese Investigation Committee [10]

Type	A	B	C-1	C-2
Steroid-induced ON	0	2	10	15
Alcohol-related ON	0	2	7	16
Idiopathic ON	0	0	3	1
Total	0	4	20	32

Date are number of cases

Etiology, preoperative stage, and preoperative type were examined to clarify the relationships with radiographic progression and occurrence of recollapse.

Operative Procedure

The operation is performed with the patient in the supine position. A sterile tourniquet is placed on the thigh, and the ipsilateral fibula, which is 15 cm in length, is harvested. The cutaneous branch of the peroneal artery is identified, and a 4 × 2 cm flap is designed. After harvesting of a fibular segment, a slightly curved (medial convex) 10-cm skin incision is made in the inguinal area. After retracting the sartorius, the attachment of the rectus femoris muscle from the ilium is detached, leaving a few centimeters of tendon. The rectus femoris muscle is then retracted distally. The lateral femoral circumflex artery and the concomitant veins are then identified. We usually use the transverse or descending branch of the lateral femoral circumflex vessels for anastomosis. The lateral aspect of the proximal part of the femur is exposed through the separated tensor fasciae latae and the vastus lateralis with a lateral approach. Under fluoroscopic control, a guide-pin is inserted into the anterolateral part of the necrotic lesion with 145° to 150° of inclination, because Ohzono's study suggested that the most lateral area of the weight-bearing area is the most important part for collapse [12]. A tunnel 15 to 19 mm in diameter is created with reamers of gradually increasing size. The diameter of the vascularized fibula graft is measured in the proximal, middle, and distal portions within the vascular pedicle and soft tissue, and the diameter of the tunnel is prepared 1 to 2 mm larger than the diameter of the fibula. With the use of a high-speed burr and fluoroscopic imaging, the remaining necrotic bone to the subchondral bone is excised and the tunnel is prepared. Then, cancellous bone graft is packed into the cavity. Before insertion into the tunnel , the tip of the fibular graft is shaved as round as possible using a high-speed burr. The vascularized fibula is then positioned beneath the subchondral bone of the femoral head, with the cancellous bone graft. The fibula is stabilized to the proximal part of the femur with a small cannulated titanium screw or a Kirschner wire. The peroneal vascular bundle is introduced anteriorly through the vastus intermedius muscle. With the use of an operating microscope, the arterial and venous anastomoses are performed.

Postoperative monitoring is performed using skin flaps. Urbaniak et al. performed digital subtraction angiography on the fifth postoperative day [13]. We believe it is not necessary to perform angiography for postoperative monitoring. If vascular occlusion occurs by the fifth day, reexploration cannot rescue the grafted fibula, and reexploration should therefore be performed as soon as possible after vascular occlusion occurs. A short leg cast is applied to prevent hammer toe for 2 weeks to the leg from which the fibula was harvested. After removal of the cast, the patient begins touch-down weight-bearing. When bony union at the distal end of the fibula is confirmed, it is generally 3 months postoperatively, and partial weight-bearing is then allowed. During the next month, the amount of weight-bearing is gradually increased to 50% weight-bearing. Full unassisted weight-bearing is allowed 6 months postoperatively.

Statistical Analysis

The Mann–Whitney *U* test was used to evaluate the significance between preoperative score and the latest score. Statistical analysis was performed with the Kruskal–Wallis test to evaluate the relationship between etiology and JOA score, between etiology and radiographic progression, and between etiology and survival rate. Fisher's exact probability test was used to evaluate the relationship between preoperative stage and radiographic progression and between type and radiographic progression. Findings were considered significant at $P < 0.05$.

Results

Clinical Evaluation

The mean preoperative JOA score was 57 (range, 21–96) and the mean latest score was 79 (range, 26–100). There was a significant difference between preoperative scores and the latest scores ($P = 0.0000015$).

At the latest follow-up, 38 hips (68%) were rated good to excellent. Of 27 hips with steroid-induced osteonecrosis, 14 (52%) were rated good to excellent. Of 25 hips with alcohol-related osteonecrosis, 20 (80%) were rated good to excellent. Of 4 hips with idiopathic osteonecrosis, 4 (100%) were rated good to excellent. There was a significant relationship between clinical results and etiology ($P = 0.04$). The clinical outcomes of steroid-induced osteonecrosis were worst among the etiologies.

Radiographic Evaluation

Twenty-four hips (43%) collapsed or progressed radiographically during the follow-up period. Of 27 hips with steroid-induced osteonecrosis, 14 (52%) progressed radiographically (Fig. 1). Of 25 hips with alcohol-related osteonecrosis, 10 (40%) progressed radiographically. All 4 hips with idiopathic osteonecrosis improved or were unchanged. There was no significant relationship between etiology and radiographic progression ($P = 0.14$).

Of 38 hips with stage 1, 2, or 3A, 27 (71%) improved or were unchanged. However, of 18 hips with stage 3B or 4, only 5 (28%) improved or were unchanged. Thirteen hips (72%) worsened during the follow-up period. There was a significant relationship between preoperative stage and radiographic progression ($P = 0.003$) (Fig. 2).

Of 24 hips with type B or C-1, 19 (79%) improved or were unchanged. However, of 32 hips with type C-2, 13 (41%) improved or were unchanged. Nineteen hips with type C-2 (59%) worsened during the follow-up period. There was a significant relationship between preoperative type and radiographic progression ($P = 0.004$).

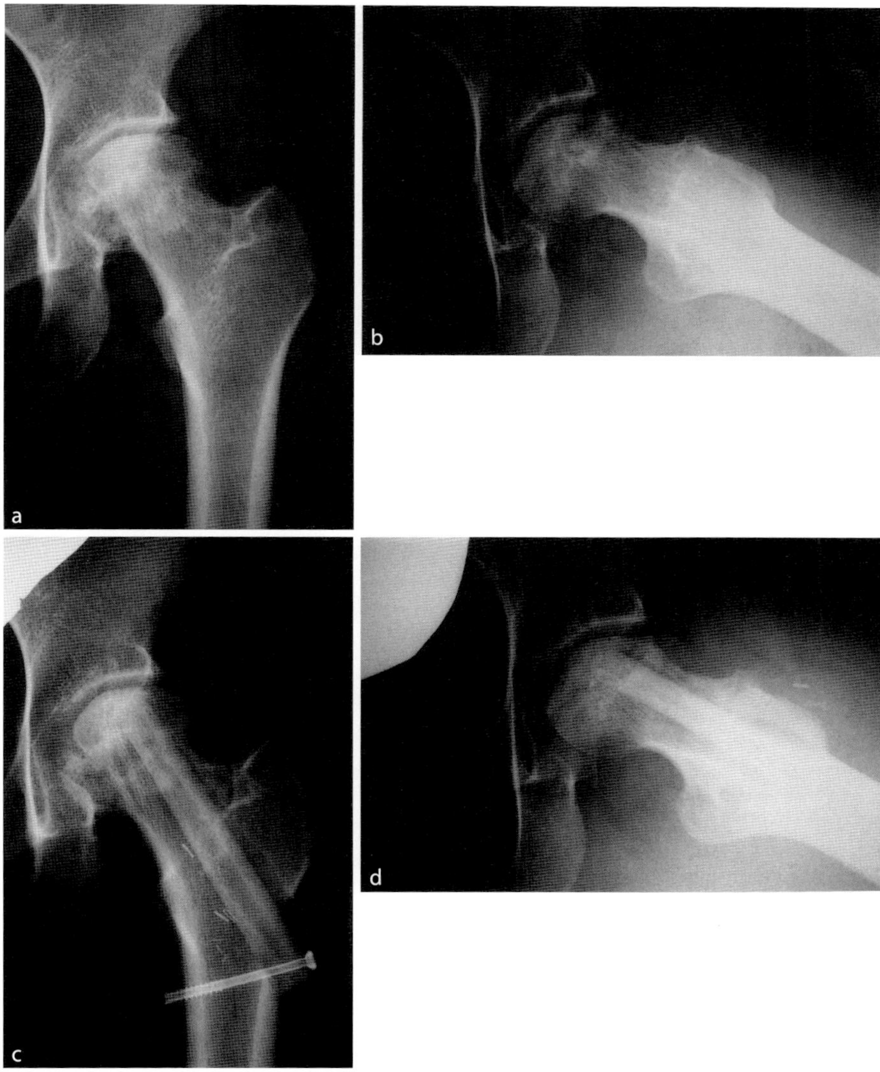

FIG. 1. A 32-year-old woman with steroid-induced osteonecrosis. **a, b** Preoperative radiographs show stage 3B osteonecrosis. **c, d** Radiographs immediately postoperative. **e, f** Radiographs at 28 months postoperatively show the collapse

Survival Rate

Eleven of the 56 hips (20%) were converted to THA during the follow-up period. Nine of these 11 hips were steroid-induced osteonecrosis and the other 2 were alcohol-related osteonecrosis. There was a significant relationship between etiology and survival rate ($P = 0.045$). Average duration was 3.5 years (range, 1.5–10) from fibular grafting to THA.

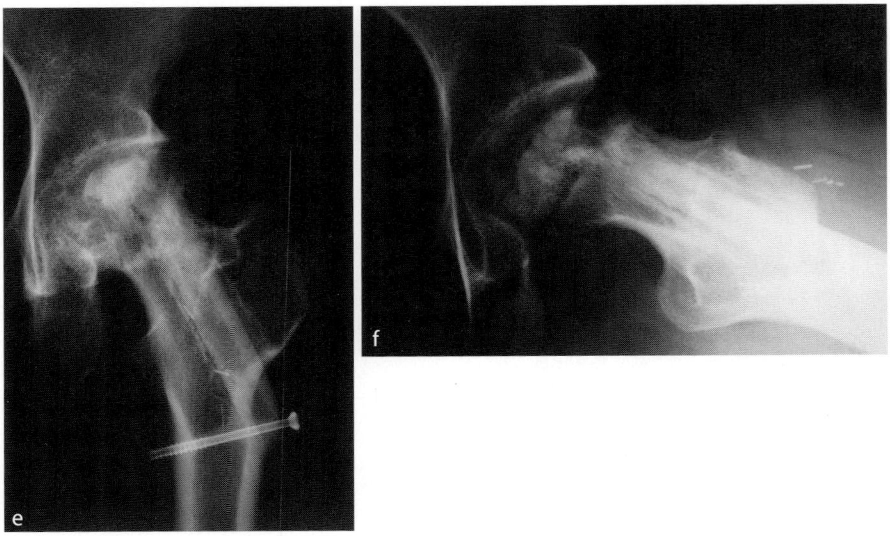

FIG. 1. *Continued*

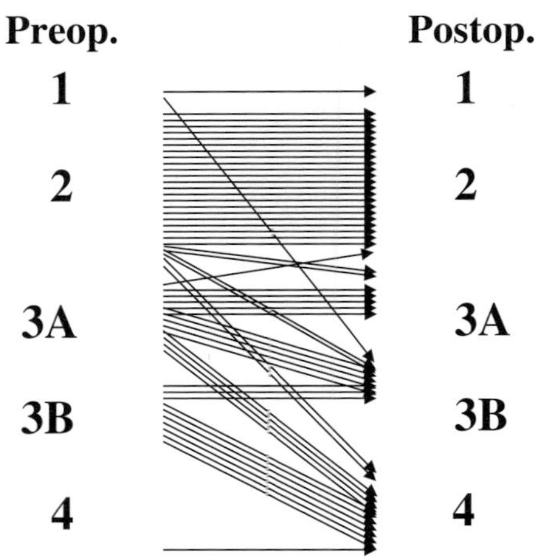

FIG. 2. Radiographic progression during follow-up period

Complications

Eleven of 56 hips (20%) required reoperation because of venous and 1 because of arterial occlusions. Ten hips with venous occlusions were recovered. The hip with arterial occlusion could not be recovered and required THA 3.5 years after surgery. Hammer toes was detected in 11 patients (20%). These patients were treated by cutting off the flexor hallucis longus muscle [14]. Two subtrochanteric oblique fractures occurred from the site of the tunnel to the shaft as the result of a fall 1 month after operation. One patient was treated with open reduction and internal fixation with three screws and casting. The other was treated with open reduction and internal fixation with a plate and cast. No vascular damage was detected, and the results of both free vascularized fibular graftings were excellent at the latest follow-up.

Discussion

Urbaniak et al. reported that the average Harris hip score improved significantly for all stages of Marcus et al. [13,15]. Sotereanos et al. reported excellent or good results in 69.3% of hips, fair for 8%, and poor for 22.7% of hips [16]. Yoo et al. reported excellent or good results for 91%, fair for 7%, and poor for 2% of hips [9]. They reported no significant relationship could be detected between etiology and clinical results. In the present study, the results were excellent or good for 68% of hips. There was a significant relationship between etiology and clinical results. The clinical results of steroid-induced osteonecrosis were poorest among the etiologies.

On radiographic evaluation, radiographic progression was observed in 73% of hips in the study by Urbaniak et al. [13] and in 42% in that by Sotereanos et al. [16]. Yoo et al. reported very low rates of progression (11%) in their study [9]. Radiographic progression was observed in 43% of hips in the present study. Significant relationships were detected between radiographic results and stage or type.

Magnussen reported that articular cartilage that appears macroscopically normal remained mechanically functional even in patients with large osteonecrotic lesions or a late radiographic stage of the disease [17]. However, the present study indicated that most hips with stage 3B progressed during the follow-up period. Severe collapse was not recovered by vascularized fibular grafting.

Regarding etiology, Berend et al. reported that results of idiopathic or alcohol-induced hips with preoperative collapse were worse than hips with other causes [18]. The present study indicated that patients with larger lesions, preoperative collapse, and a history of high-dose steroids had poor results.

Conclusion

The current results show that vascularized fibular grafting is a good procedure for the precollapse stages and a valuable alternative for patients with stage 3A.

References

1. Dorr LD, Luckett M, Conaty JP (1990) Total hip arthroplasties in patients younger than 45 years: a nine- to ten-year follow-up study. Clin Orthop 260:215–219
2. Barrack RL, Mulroy RD Jr, Harris WH (1992) Improved cementing technique and femoral component loosening in young patients with hip arthroplasties: a 12-year radiographic review. J Bone Joint Surg 74B:385–389

3. Kobayashi S, Eftekhar NS, Terayama K, et al (1997) Comparative study of total hip arthroplasty between younger and older patients. Clin Orthop 339:140–151
4. Bozic KJ, Zurakowski D, Thornhill T (1999) Survivorship analysis of hips treated with core decompression for nontraumatic osteonecrosis of the femoral head. J Bone Joint Surg [Am] 81:200–209
5. Mont MA, Fairbank AC, Krackow KA, et al (1996) Corrective osteotomy for osteonecrosis of the femoral head. J Bone Joint Surg [Am] 78:1032–1038
6. Sugioka Y, Hotokebuchi T, Tsutsui H (1992) Transtrochanteric anterior rotational osteotomy for idiopathic and steroid-induced necrosis of the femoral head. Clin Orthop Relat Res 277:111–120
7. Buckley PD, Gearen PF, Petty RW (1991) Structural bone-grafting for early atraumatic avascular necrosis of the femoral head. J Bone Joint Surg [Am] 73:1357–1364
8. Hori Y, Tamai S, Okuda H, et al (1979) Blood vessel transplantation to bone. J Hand Surg 4:23–33
9. Yoo MC, Chung DW, Hahn CS (1992) Free vascularized fibula grafting for the treatment of osteonecrosis of the femoral head. Clin Orthop 277:128–138
10. Sugano N, Atsumi T, Ohzono K, et al (2002) The 2001 revised criteria for diagnosis, classification, and staging of idiopathic osteonecrosis of the femoral head. J Orthop Sci 7:601–605
11. Ogawa R, Imura S (1995) Evaluation chart of hip joint functions. J Jpn Orthop Assoc 69:860–867
12. Ohzono K, Saito M, Takaoka K, et al (1991) Natural history of nontraumatic avascular necrosis of the femoral head. J Bone Joint Surg [Br] 73:68–72
13. Urbaniak JR, Coogan PG, Gunneson EB, et al (1995) Treatment of osteonecrosis of the femoral head with free vascularized fibular grafting. A long-term follow-up study of one hundred and three hips. J Bone Joint Surg [Am] 77:681–694
14. Takakura Y, Yajima H, Tanaka Y, et al (2000) Treatment of extrinsic flexion deformity of the toes associated with previous removal of a vascularized fibular graft. J Bone Joint Surg [Am] 82:58–61
15. Marcus ND, Enneking WF, Massam RA (1973) The silent hip in idiopathic aseptic necrosis. J Bone Joint Surg [Am] 55:1351–1366
16. Sotereanos DG, Plakseychuk AY, Rubash HE (1997) Free vascularized fibula grafting for the treatment of osteonecrosis of the femoral head. Clin Orthop 344:243–256
17. Magnussen RA, Guilak F, Vail TP (2005) Articular cartilage degeneration in post-collapse osteonecrosis of the femoral head. J Bone Joint Surg [Am] 87:1272–1277
18. Berend KR, Gunneson EE, Urbaniak JR (2003) Free vascularized fibular grafting for the treatment of postcollapse osteonecrosis of the femoral head. J Bone Joint Surg [Am] 85:987–993

Treatment of Large Osteonecrotic Lesions of the Femoral Head: Comparison of Vascularized Fibular Grafts with Nonvascularized Fibular Grafts

Shin-Yoon Kim

Summary. To date, it has been recognized that large osteonecrotic lesions of the femoral head are the most difficult to treat effectively, regardless of the technique used. We compared vascular fibular grafting (VFG) with nonvascular fibular grafting (NVFG) in 19 patients (23 hips: 10 stage IIc hips, 2 stage IIIc hips, and 11 stage IVc hips) matched on the basis of stage, extent of lesions, etiology of the lesions, average age, and preoperative Harris hip score (HHS). The mean duration of follow-up was 4 years (minimum, 3 years; range, 3–5 years). Mean HHS of the stage IIc and IVc hips was significantly better in the VFG group. The rate of radiographic signs of progression and mean dome depression in all hips was significantly less in the VFG group. The conversion rate to total hip replacement (THR) in the VFG group was 13%; in the NVFG group, it was 24%. The Kaplan–Meier survivorship analysis revealed a 3-year survival rate of 91.3% (95% confidence interval, 85.4%–92.2%) for the VFG group and 78.3% (95% confidence interval, 69.7%–86.9%) for the NVFG group.

Key words. Osteonecrosis, Femoral head, Comparison, Vascularized fibular grafting, Nonvascularized fibular grafting

Introduction

Osteonecrosis (ON) of the bone is a disease in which cell death in components of bone occurs as a result of an interrupted blood supply, probably because of restricted perfusion. The most common site is the femoral head. Extravascular pressure and subsequent tamponade of the arterial vessels or intravascular thrombosis has been involved [1]. Untreated osteonecrosis of the femoral head (ONFH) generally results in a progressive course of subchondral fracture, collapse, and painful disabling arthrosis [2]. The ultimate goal of treatment is to preserve the femoral head because this condition occurs primarily in young adults. The development of successful strategies in treating this disease, however, has been difficult because ON is associated with numerous diseases and neither its etiology nor its natural history has been delineated

Department of Orthopedic Surgery, Kyungpook National University Hospital, Samduck 2-ga, 50 Jung-gu, Daegu 700-721, Korea

clearly [3]. Therefore, the management of ON is primarily palliative, which does not necessarily halt or retard the progression of the disease [4].

Classification and Staging System

Several methods have been proposed for staging and classification that will assist in the following: help clinicians establish a prognosis; track improvement or progression; compare the effectiveness of different methods of treatment; and determine the best method of management for patients with different stages of osteonecrosis. The staging systems of Ficat [5] and Marcus et al. [6] depended on the collapse of the femoral head, and there was no attempt to quantitate the extent of involvement. The University of Pennsylvania staging system (Steinberg system) [7] was the first to use magnetic resonance imaging (MRI) as a specific modality for determining stage; in addition, it was the first to include measurement of lesions and surface involvement as an integral part of the system. Mild lesions are characterized as having less than 15% of head involvement or/and depression of less than 2 mm; moderate lesions have a 15%–30% head involvement and/or 2–4 mm depression; and severe lesions have more than 30% of head involvement and/or a depression of more than 4 mm. According to Kerboul et al. [8], in combined necrotic angle, which was measured on anteroposterior and lateral pelvic radiographs, the extent of necrosis is considered large if the angle is greater than 200°, medium if the angle is between 160° and 200°, and small if the angle is less than 160°. Koo and Kim [9] used similar angular measurements taken from the midcoronal and midsagittal images as the index of necrosis. The Japanese Investigation Committee (JIC) [10] subdivided only Ficat and Alert classification stages II and III according to the type and location of the lesion, as seen on anteroposterior radiographs (types 1A, 1B, 1C, 2, 3A, and 3B). Recently, they revised the classification criteria based on the central coronal section of the femoral head on T_1-weighted images or anteroposterior radiographs (types A, B, C1, C2) [11]. ARCO (Association for Research in Bone Circulation) designed a uniform staging and classification system that combined the University of Pennsylvania staging system and the JIC classification system [12].

Natural Course and Prognosis

The prognosis of ONFH is usually influenced by the diverse stage, the size of the lesion, and the location of the lesion. Before the availability of MRI, little was known about the preradiologic stage of the disease, particularly with regard to the size and location of lesions. The natural course of ONFH varies. Determining the degree of involvement helps select the optimal treatment and provides a correlation between the size of the necrotic segment and outcome. Staging also provides standards to compare the morbidity and long-term results of different treatment modalities. Recently, it has been reported that some lesions do not progress clinically or radiographically [13–15]. Several investigators have shown that some lesions may decrease in size over time or that the spontaneous resolution of ONFH can occur in early, asymptomatic disease that has small lesions [16]. Ohzono et al. [10] reported the incidences of collapse was 0% for type 1A, 19% for type 1B, 94% for type 1C, 100%

for type 2, 12% for type 3A, and 100% for type 3B, according to the JIC classification system. Koo et al. [17] reported that cases of hips with a necrosis index of less than 30% are at low risk for collapse. Nishii et al. [15] reported that even after a collapse occurs, hips with a collapse of 2 mm or less and necrotic lesions that occupy less than the medial two-thirds of the weight-bearing area have a high chance of cessation of collapse and improvement of symptoms with no surgical intervention. Therefore, it is important to determine the type of patient who may be at risk for progression of the lesion [8,14,18].

Head-Preserving Surgery

Although surgical interventions are superior to conservative treatment [19,20], they should be avoided in cases with little risk of collapse. Conservative measures may be beneficial when the involved segment is smaller than 15% and when it is far from the weight-bearing region, even though there have been contradictory reports [21]. There is no general consensus as to which procedure is the best, under what circumstances the results of one technique are sufficiently superior to another, and what the specific indications for the several treatment methods and procedures are. Long-term clinical experience and results, however, support positive data in which certain procedures are indicated for cases identified as being specific as to stage and extent of the osteonecrotic lesions. The decision of hip treatment for ON should be made on a personalized basis (tailored medicine) after the lesions have been accurately classified according to staging, extent, and location.

Core decompression has been found to be most efficacious in patients who have hips with small- or medium-sized precollapsed lesions. Results were not as favorable when lesions were large and a collapse had occurred [18,21–23].

The outcome of a transtrochanteric rotational osteotomy is chiefly dependent on the ratio of the transposed intact posterior articular surface to the acetabular weight-bearing area. Sugioka et al. [24,25] suggested that the transposed intact area should occupy more than 36% of the acetabular weight-bearing area by adequate rotation and intentional varus positions, especially for extensive lesions. Koo et al. [26] have used three criteria for the selection of transtrochanteric rotational osteotomy to achieve better results. This procedure has shown favorable results in Japan and Korea; however, the results from Europe and America are disappointing [27,28].

The use of nonvascularized bone grafting, as originally described by Phemister [29], and modifications of the original technique [30,31] to treat osteonecrosis have had a wide range of success rates. In a short-term follow-up study [31–34], satisfactory clinical results were obtained. In long-term evaluation, however, the method showed deteriorating results [35,36]. Also, this technique was not effective once a collapse had occurred, and it is not used commonly now [37].

Animal studies and histopathological analysis of failed vascularized fibular grafts in ONFH have suggested that vascularized grafts are more effective than nonvascularized grafts [38,39]. One of the major advantages of VFG is believed to be the direct and immediate introduction of a viable, vascularized graft into a necrotic region of the femoral head, thus enhancing the healing process. Advocates of this procedure believe that this procedure is superior to most other surgical approaches [40–42], and they have described excellent results [43–49]. The long-term results of VFG showed that a vascularized fibula that was implanted before collapse had the potential to restructure the major segment of the affected head and delay joint degeneration for many years, if a circumferential graft–host union was established [43,45,50,51]. To date, it has been recognized that large (>30%), lateral (C1 and C2) lesions are the most difficult to treat effectively, regardless of the technique used. Rijnen et al. [52] reported good clinical and radiographic success in hips with extensive osteonecrotic lesions (combined necrotic angle >200°) in young patients by using impaction bone grafting. Patients who had preoperative collapse and who used corticosteroids had disappointing results. Recently, Lai et al. [53] and Nishii et al. [54] showed that alendronate could prevent the early collapse of the femoral head in hips with extensive lateral lesions. These studies, however, have limitations in the number of patients as well as a too-short follow-up period.

VFG Versus NVFG

Plakseychuk et al. [42] evaluated the results of VFG (220 hips) and NVFG (123 hips) in a retrospective biinstitutional cohort study. They matched the hips (50 hips, respectively) according to the stage, size, and etiology of the lesions and by the mean preoperative HHS and with a minimum follow-up period of 3 years (average, 5 years). The mean HHS improved in 70% of the hips treated with VFG and in 36% of the hips treated with NVFG. The rate of survival at 7 years for stage I and II hips (precollapse) was 86% after treatment with VFG, compared with 30% after treatment with NVFG. The authors concluded that VFG is associated with better clinical and radiographic results, especially in hips with precollapsed lesions.

No significant differences were noted in the hips that were treated after a collapse, and poor results were noted in both groups. Unfortunately, the two groups were not entirely comparable because all vascularized grafting was performed in the United States and all nonvascularized grafting was done in Korea. Hence, the strength of their conclusions was limited by many variables, including differences in population demographics, surgical techniques, method of evaluation, and indications for total hip replacement (THR). After this study, we performed a study to compare the effectiveness of VFG with that of NVFG for preventing collapses and the progression of large osteonecrotic lesions in two groups of patients who were prospectively matched by etiology, stage, and extent of the lesions [55]. Forty-four patients (50 hips) with large osteonecrotic lesions of the femoral head underwent VFG, and 24 patients (30 hips) with large osteonecrotic lesions of the femoral head underwent NVFG at Kyungpook National University Hospital between March 1998 and April 2000. From this group, 19 patients (23 hips) who had been treated with VFG were matched with 19 patients (23 hips) who had undergone NVFG on the basis of stage, extent of lesions, etiology of the lesions, average age, and preoperative HHS. The data included 10 stage IIC hips, 2 stage IIIC hips, and 11 stage IVC hips. With the numbers available, there were no significant preoperative differences between the groups regarding sex, age, or duration of follow-up (minimum, 3 years; range, 3–5 years).

We modified the procedure of the traditional VFG by packing local autologous cancellous bone into the defect, anastomosing the peroneal vessels to the first or second perforating branch of the profunda femoris by using the surgical technique described by Yoo et al. [49], and attaching the buoy flap, which was vascularized by the circular periosteal vessels of the fibula, to the lateral aspect of the proximal thigh. This step was done to monitor the vascular patency of the grafted fibula after suturing the vessel by using the surgical technique described by Gilbert et al. [56] (Fig. 1). The vascularity of the graft was also assessed by noninvasive color Doppler ultrasonography, magnetic resonance angiography (Fig. 2), and serial bone scintigraphy. The mean HHS of the stage IIc and IVc hips was significantly better and the rate of

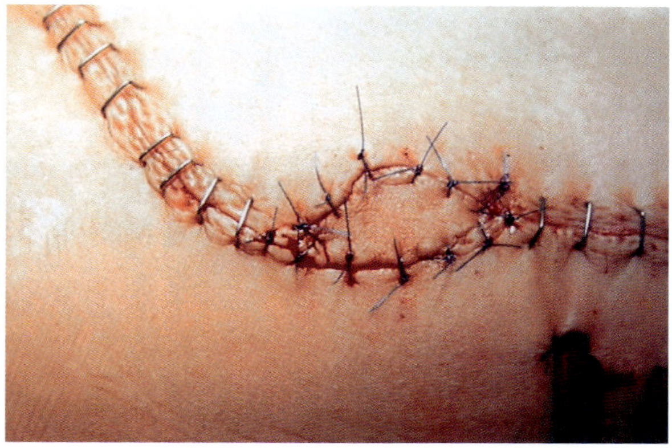

Fig. 1. The intact patency of vessels monitored using a buoy flap is shown by normal skin color without bluish discoloration

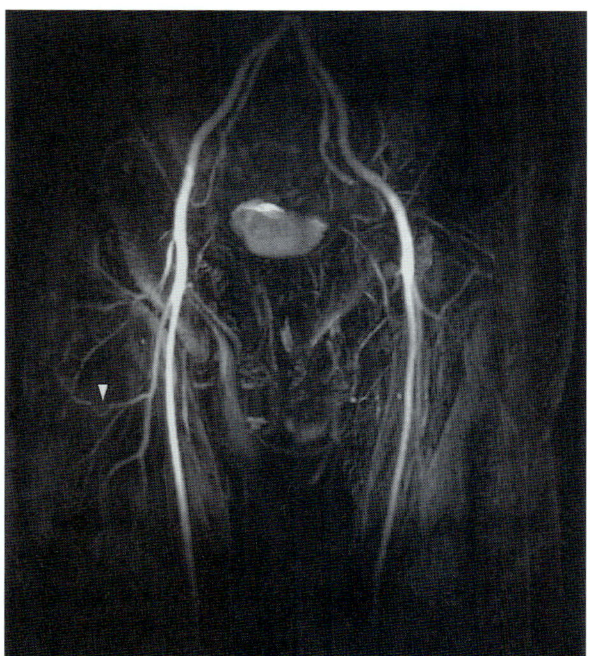

Fig. 2. Magnetic resonance angiography shows the continuation at the anastomosis site (*arrowhead*) when the anastomosed vessel was patent

radiographic signs of progression and collapse in all hips was significantly less in the VFG group when compared to the NVFG group at the time of the final follow-up (Fig. 3). The mean period to collapse of the stage IIc hips was 23 months (range, 5–50 months) in the VFG group and 24 months (range, 4–48 months) in the NVFG group. The mean dome depression was significantly less in the VFG group (2.8 mm; range, 1–7 mm) than in the NVFG group (4.3 mm; range, 1–10 mm). In stage IIc involvement, the mean dome depression was 0.8 mm (range, 0–2 mm) in the VFG group and 2.6 mm (range, 0–4 mm) in the NVFG group. The conversion rate to total hip replacement in the VFG group was 13% (3/23 hips); in the NVFG group, it was 24% (5/23 hips). The Kaplan–Meier survivorship analysis revealed a 3-year survival rate of 91.3% (95% confidence interval, 85.4%–92.2%) for the entire VFG group and 78.3% (95%

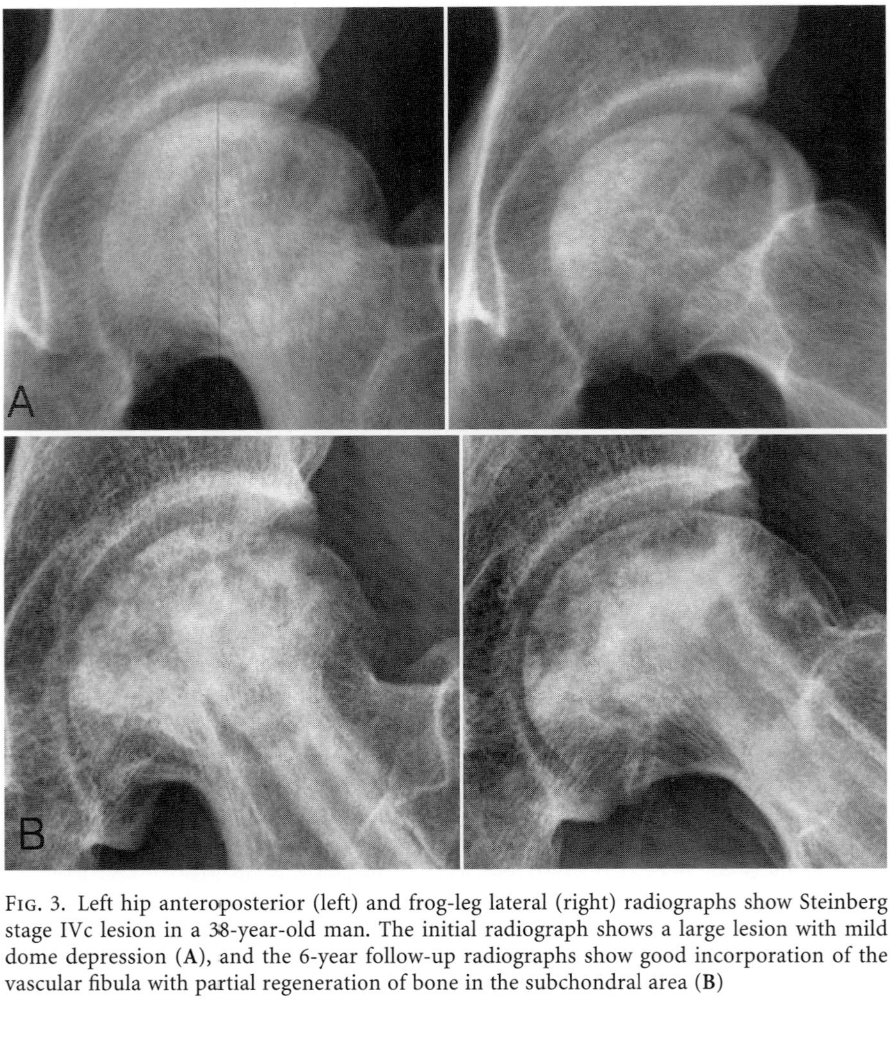

Fig. 3. Left hip anteroposterior (left) and frog-leg lateral (right) radiographs show Steinberg stage IVc lesion in a 38-year-old man. The initial radiograph shows a large lesion with mild dome depression (**A**), and the 6-year follow-up radiographs show good incorporation of the vascular fibula with partial regeneration of bone in the subchondral area (**B**)

confidence interval, 69.7%–86.9%) for the entire NVFG group. Gross and histological examinations of the cross-sectional femoral head when the hip had been converted to THR showed partially regenerated bone with a good incorporation of the fibula graft to the host bone in the VFG and absence of this effect in the NVFG. Complications occurred predominantly in the vascularized group, with clawing of the toes in 3 patients and sensory peroneal neuropathy in another 3. Only 1 complication (a sensory peroneal neuropathy) was reported in the NVFG group.

We strongly suggest that VFG is associated with better results than NVFG, particularly in young patients with precollapsed large osteonecrotic lesions. The study has obvious advantages over the previous report of Plakseychuk and Kim [42]; it is a closely matched prospective study in which both VFG and NVFG were done in parallel by the same surgeons at the same institution. Evaluation of patient outcomes did not indicate differences in ethnicity or in social and economic factors. The patency of the artery, which is critical in free vascular bone graft, was evaluated with a buoy flap, color Doppler ultrasonography, magnetic resonance angiography, and bone scintigraphy, rather than by invasive direct angiography [46,48]. We believe that the VFG had better clinical and radiographic results compared with the NVFG, particularly in Steinberg stage IIc hips of young patients, because the VFG-treated hips seemed to have less dome depression of the femoral head, retention of head sphericity associated with a more rapid osteoinduction of the primary callus formation in the subchondral bone, and more robust revascularization. Free vascularized fibular grafting is a technically difficult procedure that requires specialized training and expertise. It is costly and time consuming, and it requires a long period of recovery. In addition, it comes with a relatively high prevalence of complications [57–59].

Conclusions

Core decompression showed better clinical results than nonoperative management [19]. The VFG had significantly better results than core decompression [40]. We demonstrated that VFG had significantly better results than NVFG [42], particularly in large osteonecrotic lesions of ONFH [55]. VFG had less dome depression of the femoral head and retained sphericity of the femoral head. In addition, we think VFG can change large lesions into small ones and lateral lesions into medial or central ones, which will be less likely to progress, even though it cannot cure large necrotic lesions. Recently, surgeons have tried core decompression with autogenous bone marrow cells [60,61] and osteoinductive bone morphogenetic protein to enhance bone repair in the femoral head [62]. In an animal osteonecrosis model, osteogenic protein 1 [63] or vascular endothelial growth factor [64] were successful in regenerating bone defects.

In the future, it is believed that nonsurgical techniques [65] or minimally invasive procedures using tissue engineering will be tried. We cannot directly compare the results of the VFG with those of other techniques for treating large osteonecrotic lesion of the femoral head. Large randomized and prospective controlled trials, which can compare the efficacy of several treatment modalities regarding the specific stages, sizes, and locations of osteonecrosis, however, are needed in future.

References

1. Mankin HJ (1992) Nontraumatic necrosis of bone (osteonecrosis). N Engl J Med 326:1473–1479
2. Merle d'Aubigne R, Postel M, Mazabraud A, et al (1965) Idiopathic necrosis of the femoral head in adults. J Bone Joint Surg 47B:612–633
3. Lieberman JR (2004) Core decompression for osteonecrosis of the hip. Clin Orthop 418:29–33
4. Assouline-Dayan Y, Chang C, Greenspan A, et al (2002) Pathogenesis and natural history of osteonecrosis. Semin Arthritis Rheum 32:94–124
5. Ficat RP (1985) Idiopathic bone necrosis of the femoral head. Early diagnosis and treatment. J Bone Joint Surg 67B:3–9
6. Marcus ND, Enneking WF, Massam RA (1973) The silent hip in idiopathic aseptic necrosis. Treatment by bone-grafting. J Bone Joint Surg 55A:1351–1366
7. Steinberg ME, Hayken GD, Steinberg DR (1995) A quantitative system for staging avascular necrosis. J Bone Joint Surg 77B:34–41
8. Kerboul M, Thomine J, Postel M, et al (1974) The conservative surgical treatment of idiopathic aseptic necrosis of the femoral head. J Bone Joint Surg 56B:291–296
9. Koo KH, Kim R (1995) Quantifying the extent of osteonecrosis of the femoral head. A new method using MRI. J Bone Joint Surg 77B:875–880
10. Ohzono K, Saito M, Sugano N, et al (1992) The fate of nontraumatic avascular necrosis of the femoral head. A radiologic classification to formulate prognosis. Clin Orthop 277:73–78
11. Sugano N, Atsumi T, Ohzono K, et al (2002) The 2001 revised criteria for diagnosis, classification, and staging of idiopathic osteonecrosis of the femoral head. J Orthop Sci 7:601–605
12. Gardeniers JWM (1993) The ARCO perspective for reaching one uniform staging system of osteonecrosis. In: Schoutens A, Arlet J, Gardeniers JWM, et al (eds) Bone circulation and vascularization in normal and pathological conditions. Plenum Press, New York, pp 375–380
13. Jergesen HE, Kahn AS (1997) The natural history of untreated asymptomatic hips in patients who have non-traumatic osteonecrosis. J Bone Joint Surg 79A: 359–363
14. Kopecky KK, Braunstein EM, Brandt KD, et al (1991) Apparent avascular necrosis of the hip: appearance and spontaneous resolution of MR findings in renal allograft patients. Radiology 179:523–527
15. Nishii T, Sugano N, Ohzono K, et al (2002) Progression and cessation of collapse in osteonecrosis of the femoral head. Clin Orthop 400:149–157
16. Cheng EY, Thongtrangan I, Laorr A, et al (2003) Spontaneous resolution of osteonecrosis of the femoral head. Quantifying the extent of femoral head involvement in osteonecrosis. J Bone Joint Surg 85A:309–315
17. Koo KH, Kim R, Ko GH, et al (1995) Preventing collapse in early osteonecrosis of the femoral head. A randomized clinical trial of core decompression. J Bone Joint Surg 77B:870–874
18. Sakamoto M, Shimizu K, Iida S, et al (1997) Osteonecrosis of the femoral head: a prospective study with MRI. J Bone Joint Surg 79B:213–219
19. Mont MA, Carbone JJ, Fairbank AC (1996) Core decompression versus nonoperative management for osteonecrosis of the hip. Clin Orthop 324:169–178
20. Stulberg BN, Davis AW, Bauer TW, et al (1991) Osteonecrosis of the femoral head. A prospective randomized treatment protocol. Clin Orthop 268:140–151
21. Hernigou P, Poignard A, Nogier A, et al (2004) Fate of very small asymptomatic stage-I osteonecrotic lesions of the hip. J Bone Joint Surg 86A:2589–2593

22. Beltran J, Knight CT, Zuelzer WA, et al (1990) Core decompression for avascular necrosis of the femoral head: correlation between long-term results and preoperative MR staging. Radiology 175:533–536
23. Holman AJ, Gardner GC, Richardson ML, et al (1995) Quantitative magnetic resonance imaging predicts clinical outcome of core decompression for osteonecrosis of the femoral head. J Rheumatol 22:1929–1933
24. Sugioka Y, Hotokebuchi T, Tsutsui H (1992) Transtrochanteric anterior rotational osteotomy for idiopathic and steroid-induced necrosis of the femoral head. Indications and long-term results. Clin Orthop 277:111–120
25. Sugioka Y, Katsuki I, Hotokebuchi T (1982) Transtrochanteric rotational osteotomy of the femoral head for the treatment of osteonecrosis. Follow-up statistics. Clin Orthop 169:115–126
26. Koo KH, Song HR, Yang JW, et al (2001) Trochanteric rotational osteotomy for osteonecrosis of the femoral head. J Bone Joint Surg 83B:83–89
27. Dean MT, Cabanela ME (1993) Transtrochanteric anterior rotational osteotomy for avascular necrosis of the femoral head. Long-term results. J Bone Joint Surg 75B: 597–601
28. Rijnen WH, Gardeniers JW, Westrek BL, et al (2005) Sugioka's osteotomy for femoral-head necrosis in young Caucasians. Int Orthop 29(3):140–144
29. Phemister DB (1949) Treatment of the necrotic head of the femur in adults. J Bone Joint Surg 31A:55–66
30. Rosenwasser MP, Garino JP, Kiernan HA, et al (1994) Long term follow-up of thorough debridement and cancellous bone grafting of the femoral head for a vascular necrosis. Clin Orthop 306:17–27
31. Mont MA, Einhorn TA, Sponseller PD, et al (1998) The trapdoor procedure using autogenous cortical and cancellous bone grafts for osteonecrosis of the femoral head. J Bone Joint Surg 80B:56–62
32. Buckley PD, Gearen PF, Petty RW (1991) Structural bone-grafting for early atraumatic avascular necrosis of the femoral head. J Bone Joint Surg 73A:1357–1364
33. Boettcher WG, Bonfiglio M, Smith K (1970) Non-traumatic necrosis of the femoral head. ll. Experiences in treatment. J Bone Joint Surg 52A:322–329
34. Bonfiglio M, Voke EM (1968) Aseptic necrosis of the femoral head and non-union of the femoral neck. Effect of treatment by drilling and bone-grafting (Phemister technique). J Bone Joint Surg 50A:48–66
35. Smith KR, Bonfiglio M, Montgomery WJ (1980) Non-traumatic necrosis of the femoral head treated with tibial bone-grafting. A follow-up note. J Bone Joint Surg 62A: 845–847
36. Dunn AW, Grow T (1977) Aseptic necrosis on the femoral head. Treatment with bone grafts of doubtful value. Clin Orthop 122:249–254
37. Nelson LM, Clark CR (1993) Efficacy of Phemister bone grafting in nontraumatic aseptic necrosis of the femoral head. J Arthroplasty 8:253–268
38. Carter JR, Furey CG, Shaffer JW (1998) Histopathologic analysis of failed vascularized fibular grafts in femoral head osteonecrosis. Microsurgery 18:110–118
39. Malizos KN, Seaber AV, Glisson RR, et al (1997) The potential of vascularized cortical graft in revitalizing necrotic cancellous bone in canines. In: Urbaniak JR, Jones JP Jr (eds) Osteonecrosis: etiology, diagnosis, and treatment, 1st edn. American Academy of Orthopaedic Surgeons, Rosemont, IL, pp 361–371
40. Kane SM, Ward WA, Jordan LC, et al (1996) Vascularized fibular grafting compared with core decompression in the treatment of femoral head osteonecrosis. Orthopedics 19:869–872
41. Berend KR, Gunneson EE, Urbaniak JR (2003) Free vascularized fibular grafting for the treatment of postcollapse osteonecrosis of the femoral head. J Bone Joint Surg 85A:987–993

42. Plakseychuk AY, Kim SY, Park BC, et al (2003) Vascularized compared with nonvascularized fibular grafting for the treatment of osteonecrosis of the femoral head. J Bone Joint Surg 85A:589–596
43. Judet H, Gilbert A (2001) Long-term results of free vascularized fibular grafting for femoral head necrosis. Clin Orthop 386:114–119
44. Malizos KN, Soucacos PN, Beris AE (1995) Osteonecrosis of the femoral head. Hip salvaging with implantation of a vascularized fibular graft. Clin Orthop 314:67–75
45. Marciniak D, Furey C, Shaffer JW (2005) Osteonecrosis of the femoral head. A study of 101 hips treated with vascularized fibular grafting. J Bone Joint Surg 87A:742–747
46. Sotereanos DG, Plakseychuk AY, Rubash HE (1997) Free vascularized fibula grafting for the treatment of osteonecrosis of the femoral head. Clin Orthop 344:243–256
47. Scully SP, Aaron RK, Urbaniak JR (1998) Survival analysis of hips treated with core decompression or vascularized fibular grafting because of avascular necrosis. J Bone Joint Surg 80:1270–1275
48. Urbaniak JR, Coogan PG, Gunneson EB, et al (1995) Treatment of osteonecrosis of the femoral head with free vascularized fibular grafting. A long-term follow-up study of one hundred and three hips. J Bone Joint Surg 77:681–694
49. Yoo MC, Chung DW, Hahn CS (1992) Free vascularized fibula grafting for the treatment of osteonecrosis of the femoral head. Clin Orthop 277:128–138
50. Malizos KN, Quarles LD, Dailiana ZH, et al (2004) Analysis of failures after vascularized fibular grafting in femoral head necrosis. Orthop Clin N Am 35:305–314
51. Soucacos PN, Beris AE, Malizos K, et al (2001) Treatment of avascular necrosis of the femoral head with vascularized fibular transplant. Clin Orthop 386:120–130
52. Rijnen WH, Gardeniers JW, Buma P, et al (2003) Treatment of femoral head osteonecrosis using bone impaction grafting. Clin Orthop 417:74–83
53. Lai KA, Shen WJ, Yang CY, et al (2005) The use of alendronate to prevent early collapse of the femoral head in patients with nontraumatic osteonecrosis. A randomized clinical study. J Bone Joint Surg 87A:2155–2159
54. Nishii T, Sugano N, Miki H, et al (2006) Does alendronate prevent collapse in osteonecrosis of the femoral head?. Clin Orthop 443:273–279
55. Kim SY, Kim YG, Kim PT, et al (2005) Vascularized compared with nonvascularized fibular grafts for large osteonecrotic lesions of the femoral head. J Bone Joint Surg 87A:2012–2018
56. Gilbert A, Judet H, Judet J, et al (1986) Microvascular transfer of the fibula for necrosis of the femoral head. Orthopedics 9:885–890
57. Aluisio FV, Urbaniak JR (1998) Proximal femur fractures after free vascularized fibular grafting to the hip. Clin Orthop 356:192–201
58. Dailiana ZH, Gunneson EE, Urbaniak JR (2003) Heterotopic ossification after treatment of femoral head osteonecrosis with free vascularized fibular graft. J Arthroplasty 18:83–88
59. Vail TP, Urbaniak JR (1996) Donor-site morbidity with use of vascularized autogenous fibular grafts. J Bone Joint Surg 78A:204–211
60. Gangji V, Hauzeur JP, Matos C, et al (2004) Treatment of osteonecrosis of the femoral head with implantation of autologous bone-marrow cells. A pilot study. J Bone Joint Surg 86A:1153–1160
61. Hernigou P, Beaujean F (2002) Treatment of osteonecrosis with autologous bone marrow grafting. Clin Orthop 405:14–23
62. Lieberman JR, Conduah A, Urist MR (2004) Treatment of osteonecrosis of the femoral head with core decompression and human bone morphogenetic protein. Clin Orthop 429:139–145
63. Mont MA, Jones LC, Elias JJ, et al (2001) Strut-autografting with and without osteogenic protein-1: a preliminary study of a canine femoral head defect model. J Bone Joint Surg 83A:1013–1022

64. Yang C, Yang S, Du J, et al (2003) Vascular endothelial growth factor gene transfection to enhance the repair of avascular necrosis of the femoral head of rabbit. Chin Med J (Engl) 116:1544–1548
65. Reis ND, Schwartz O, Militianu D, et al (2003) Hyperbaric oxygen therapy as a treatment for stage-I avascular necrosis of the femoral head. J Bone Joint Surg 85B: 371–337

A Modified Transtrochanteric Rotational Osteotomy for Osteonecrosis of the Femoral Head

Taek Rim Yoon[1], Sang Gwon Cho[2], Jin Ho Lee[3], and Suk Hyun Kwon[4]

Summary. The aim of this study is to report the clinical results of modified transtrochanteric osteotomy in osteonecrosis of the femoral head. The authors used a modified transtrochanteric osteotomy for rotational osteotomy in which the greater trochanter is not detached. In 82 cases (75 patients), the mean age was 33 years; 14 were classified as Ficat stage 2, 55 as stage 3, and 13 as Ficat stage 4. We performed simple modified rotational osteotomy in 16 cases, a combination of osteotomy and simple bone grafting in 7, and a combination of osteotomy and muscle pedicle bone grafting in 59 cases. Postoperative evaluation utilized radiographic findings and the Harris hip score. Five patients underwent total hip arthroplasty. Among the 77 surviving cases, excellent results were obtained in 47 hips, good in 22, fair in 5, and poor in 3. Including 3 cases that were classed as poor, overall survival rate was 90%. Using modified transtrochanteric rotational osteotomy, we were able to obtain satisfactory results. Although this technique is difficult to perform, it is recommended particularly for young patients with stage 2 or 3 and some selected patients with stage 4.

Key words. Femoral head, Avascular necrosis, Modified transtrochanteric osteotomy

Introduction

Avascular necrosis of the femoral head is characterized by impairment of blood circulation to the femoral head and progressive femoral head collapse. Secondary degenerative changes induce pain and limitation of joint motion. Various treatments have been attempted in accordance with staging, necrotic area, and size. Surgical treatment

[1]Center for Joint Disease, Chonnam National University Hwasun Hospital, 160 Ilsimri, Hwasuneup, Hwasungun, Jeonnam 519-809, Korea
[2]Department of Orthopedics, Chonnam National University School of Medicine, Gwangju, Korea
[3]Center for Joint Disease, Chonnam National University Hwasun Hospital, Jeonnam, Korea
[4]Department of Orthopaedic Surgery, School of Medicine, Wonkwang University, Iksan, Korea

can be divided largely into head preservation procedures and total hip arthroplasty (THA). When performing THA on young patients, a high rate of failure has been reported [1–5].

On the other hand, various head preservation procedures have been reported, typically core decompression, which reduces bone marrow pressure [6,7], proximal femoral osteotomy [8], bone graft [9,10], and trochanteric or transtrochanteric rotational osteotomy [11,12]. Sugioka's transtrochanteric rotational osteotomy [13] as treatment for osteonecrosis of the femoral head in young patients is an effective head preservation procedure. We report here the clinical results of a modified transtrochanteric osteotomy for osteonecrosis of the femoral head.

Materials and Methods

Materials

We reviewed 82 hips in 75 patients with osteonecrosis of the femoral head in whom follow-up was possible for more than 1 year. The surgery was performed by one surgeon (T.R.Y.). The average age was 33 years (range, 19–51 years). The study population included 64 men and 11 women. Fourteen were classified as Ficat stage 2, 55 as stage 3, and 13 as Ficat stage 4 (Table 1). The causes of osteonecrosis were excessive alcohol consumption in 30 hips, steroid use in 26, idiopathic in 17, and posttraumatic in 9. The direction of rotation was anterior in 77 cases and posterior in 5 cases. We performed a simple modified rotational osteotomy in 16 cases, a combination of osteotomy and simple bone grafting in 7 (Fig. 1), and a combination of osteotomy and muscle-pedicle-bone grafting in 59 (Fig. 2). The average follow-up was 1.8 years (range, 1–3.3 years).

Surgical Technique

The lateral approach was used with dissection of the joint capsule to expose the femoral head. The short external rotator muscles were completely transected, preserving the quadratus femoris, and being wary of injury to the medial circumflex artery above the lesser trochanter, and then the joint capsule was exposed. A line on the osteotomy site was drawn. A Kirschner wire was driven into the femur perpendicular to its neck. Using the Kirschner wire as a guide, the osteotomy was performed.

TABLE 1. Classification of cases on the basis of the Ficat stage and operation procedure

Stage	Only transtrochanteric rotational osteotomy	Transtrochanteric rotational osteotomy with bone graft	Transtrochanteric rotational osteotomy with MPBG	Total
II	4	3	7	14
III	12	4	39	55
IV	0	0	13	13
Total	16	7	59	82

MPBG, muscle-pedicle-bone graft

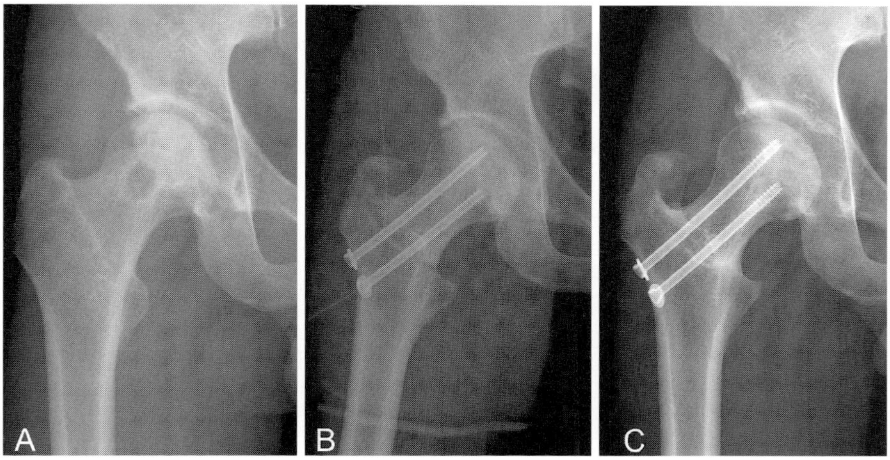

FIG. 1. Radiographs of a 42-year-old man who had transtrochanteric rotational osteotomy with bone graft for osteonecrosis of the femoral head (Ficat stage II) (**A**, **B**). Radiographs 14 months postoperatively show good union of the osteotomy site and good incorporation of grafted bone at the necrotic area (**C**)

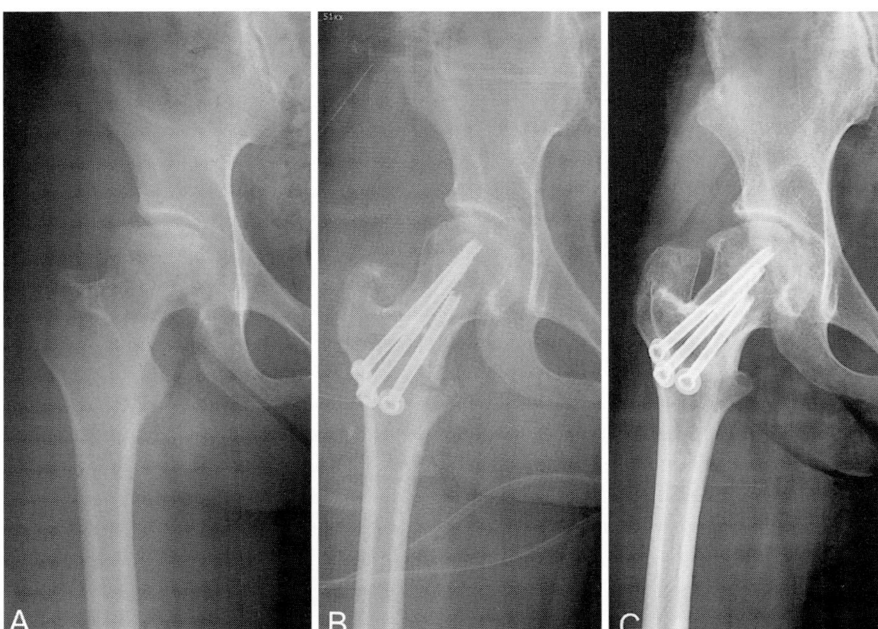

FIG. 2. Radiographs of a 19-year-old woman who had transtrochanteric rotational osteotomy with muscle-pedicle-bone graft for osteonecrosis of the femoral head (Ficat stage IV) (**A**, **B**). Radiographs 18 months postoperatively show no progression to degenerative osteoarthritis (**C**)

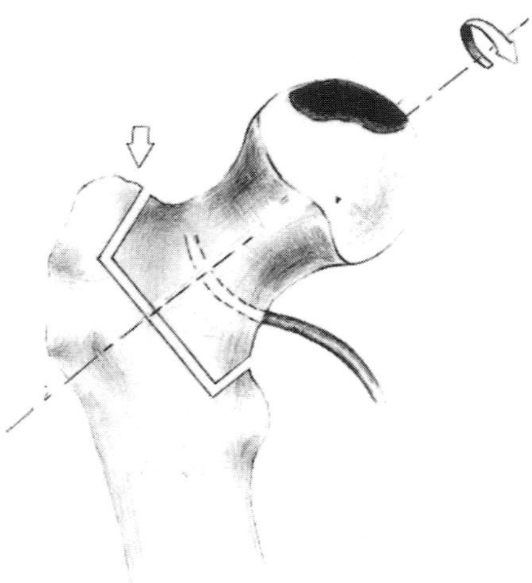

FIG. 3. The site of osteotomy (*arrow*), sparing the greater trochanter

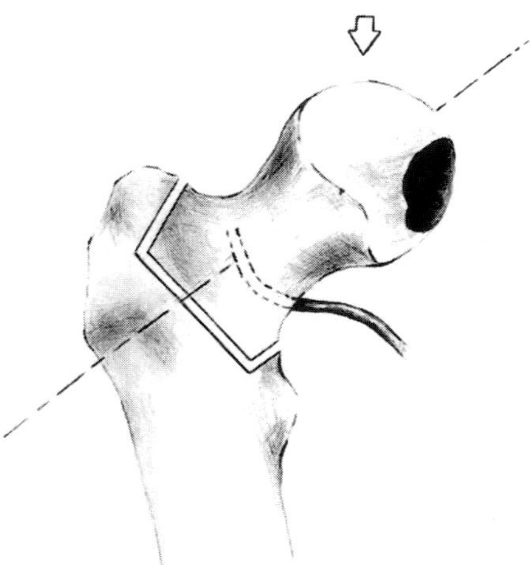

FIG. 4. The femoral head (*arrow*) was rotated anteriorly depending on the necrotic area in this case

In contrast to Sugioka's traditional technique, the greater trochanter is not detached (Fig. 3); only the femoral neck is osteotomized. The femoral head was then rotated anteriorly or posteriorly, depending on the location of necrotic area, and stabilized using two or three cannulated screws (Figs. 4, 5).

Methods

Clinical evaluation was performed with use of the Harris hip score (HHS). A clinical score was considered to be excellent if it was above 90 points, good if between 89 and 80 points, fair if between 79 and 70 points, and poor if 69 points or less. If there was progression of osteonecrosis or THA was performed in the follow-up period, the results were considered as a "failure."

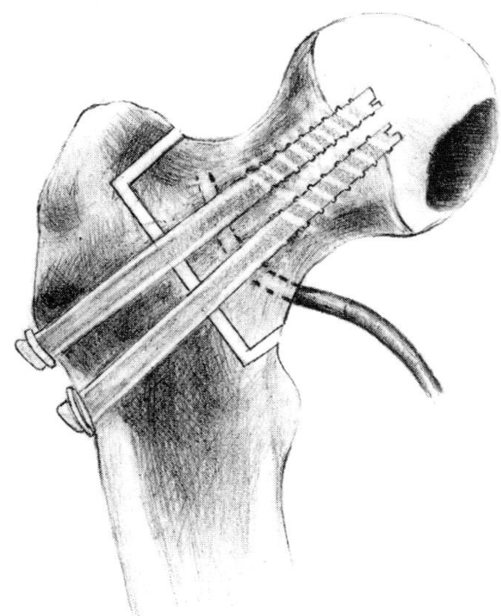

Fig. 5. Fixation for the rotational osteotomy was accomplished by two cannulated screws

Radiologic evaluation was performed with bone scan 3 weeks after the operation to assess revascularization or vascular injury. Also, periodic anteroposterior and lateral roentgenograms were taken to monitor for femoral head collapse or degenerative change. If there was no progression of necrosis on the newly formed weight-bearing surface, evidence of union could be found on the osteotomized site, and no collapse of femoral head greater than 2 mm and no degenerative change of joint space narrowing occurred, we defined the operation as a radiologic success; otherwise, it was considered a failure.

Results

Five of 82 cases who underwent modified transtrochanteric rotation osteotomy were revised by THA at final follow-up and were thus considered to be clinical failures; overall viability was 94%. Among the failed 5 cases, 3 cases failed because of severe pain related to further collapse of the head, 1 case failed because of a pathologic subcapital fracture, and 1 case failed due to fixation failure. Among the surviving 77 cases, the average HHS was 72 points (61–84) preoperatively and improved to 91 points (69–100) at last follow-up. Excellent results were obtained in 47 hips, good in 22, fair in 5, and poor in 3. The 3 hips with a poor result were the result of inadequate blood supply to the femoral head. Including the 3 cases that were classified as poor, the overall clinical survival rate was 90%.

All Ficat stage II, 52 (96%) of 55 stage III, and 8 (62%) of 13 stage IV had no progression of osteonecrosis. The overall radiologic success rate was 90%; 28 (93%) of 30 patients with alcoholic abuse and 23 (88%) of 26 patients who had used steroids were prevented from progression.

The five THAs that were treated previously by modified transtrochanteric rotational osteotomy combined with muscle-pedicle-bone graft were classified as Ficat stage IV initially. There was no need to revise to hip replacement in 16 cases in which modified transtrochanteric rotational osteotomy alone was performed and in 7 bone grafting cases.

The complications were varus angulation in two cases, sensory disturbance on the lateral thigh in two cases, osteophyte formation in five cases, and deep vein thrombosis in one case. There was no infection. In the two cases with varus angulation, postoperatively measured neck–shaft angle was 118°, but no additional treatment was required. Two cases had lateral thigh paresthesia resulting from lateral femoral cutaneous nerve injury, but their condition improved as time passed. Five cases had shown subcapital osteophyte formation on radiography but were free of pain and had little limitation of motion. One patient had heterotopic ossification with mild limitation of motion, and no further treatment was done. Deep vein thrombosis occurred in one patient, who improved after medical management.

Discussion

The etiology of osteonecrosis of the femoral head has been unclear, although young patients under 40 years of age are frequently affected, with progression to femoral head collapse and degenerative arthritis. Options for treatment range from simple observation to surgical procedures. Surgical treatment can be largely categorized into joint salvage procedure and THA. THA has been known to be the one and only definitive treatment for osteonecrosis of the femoral head that directly removed the lesion and renewed the articular surface. Nevertheless, THA is not a permanent treatment. It should not be a final choice in young patients because new problems such as prosthetic wear, osteolysis, and loosening have developed in THA, requiring later revision surgery. Therefore, it is reasonable to perform a salvage procedure for those patients who are young and are diagnosed early.

Core decompression, nonvascularized or vascularized bone graft, and transtrochanteric rotational osteotomy were developed and performed as head preservation procedures. Core decompression has its theoretical basis in the following principles: first, pain relief from decreasing intraosseous pressure; second, decompression of interstitial edema; and third, neovascularization that eventually alleviates femoral head necrosis [15]. Many investigators believe that temporary symptom relief can be expected from core decompression, but it is hard to prevent femoral head collapse if the necrotic lesion is large [16,17]. Vascularized bone grafting was introduced by Judet and associates [18] and popularized by Urbaniak and associates [19]. However, Urbaniak reported that vascularized bone grafting requires a surgeon experienced in microsurgical technique, and because fibular bone is sacrificed, weight-bearing is restricted for 6 months, eventually leading to weakness of ankle dorsiflexion, sensory deficit, and progressive foot pain.

In 1980, Wagner and Zeiler proposed transtrochanteric rotational osteotomy, but compared to classical procedures it was difficult and the results were quite similar or unsatisfactory [20]. Sugioka [12] introduced a new method of transtrochanteric rotational osteotomy, and it has been performed as one of the procedures for osteonecrosis of femoral head. Sugioka transtrochanteric rotational osteotomy is applied to young patients with an intact posterior femoral area so that the necrotic zone is shifted to a lesser weight-bearing portion of the posteroinferior aspect. The weight-bearing surface is replaced by healthy bone or cartilage, aiming at elimination of shearing forces in the femoral head and progressive collapse and realignment of the articular surface of the subluxated femoral head [13,17].

Sugioka reported a 86% success rate in 11 years of follow-up study; not only the early necrotic stage but also Ficat stage III and IV with advanced collapse and arthritic change had 73% and 68% success rates, respectively [13]. Maistrelli and associates [21] reported transtrochanteric rotational osteotomy is not permanent, but those young patients who have neither metabolic bone disease nor articular destruction can gain enough time to delay THA. Although successful results were seen on short-term follow-up, long-term follow-up results were variable and not quite satisfactory [21,22]. Some authors reported a 50% success rate after transtrochanteric osteotomy [23], and Ohzono and associates [4] proposed that lack of skilled surgical technique or inappropriate patient selection or fixation causes a high failure rate. Our modified transtrochanteric osteotomy for rotational osteotomy in which the greater trochanter is not detached has several advantages: no greater trochanteric fixation is needed, operation time is shortened, additional procedures such as muscle pedicle vascularized or nonvascularized bone graft can be combined, early rehabilitation is possible because shear force is reduced, and subsequent THA is not affected because the greater trochanter anatomy is not altered. However, our modification is also technically demanding. It may be reasonable that it is performed by only experienced surgeons if a good outcome is to be expected.

In our study, overall early survival rate was 90%. Although this study had a short-term follow-up, we had 62% success rate even in stage IV patients, in whom joint preservation is usually known to be impossible, thus effectively delaying performing THA.

Conclusions

We were able to get satisfactory results even in advanced cases using the modified transtrochanteric rotational osteotomy. Particularly, it has advantages in that operation time is reduced, rehabilitation as well as the surgical technique is easier, additional procedures such as bone graft can be combined, and a stage IV patient can be treated with acceptable results. Therefore, it is recommended particularly for young patients with stage 2 or 3 and some selected patients with stage 4.

References

1. Brinker MR. Rosenberg AG, Kull L, Galante JO (1994) Primary total hip arthroplasty using noncemented porous coated femoral components in patients with osteonecrosis of the femoral head. J Arthroplasty 9:457–468
2. Coventry MB, Beckenbaugh RD, Nolan DR, Ilstrup DM (1974) 2012 total hip arthroplasties: a study of postoperative course and early complications. J Bone Joint Surg 56A:272–284

3. Krackow KA, Mont MA, Maar DC (1993) Limited femoral endoprosthesis for avascular necrosis of the femoral head. Orthop Rev 12:457–163
4. Saito S, Saito M, Nishina T, Ohzono K, Ono K (1989) Long-term results of total hip arthroplasty for osteonecrosis of the femoral head: a comparison with osteoarthritis. Clin Orthop 244:198–207
5. Stauffer RN (1982) Ten-year follow-up study of total hip replacement. J Bone Joint Surg 64A:983–990
6. Fairbank AC, Bhatia D, Jinnah RH, Hungerford DS (1995) Long-term results of core decompression for ischaemic necrosis of the femoral head. J Bone Joint Surg 77B: 42–49
7. Rosenwasser MP, Gartino JP, Kiernan HA, Michelsen CB (1994) Long term follow-up of through debridement and cancellous bone grafting of the femoral head for avascular necrosis. Clin Orthop 306:17–27
8. Fuchs B, Knothe U, Hertel R, Ganz R (2003) Femoral osteotomy and iliac graft vascularization for femoral head osteonecrosis. Clin Orthop 412:84–93
9. Bonfiglio M, Bardenstein MB (1958) Treatment by bone grafting of aseptic necrosis of the femoral head and nonunion of the femoral neck (Phemister technique). J Bone Joint Surg 40A:1329–1346
10. Buckley PD, Gearen PF, Petty RW (1991) Structural bone grafting for early atraumatic avascular necrosis of the femoral head. J Bone Joint Surg 73S:1357–1364
11. Ohzono K, Saito M, Takaoka K, et al (1991) Natural history of nontraumatic avascular necrosis of the femoral head. J Bone Joint Surg 73B:68–72
12. Sugioka Y (1978) Transtrochanteric anterior rotational osteotomy of the femoral head in the treatment of osteonecrosis affecting the hip: a new osteotomy operation. Clin Orthop 130:191–201
13. Sugioka Y (1984) Transtrochanteric rotational osteotomy in the treatment of idiopathic and steroid induced femoral head necrosis, Perthes disease, slipped capital femoral epiphysis, and osteoarthritis of the hip: indications and results. Clin Orthop 184:12–23
14. Harris WH (1969) Traumatic arthritis of the hip after dislocation and acetabular fractures: treatment by mold arthroplasty. J Bone Joint Surg 51A:737–755
15. Mont MA, Hungerfold DS 1995) Current concept review. Non-traumatic avascular necrosis of the femoral head. J Bone Joint Surg 77A:459–474
16. Koo KH, Kim R, Ko GH, Song HR, Jeong ST, Cho SH (1995) Preventing collapse in early-stage osteonecrosis of the femoral head: a randomized clinical trial of core decompression. J Bone Joint Surg 77B:870–874
17. Lafforgue P, Dahan E, Chagnnaud C, Schiano A, Kasbarian M, Acquaviva PC (1993) Early-stage avascular necrosis of the femoral head: MR imaging for prognosis in 31 cases with at least 2 years of follow-up. Radiology 187:199–204
18. Judet H, Judet J, Gilbert A (1981) Vascular microsurgery in osthopaedics. Int Orthop 5:61–68
19. Urbaniak JR, Coogan PG, Gunneson EB, Nunley JA (1995) Treatment of osteonecrosis of the femoral head with free vascularized fibular grafting: a long-term follow-up study of one hundred and three hips. J Bone Joint Surg 77A:681–694
20. Wagner H, Zeiler G (1980) Idiopathic avascular necrosis of the femoral head. Results of intertrochanteric osteotomy and resurfacing (author's transl). Orthopaede 9:290–310
21. Maistrelli G, Fusco U, Avai A, Bombelli R (1988) Osteonecrosis of the hip treated by intertrochanteric osteotomy: a four to 15 year follow-up. J Bone Joint Surg 70B: 761–766
22. Ganz R, Buechler U (1983) Overview of attempts to revitalize the dead head in aseptic necrosis of the femoral head: osteotomy and revascularization. In: Hungerford DS (ed) The hip. Mosby, St. Louis, pp 96–305
23. Dean MT, Cabenela ME (1993) Transtrochanteric anterior rotational osteotomy for avascular necrosis of the femoral head. J Bone Joint Surg 75B:597–602

Vascularized Iliac Bone Graft Using Deep Circumflex Iliac Vessels for Idiopathic Osteonecrosis of the Femoral Head

Kunihiko Tokunaga, Muroto Sofue, Youichirou Dohmae, Kenji Watanabe, Masaki Ishizaka, Yutaka Ohkawa, Toshio Iga, and Naoto Endo

Summary. This study aimed to analyze the clinical and radiologic findings of 59 hips from 46 patients who underwent vascularized iliac bone graft (VIBG) using the deep circumflex iliac artery and vein for idiopathic osteonecrosis of the femoral head (ION). Progress rate of femoral head collapse was 76.3% after VIBG. More than half of the femoral heads collapsed even though they did not show preoperative collapse. Average Japanese Orthopedic Association (JOA) score was 73.3 points, and there was no significant difference between preoperative and postoperative JOA scores. In males, preoperative collapse of the femoral head, bone graft with total curettage of the osteonecrotic lesion, and bilateral VIBG reduced JOA scores. For patients over 30 years old, preoperative collapse, bone graft with total curettage of the osteonecrotic lesion, and abuse of alcohol reduced survival rate after VIBG when the endpoint was set as collapse of the femoral head. These data suggest that young patients suffering from early-stage ION without collapse of the femoral head should be indicated to undergo VIBG. However, VIBG is only a time-saving surgery to postpone performing total arthroplasty or hemiarthroplasty for patients with early-stage ION because VIBG cannot always improve hip function and femoral head deformity.

Key words. Idiopathic osteonecrosis, Femoral head, Vascularized iliac bone graft, Collapse, Time-saving surgery

Introduction

Since 1982, vascularized iliac bone graft (VIBG) has been performed using the deep circumflex iliac vessels in patients suffering from idiopathic osteonecrosis of the femoral head (ION) [1,2]. The concepts of our VIBG method are based on the aim to

Division of Orthopedic Surgery, Department of Regenerative Transplant Medicine, Niigata University Graduate School of Medical and Dental Sciences, 1-757 Asahimachi-dori, Niigata 951-8510, Japan

revascularize the necrotic lesion and to prevent collapse of the femoral head during the repair process after osteonecrosis. VIBG is indicated for IONs of types B, C-1, and C-2 according to a system devised by the Japanese Investigation Committee for ION [3]. Because other bone- and cartilage-preserving surgeries for the treatment of ION were also available, including transtrochanteric varus osteotomy and transtrochanteric anterior rotational osteotomy, our VIBG was often indicated for IONs with a relatively wide necrotic area. We initially carried out VIBG for advanced cases with severe femoral head collapse such as stage 3-B or 4 according to the system devised by the Japanese Investigation Committee for ION [3]. The objectives of this study were (1) to analyze radiologic and clinical findings of our VIBG method, (2) to investigate factors affecting radiologic and clinical results, and (3) to determine the indication of VIBG for patients with ION.

Patients and Methods

We performed VIBG using the deep circumflex iliac artery and vein using the Smith-Petersen approach (Fig. 1). For initial cases, the entire necrotic lesion was curetted, and bone chips were harvested from the ilium and packed with the pedicular bone graft ("old method"). The more-recent method included curettage of the region where the pedicular bone was grafted ("current method").

We analyzed 59 hips from 46 patients (18 women and 28 men) with ION who underwent VIBG from 1982 to 2001. Average follow-up period was 9 years, and average patient age at surgery was 34 years. Etiological factors in the VIBG group were steroid related (62.7%), alcohol related (28.8%), and idiopathic (8.5%). To assign grades to each type of ION, a system devised by the Japanese Investigation Committee for ION was used, as follows [3]. Types A and B corresponded to cases with a necrotic area less than two-thirds of the weight-bearing surface of the acetabulum. Type C-1 corresponded to cases with a necrotic area greater than two-thirds of the weight-bearing surface of the acetabulum, but the lateral edge never exceeded the most lateral edge of the acetabulum. Type C-2 corresponded to cases with a necrotic area greater than two-thirds of the weight-bearing surface of the acetabulum and a lateral edge exceeding the most lateral edge of the acetabulum. The investigated hip joints were of type C-1 (22%) and type C-2 (78%). To grade the stage of each ION, a system devised by the Japanese Investigation Committee for ION was also used, as follows [3]. Stage 1 corresponded to a preadiographic stage that was detectable only by one scintigram, magnetic resonance imaging (MRI), or core biopsy. Stage 2 corresponded to an early stage with radiographic evidence of necrosis without collapse. Stage 3A corresponded to an advanced stage with less than 3 mm collapse and stage 3B also corresponded to an advanced stage with more than 3 mm collapse. Stage 4 defined a late advanced stage associated with osteoarthritic changes. The investigated hip joints consisted of stage 2 (49.2%), stage 3A (40.7%), and stage 3B (10.2%) at surgery (Fig. 2A).

We evaluated clinical hip functions of each joint according to a chart of hip joint functions from the Japanese Orthopedic Association score (JOA score) [4]. Survival rates were evaluated with Kaplan–Meier analysis in the VIBG groups using clinical and radiologic endpoints. The clinical endpoint was set at the time when patients

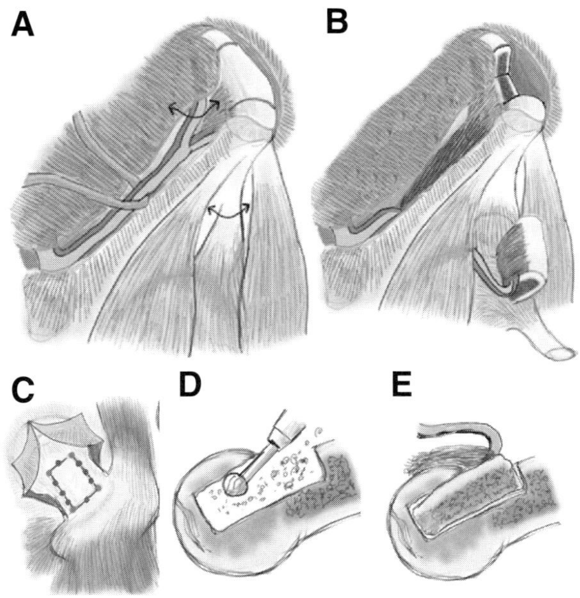

FIG. 1. Surgical procedure for vascularized iliac bone graft (VIBG). Since 1982, the deep iliac circumflex artery and vein for VIBG have been used for idiopathic osteonecrosis of the femoral head (ION). **A** An iliac bone block of about 45 × 25 × 15 mm is harvested from the iliac crest, preserving a vascular bundle containing the deep circumflex iliac artery and vein with the surrounding iliac muscle. The muscular branches of the deep circumflex iliac artery and vein must be ligated and severed. The affected hip joint is exposed using an anterior approach after the Smith-Petersen technique. The tendon of the rectus femoris muscle is detached from the inferior anterior iliac spine and is reflected caudally. **B** The harvested iliac bone is passed beneath the iliopsoas muscle to bring it anteriorly to the hip joint. **C** A bony window of about 20 × 15 × 30 mm is made on the anterior aspect of the femoral neck using a drill point and a chisel. **D** A bony gutter is made using a high-speed drill. **E** The harvested iliac bone is inserted into the bony gutter

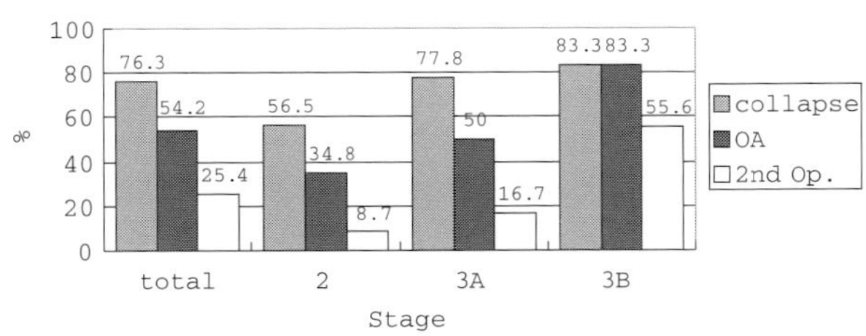

FIG. 2. Percentages of femoral head collapse, osteoarthritic changes (*OA*), and need for second operation at each stage at initial diagnosis were 76.3%, 54.2%, and 25.4%, respectively, in total joints that underwent VIBG. Joints with further collapse at initial diagnosis showed more progression of collapse, osteoarthritic changes, and need for second operation. More than half (56.5%) of the joints showed progress of collapse, even though they did not collapse at initial diagnosis (stage 2). When joints had collapse of more than 3 mm at initial diagnosis, more than 80% showed progression of collapse and osteoarthritic changes and more than half (55.6%) required a second operation

underwent additional surgery such as total hip arthroplasty, hemiarthroplasty, or arthrodesis because of failure of the initial treatment. The radiologic endpoint was set at the time when femoral collapse occurred or advanced after VIBG. We analyzed the effects of age, gender, body mass index (BMI), side of ION, side of VIBG, method of bone graft, and preoperative collapse of the femoral head on JOA scores and survival rates. A Mann–Whitney *U* test and a Kaplan–Meier analysis were used for statistical analyses using Stat View version 5.0 (SAS Institute, Cary, NC, USA). A *P* value less than 0.05 was considered statistically significant.

Results

Radiologic Changes After VIBG

Radiologic changes and rate of second operation are shown in Fig. 2. Collapse of the femoral head occurred or progressed in 76.3% of hips that underwent VIBG. Osteoarthritic changes were observed in 52.2% of hips, and additional surgical treatment was required for 25.4% of hips. Percentages of femoral head collapse progression and osteoarthritic changes were 56.5% and 34.8% in stage 2 cases at initial diagnosis, respectively; 77.8% and 50% in stage 3A cases, respectively, at initial diagnosis; and both were 83.3% in stage 3B cases at initial diagnosis. Average time period until collapse occurred or advanced was 13 ± 11 months. Time period until additional surgical treatment such as total hip arthroplasty, hemiarthroplasty, or arthrodesis was required was 117.6 ± 78.6 months.

Clinical Effects of VIBG on ION

Average total points of pre- and postoperative JOA scores were 70 and 73.3, respectively. There was no significant difference between pre- and postoperative JOA scores (Fig. 3).

Factors Affecting the JOA Score

To identify factors affecting the JOA score and survival rate after VIBG, we analyzed operative age, sex, body mass index (BMI), side of ION, side of VIBG, method of bone

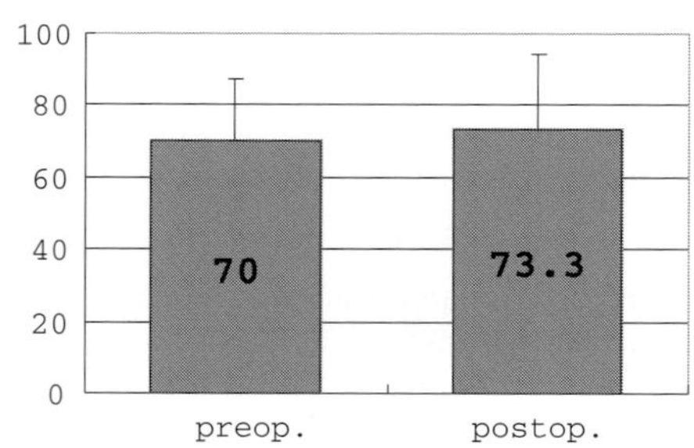

Fig. 3. Japanese Orthopedic Association (JOA) scores before and after VIBG. Averages of pre- and postoperative total JOA scores were 70 and 73.3 points, respectively, and there was no significant difference between them

graft, and preoperative collapse of the femoral head. Factors affecting postoperative JOA score are shown in Figs. 4 and 5. The JOA score of the total pain category in joints with preoperative collapse was significantly lower than that in joints without preoperative collapse (Fig. 4A,B). The score of range of motion (ROM) was lower in men (Fig. 5A). The old method of bone graft, in which the osteonecrotic lesion was completely curetted and the vascularized iliac bone was grafted using iliac bone chips, also negatively affected the JOA score of ROM (Fig. 5B). The score of walking activity was lower in joints that underwent bilateral VIBG than that in joints which underwent unilateral VIBG (Fig. 5C).

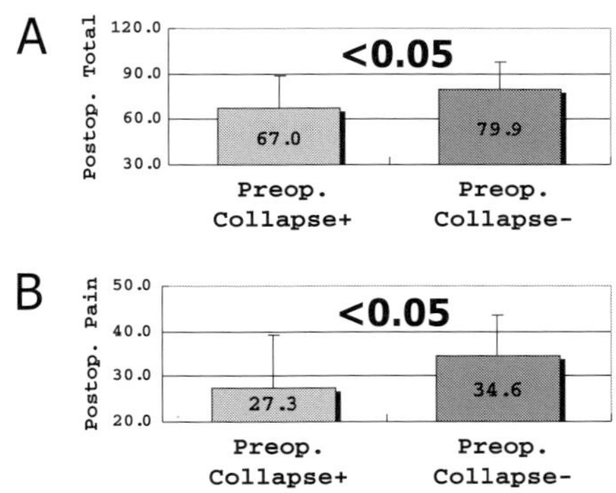

FIG. 4. When joints had preoperative collapse, total (**A**) and pain (**B**) points of JOA scores significantly decreased

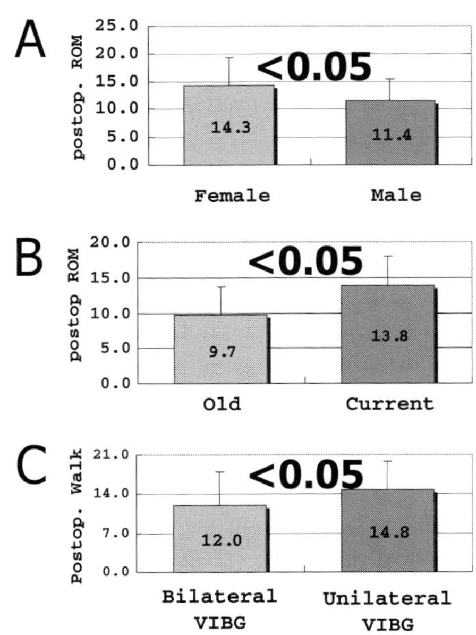

FIG. 5. Factors affecting range of motion of hip joints and walking ability. JOA scores for range of motion (*ROM*) for male sex (**A**) and the old procedure for bone graft (**B**), in which the osteonecrotic lesion was completely resected and the vascularized iliac bone was grafted with iliac chip bones, were significantly reduced. **C** JOA scores for walking ability were significantly decreased when VIBG was performed on both sides of the hip joint

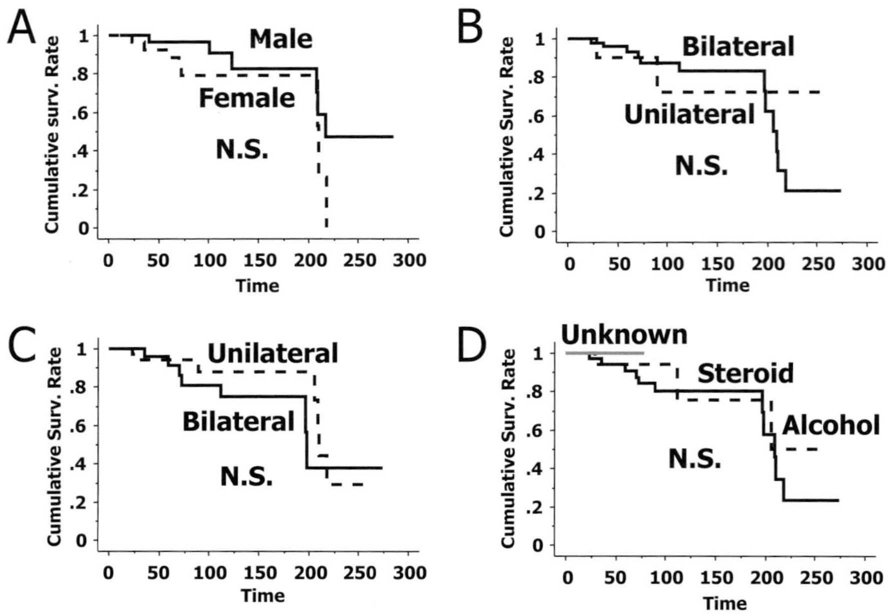

FIG. 6. Sex (**A**), side of affected hip joints (**B**), side of VIBG (**C**), and inducer of ION (**D**) did not affect survival (*Surv.*) rate when the endpoint was set as a second operation such as total hip arthroplasty, hemiarthroplasty, or arthrodesis. *N.S.*, not significant

Factors Affecting Survival Rate After VIBG

When the endpoint was set as the second operation, including total hip arthroplasty, hemiarthroplasty, and arthrodesis, sex, side of ION, side of VIBG, and inducer did not affect survival rate (Fig. 6A–D). In addition, sex, side of ION, and side of VIBG never affected survival rate after VIBG when the endpoint was set as collapse of the femoral head (Fig. 7A–C). However, for operative age over 30 years, the old bone graft method and preoperative collapse of the femoral head reduced survival rate when the endpoint was set at collapse (Fig. 8A–C). Abuse of alcohol also reduced survival rate (Fig. 8D).

Discussion

The concepts of VIBG are based on two goals: (1) to revascularize the necrotic lesion by using vascularized iliac bone, and (2) to prevent femoral head collapse by the iliac strut. Previous reports showed acceptable clinical results after VIBG; however, stages progressed in 40%–50% of cases after VIBG [1,2,5–10]. In our study, more than 70% of joints showed progression of femoral head collapse after VIBG. Collapse rate of joints without preoperative collapse was 56.5%. In addition, the progression rate of joints with preoperative collapse after VIBG was more than 80%. Therefore, we

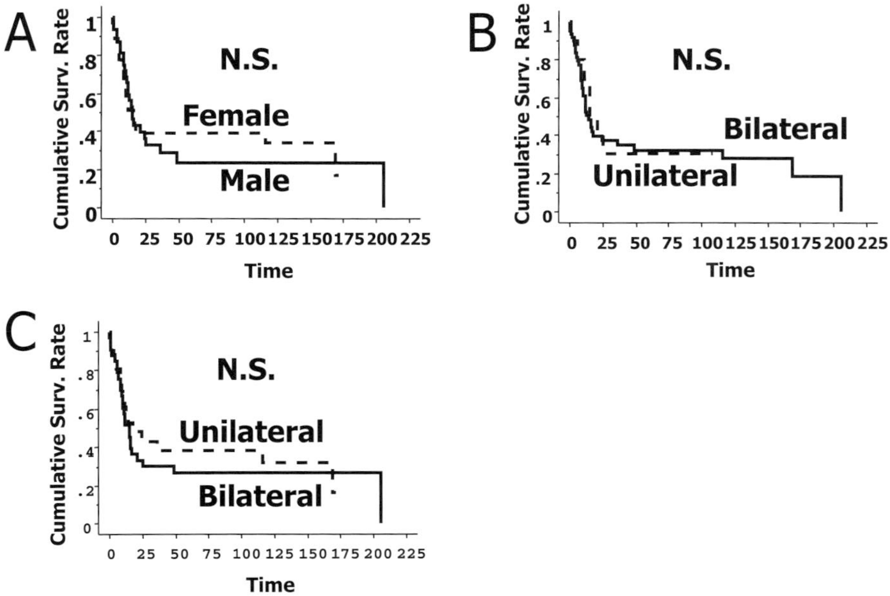

FIG. 7. Survival rates when endpoint was set at progress of collapse of the femoral head apparently were not affected by the factors thought to affect clinical results of VIBG such as sex (**A**), side of ION (**B**), and side of VIBG (**C**)

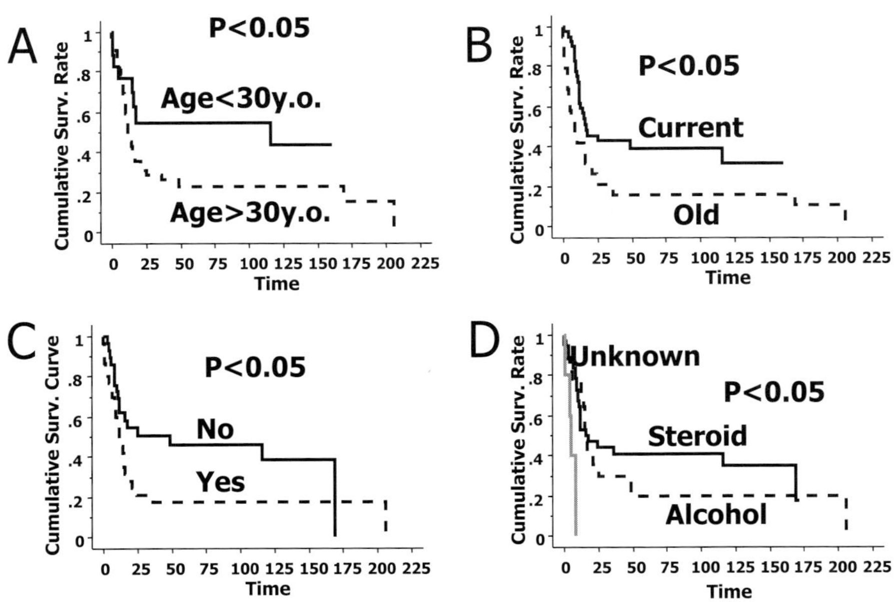

FIG. 8. When the endpoint was set at progress of femoral head collapse, age over 30 years (*y.o.*, years old) (**A**), the old method of bone graft (in which the osteonecrotic lesion in the femoral head was completely resected and the vascularized iliac bone was grafted with iliac bone chips) (**B**), preoperative collapse of the femoral head (**C**), and abuse of alcohol (**D**) significantly reduced the survival rate

concluded that VIBG could not always prevent femoral head collapse. We confirmed vascularization in the grafted iliac bone for a couple of years after surgery using dynamic MRI (unpublished data). However, we did not show histologically whether the grafted iliac bone could be incorporated in the host necrotic bone around the necrotic lesion.

During the repair process following osteonecrosis, new bones are formed by additional bone formation in which the new bone is directly added on the dead bone surface without osteoclastic resorption [11]. Dead bones remain for a long time, and it takes more than a couple of years to completely replace the dead bone in human osteonecrotic lesions. Therefore, it will take a long time for the vascularized grafted bone to be incorporated into the host osteonecrotic bone. Patients were restricted to partial weight-bearing for about 6–12 months after VIBG in our series; however, this time period might be too short to allow incorporation of the grafted bone into the host bones. These data indicate that it is difficult to prevent collapse of the femoral head because of the remnants of necrotic tissue in the weight-bearing area. Noguchi et al. reported that stage progression was observed in three of four joints in a group who underwent VIBG alone, whereas stage progression was noted in two of ten joints in a group who underwent combined VIBG with transtrochanteric anterior rotational osteotomy [12]. To prevent complete collapse, displacement of the necrotic lesion out of the weight-bearing area such as is done in transtrochanteric anterior rotational osteotomy of the femoral head is needed [13,14].

The mechanical property of an iliac bone block is inferior to other harder struts such as that from a fibula. Our bone block consisted of a solid rectangle, and only three of its six faces were covered with cortical bone. In addition, the cross-sectional area of our bone block was usually $1.5\,\text{cm} \times 2.5\,\text{cm}$. This area was not sufficient to support the weight of a human body. These data indicated that VIBG cannot always meet the original goal of regenerating bones and supporting body weight. The position of the grafted bone is also important. Nakamura et al. reported that the bony strut should be placed at $5°$–$10°$ of the valgus position relative to the neck–shaft angle [9,15]. They also emphasized that the distance between the subchondral bone and the tip of the grafted bone should be less than 5 mm [15]. Because the femoral head is spherical, it is quite difficult to place the graft in that position. Indeed, the average distance between the grafted bones and the subchondral bones was more than 5 mm in our series (data not shown). We recently developed a metal cast of grafted bone that is used to confirm the direction and depth of the bony gutter in the femoral head by fluoroscopy during VIBG to secure graft position.

Little is known about factors affecting the clinical results of VIBG except for the position of the grafted bone [9]. Our previous study concluded that risk factors for VIBG were female sex, systemic lupus erythematosis (SLE), steroid administration, and bilateral cases by investigating unsuccessful cases after VIBG [16]. However, the present study demonstrated that female sex and steroids did not always affect JOA score and survival rate after VIBG. The other risk factor that we should further consider is preoperative collapse, which affects JOA score and survival rate. Once collapse occurs, the vascularized iliac bone cannot support the destroyed bone structure in the femoral head. Male sex and abuse of alcohol were also found to be risk factors for survival rate after VIBG. This finding might be explained by the fact that most osteonecrosis-affected patients with abuse of alcohol are men.

Taken together, VIBG should be indicated in limited cases with early-stage ION. Hip joints without collapse should be treated with VIBG. However, we found that patients with pain in the affected hip always showed a certain degree of collapse of the femoral head. Therefore, actual indications of VIBG should be restricted. In addition, VIBG cannot always prevent progress of femoral head collapse or advancement of osteoarthritic changes, even though the femoral head shows no collapse. We conclude that VIBG for ION should be indicated for (1) joints without or with little collapse of the femoral head and (2) joints with a wide lesion for which transtrochanteric rotational osteotomies are never indicated. VIBG is a time-saving surgery for young patients to postpone total hip arthroplasty or hemiarthroplasty.

Conclusions

1. VIBG cannot always prevent stage progression of the femoral head after ION.
2. Preoperative collapse, sex, total curettage of the necrotic lesion for bone grafts, and bilateral ION reduce JOA score after VIBG.
3. Total curettage of the necrotic lesion, operative age over 30 years, precollapse, and abuse of alcohol reduce survival rate of ION when the endpoint is set at progress of femoral head collapse.
4. VIBG is a "time-saving surgery" for young patients with ION to postpone performance of total hip arthroplasty or hemiarthroplasty.

Acknowledgments. This work was not supported by any grant.

References

1. Solonen KA, Rindell K, Paavilainen T (1990) Vascularized pedicled bone graft into the femoral head: treatment of aseptic necrosis of the femoral head. Arch Orthop Trauma Surg 109(3):160–163
2. Cheung HS, Stewart IE, Ho KC, Leung PC, Metreweli C (1993) Vascularized iliac crest grafts: evaluation of viability status with marrow scintigraphy. Radiology 186(1): 241–245
3. Sugano N, Atsumi T, Ohzono K, Kubo T, Hotokebuchi T, Takaoka K (2003) The 2001 revised criteria for diagnosis, classification, and staging of idiopathic osteonecrosis of the femoral head. J Orthop Sci 7(5):601–605
4. Hasegawa Y, Iwata H, Mizuno M, Genda E, Sato S, Miura T (1992) The natural course of osteoarthritis of the hip due to subluxation or acetabular dysplasia. Arch Orthop Trauma Surg 111(4):187–191
5. Leung PC (1996) Femoral head reconstruction and revascularization. Treatment for ischemic necrosis. Clin Orthop Relat Res 323:139–145
6. Pavlovcic V, Dolinar D, Arnez Z (1999) Femoral head necrosis treated with vascularized iliac crest graft. Int Orthop 23(3):150–153
7. Eisenschenk A, Lautenbach M, Schwetlick G, Weber U (2001) Treatment of femoral head necrosis with vascularized iliac crest transplants. Clin Orthop Relat Res 386: 100–105
8. Feng CK, Yu JK, Chang MC, Chen TH, Lo WH (1998) Vascularized iliac bone graft for treating avascular necrosis of the femoral head. Zhonghua Yi Xue Za Zhi (Taipei) 61(8):463–469

9. Nagoya S, Nagao M, Takada J, Kuwabara H, Wada T, Kukita Y, Yamashita T (2004) Predictive factors for vascularized iliac bone graft for nontraumatic osteonecrosis of the femoral head. J Orthop Sci 9(6):566–570
10. Hasegawa Y, Iwata H, Torii S, Iwase T, Kawamoto K, Iwasada S (1997) Vascularized pedicle bone-grafting for nontraumatic avascular necrosis of the femoral head. A 5- to 11-year follow-up. Arch Orthop Trauma Surg 116(5):251–258
11. Norman D, Reis D, Zinman C, Misselevich I, Boss JH (1998) Vascular deprivation-induced necrosis of the femoral head of the rat. An experimental model of avascular osteonecrosis in the skeletally immature individual or Legg–Perthes disease. Int J Exp Pathol 79(3):173–181
12. Noguchi M, Kawakami T, Yamamoto H (2001) Use of vascularized pedicle iliac bone graft in the treatment of avascular necrosis of the femoral head. Arch Orthop Trauma Surg 121(8):437–442
13. Sugioka Y (1978) Transtrochanteric anterior rotational osteotomy of the femoral head in the treatment of osteonecrosis affecting the hip: a new osteotomy operation. Clin Orthop Relat Res 130:191–201
14. Sugioka Y, Hotokebuchi T, Tsutsui H (1992) Transtrochanteric anterior rotational osteotomy for idiopathic and steroid-induced necrosis of the femoral head. Indications and long-term results. Clin Orthop Relat Res 277:111–120
15. Nakamura H, Watanabe Y, Hasegawa K, Tanabe H, Yoshino K, Fukuda T, Katsuro T (2002) Analysis of vascularized iliac bone graft using superficial circumflex iliac artery and vein. Relationship between bone strut and collapse of the femoral head (in Japanese). J Musculoskel Syst 15(4):355–361
16. Endo N, Kitahara H, Ohkawa Y, Ogawa T, Matsuba A, Tokunaga K, Dohmae Y, Sofue M, Minato I (2000) Analysis of patients underwent vascularized iliac bone graft with poor clinical results and required additional surgeries (in Japanese). Hip Joint 26: 373–375

Part III
Osteoarthritis of the Hip: Joint Preservation or Joint Replacement?

Joint-Preserving and Joint-Replacing Procedures: Why, When, and Which? A Challenging and Responsible Decision

Siegfried Weller

Summary. The decision-making process in context with the treatment of hip joint diseases and posttraumatic conditions more than ever has to be respected. Multifold experiences—especially long-term results after hip joint replacement—during the past 46 years since Charnley justify and require detailed discussion and evaluation in respect to the borderline between a joint-preserving and a joint-replacing procedure. We must remember and respect the progress made in connection with bone and joint preservation techniques and the importance of the factor of gaining time for our patients—preferably the younger patient cohort—with a longer age expectancy.

Introduction

The Joint-Preserving Procedure

Charnley's idea, almost 46 years ago, about the use of cement to anchor prosthetic components, together with his low-friction principle, profoundly influenced arthroplasty of the hip joint and promoted its clinical application.

Despite all the blessings that joint replacement has brought to many people throughout the world in the past few decades, we must remember and admit that neither the implants nor the techniques available to us today, particularly with respect to long-term results—and also and especially in younger and active people—can yet fulfill all our wishes and requirements. Therefore, they are still not an ideal and long-term solution.

Facing an increasing number of problems in context with aseptic loosening after primary or secondary joint replacement (that is, revision), it is necessary to improve and make use of all possible joint-preserving measures to prevent or at least delay joint replacement. In many cases it might be easier, faster, spectacular, and also "economically more advantageous" for the surgeon to select a prosthesis as a primary intervention rather than to perform a more or less demanding joint reconstruction or correction with all its long and detailed postoperative procedures.

We, however, should not focus on short- or medium-term results, but must look much more these days for good long-term solutions, especially when dealing with a

Engelfriedshalde 47, D-72076 Tuebingen, Germany

rising number of younger age patients from a continuously growing community of people active in sports. It is this group of patients, who have a constant desire and demand—for whatever reason—after an injury or any joint disease to return to their athletic as well as social activities as soon as possible. More and more, the demands and expectations of our so-called modern treatment results (as repeatedly advertised in the media (e.g. "an artificial joint for the young sportsman?" etc.) are rising.

It seems that in our technically orientated and fast-changing world people think everything is possible and sometimes we forget that there are still "unsolved problems," especially biological barriers, which we cannot overcome. Joint replacement, therefore, still deserves critical observation and evaluation in respect to indication and technique (Fig. 1).

We can make the following statement: "Sometimes it is good to remember where we have come from to recognize where we must go!"

In this aspect, it is therefore advisable and useful, before making our therapeutic decision, to take some time for a careful thought about, which procedure is best for the individual situation, and also from a prognostic point of view, which we should select. In this context, the "time-saving factor" for our young-generation patients, who have a longer life expectancy, must be an important issue.

So, for a joint-preserving procedure, the following techniques [1–3], in exceptional cases are, or must not be considered, old-fashioned or unmodern:

1. Osteotomy of the proximal femur and the acetabular-pelvic area (posttraumatic conditions, dysplastic deformities and changes, etc.)
2. Bone grafting, cartilage transplantation (for posttraumatic and benign bone lesions and diseases, etc.)
3. Hip fusion and "Girdlestone situation" (septic conditions)

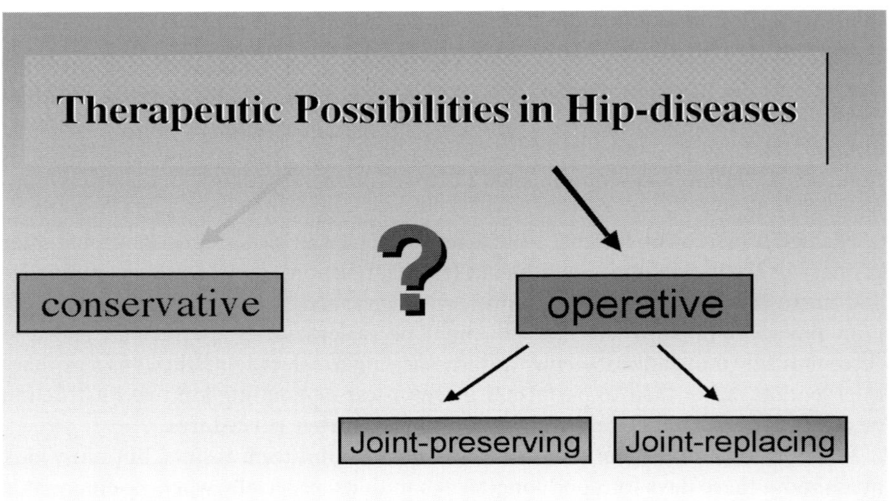

FIG. 1. The individual decision

All these procedures still must be critically and advantageously regarded, evaluated, and selected.

Experiences in the past have demonstrated in many cases that, with an adequate indication and correct technique, remarkable time savings can be achieved until a joint replacement becomes necessary as a subsequent procedure (Fig. 2).

Last but not least, the surgeon in our age also has to remember that osteoporotic bone deficiencies must receive additional drug therapy as a prophylactic and therapeutic measure to stop osteoclast production and progressive bone loss (Raloxifen, Biphosphonates, etc.).

Therefore, the orthopaedic surgeon must remember that the treatment of a hip disease (including posttraumatic defects) does not end with the surgical intervention!!

Bone and joint diseases (including trauma) require comprehensive treatment, starting with a detailed diagnosis and careful decision making. They cannot be solved exclusively by surgical interventions, especially joint replacement alone. (This is the so-called Bone and Joint Decade.)

If a necessary and justified joint-replacement remains the only and best solution, then all our technical improvements (such as surgical techniques, implant design, and materials, as well as adequate revision techniques), based on actual progress, the experience of the surgeon, and the equipment and facilities of the institution, in conjunction with necessary additional drug therapy and a critical long-term clinical follow-up (evidence based), must be considered.

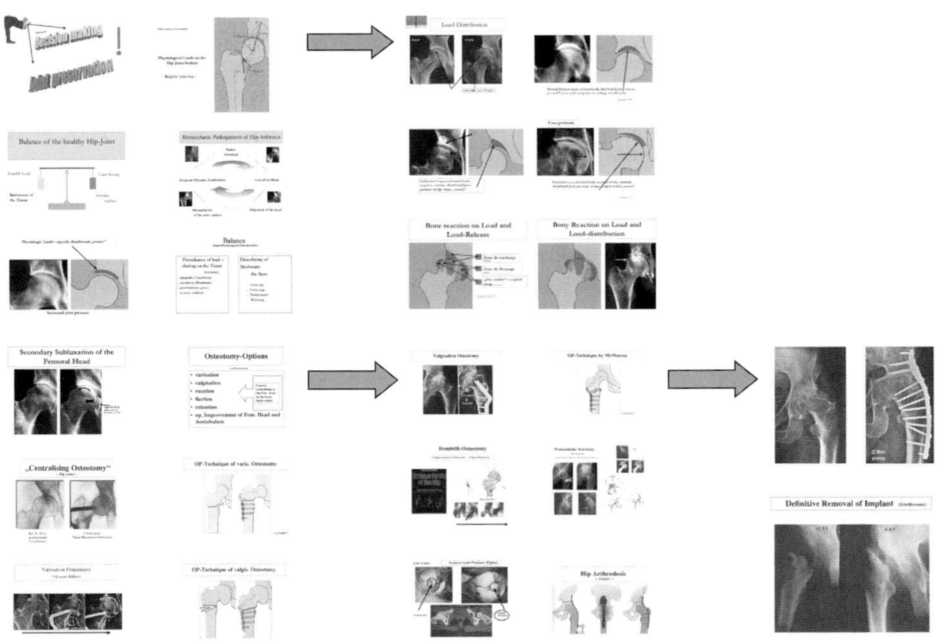

FIG. 2. Biomechanical considerations and therapeutic solutions

The Joint-Replacing Procedure

If our joint-preserving methods have reached their limits and, because of unbearable pain and growing disability, further therapeutic steps have to be selected, joint replacement becomes a good and advantageous solution. Our initial concept and technique over many years have remained unchanged. We have studied and looked into the problems of biological fixation with the goal of improving our long-term results in hip joint replacement.

Still, we must consider the relative merits of cemented and cementless technique for each patient, but in the case of the cementless primary hip replacement, proximal load transfer and high axial and rotational stability were defined as the key characteristics for our "Bicontact"-philosophy. These requirements meanwhile, after 19 years experience, are well accepted today and we use them before many others. We have added to our earlier concepts the methods of contemporary cementing techniques, press-fit cup arthroplasty, and advanced hip joint articulation. Implant extensions also met additional requirements of implant sizing in primary and revision surgery. We have seen remarkable change within our patient community, with an increase of elderly people—and a more disadvantageous increase of many young patients—receiving total replacement as a first and primary choice. This change must lead our attention to an individual decision, that is, whether to select the cemented or noncemented technique, which choice quite often has to be made intraoperatively. The Bicontact Hip System fulfills all these aspects and thus justifies the catalogue of requirements we initially have laid down.

After more than 19 years of Bicontact hip replacement, a statement on the correctness of our considerations relating to design and performance of the entire Bicontact philosophy can be made. This self-critical appraisal is based on the experiences of our own prospective study results, other published Bicontact results, and multiple worldwide experience reports. Many constructive thoughts and developments in the field of hip arthroplasty have been communicated, implemented, and introduced in clinical practice during the last few decades (46 years since Charnley). In many respects, these have resulted in visible and fundamental improvements concerning basic implant design, materials, and clinical results [4–10].

The cemented fixation of the prosthetic components introduced by Charnley (1959/1960) with his low-friction principle of the joint implant had a fundamental influence and promoted its growing use in clinical medicine. Over the years, however, we had to realize and observe certain disadvantages in context with the extended use of cement, especially in the increasing numbers of revisions.

The introduction of so-called cementless, "biological implantation" techniques during the past two decades has heralded a new era in hip replacement. With the development and introduction of the "Bicontact Hip Endoprosthesis System" in 1986–1987, we, at that time, did not intend to add another version to the numerous innovations of the most diverse types of hip implants. Much more, it has been our intention to react adaequately to the demands imposed with regard to the overall concept of a hip joint replacement, which had and still have changed considerably during recent years under the effect of modified initial conditions as a result of changes in demographic structures such as the aging population, an increasingly younger patient stock, and, in some cases, long-term results with many complications.

Looking back, we distinguish two time periods (Figs. 3, 4). According to a large number of communications, both personal and those from the literature, the pendulum of opinion concerning the advantages and disadvantages of cementless and cemented surgical methods for hip and other prostheses in certain countries still continues to swing in favour of the cemented technique (above all, in Anglo-American countries). In the majority of central European countries, in Asia, and in more and more other regions worldwide, however, the situation has changed and is still changing.

Many challenging experiences with difficult situations following cement-anchored hip endoprostheses, especially among younger patients, speak in favour of a cementless implantation whenever possible because of their greater life expectancy and potential for several future revisions.

The basic problem of long-term survival of endoprostheses, especially regarding a long-term bond between living tissue and a nonorganic (dead) material in principle, has not yet been solved. Therefore, we are still obliged in the future to decide individually and, insofar as possible, intraoperatively between a cementless and cemented implantation method depending on the particular case, especially according to the patient's age and life expectancy and the quality and load-bearing capacity of the bone stock (osteoporosis).

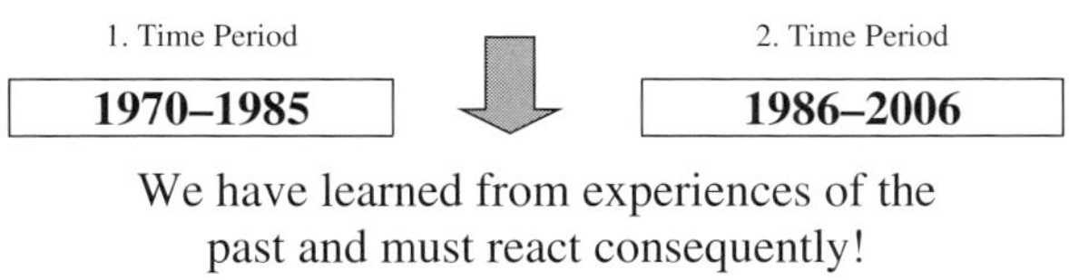

FIG. 3. Two time periods that demonstrate "learning from experiences" with consequent reaction

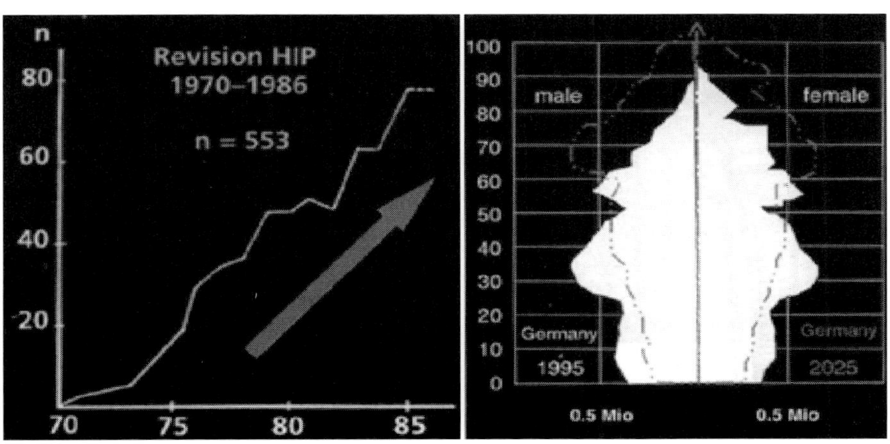

FIG. 4. First period (1970–1986): increasing number of hip revision procedures after aseptic implant loosening, and changes in demographic structure towards elderly patients, but also younger and more active patients who received total hip arthroplasty (THA)

While discussing a new concept and philosophy from a clinical point of view, following the demands for an endoprosthetic system based on earlier experiences and socioeconomic constraints (1970–1986), we set up a list of priorities to be achieved and fulfilled. These points include the following general objectives.

1. List of priorities:
   - Medical experience and facts (results and studies)
   - Medicotechnical progresses (decision-making, biological, and material aspects)
   - Demographic changes (age distribution)
   - Expectations and demands of patients (society)
   - Socioeconomic aspects (expenses, etc.)
2. Clinical and surgical demands:
   - Universal applicability (cemented, cementless, revision, etc.)
   - Simple instrumentation for all surgical techniques
   - Optimal implant design with proximal load transfer
   - Bone-preserving implant design-"biological implantation technique" (profiler)
   - High primary stability (rotation!)
   - Improvement of joint articulation with reduced wear (ceramic, metal, polyethylene, etc.)
   - Economically defensible solution (healthcare expenditure)
   - Overall improvement of long-term results (multicenter studies "evidence based")
3. In addition and as a future perspective of our focus, the following factors have been adopted to improve implant survival results:
   - Improvement of direct, cementless anchorage of the endoprosthesis in living bone stock (interface aspects, osseointegration)
   - Improvement of cement composition, chemical hardening process, and cementing techniques
   - Surgical performance (e.g., navigation for correct positioning of the implant, acetabular socket, etc.)

We have learned that the assessment of the implant and the respective surgical and anchorage technique will continue to pose a major problem, because aseptic loosening does not generally occur and become clinically symptomatic until after medium-term implantation time (approximately 10–15 years).

It is assumed today, and can be underlined by literature reports, that an endoprosthetic system—on the basis of comprehensive and detailed follow-up examination of a maximum number of cases—allows a statement of quality after around 10 to 15 years at the earliest.

Stability (primary stability) and biology (bone perfusion and osseointegration of the implant) are indispensable prerequisites to be considered. Possible factors to optimize the stability of endoprostheses after cementless implantation are:

- Surface design (coating with enlargement of surface)
- Press-fit design of the implant (interface)
- Additional fixation features (primary implantation and revision)

These points explain why prostheses implanted without cement react far more sensitively to modifications and design, to force introduction, and to bonding of the implant to bone (osseointegration). With regard to their stability in living bone compared to cemented prostheses, cementless prostheses are required to prove their advantages over and over again.

Implant Characteristics

The Bicontact Family

The Bicontact hip stem (Fig. 5) belongs to the group of so-called straight stem prostheses with a flat, tapered, square-shaped stem. Bilateral flanges and the characteristic antirotation wing make use of the greater trochanter area and provide the implant with a high level of primary stability in the sense of proximal load transmission. The outward expression of rotational stability in particular is the absence of tiresome, occasionally intolerable, thigh pain. As a modular system with different implant sizes and stem shapes, the Bicontact system also meets the requirements of dysplastic deformities with the possibility of deciding on cementless or cemented anchorage of the prosthetic components during the intervention. Therefore, the Bicontact system meets all the requirements for universality [4–6].

In this context, it is necessary to remember that:

- The external design of the Bicontact implant for different implantation types has remained unchanged since its introduction.
- The cementless anchorage is supported by a microporous, biocompatible pure titanium coating (Plasmapore) applied at the proximal part only (proximal load transfer).
- The surgeon has the possibility of adapting the type of anchorage to the local and individual condition right up to the time of final implantation.
- The bone-preserving and biological implantation technique is in accordance with the fundamental requirements of our philosophy.

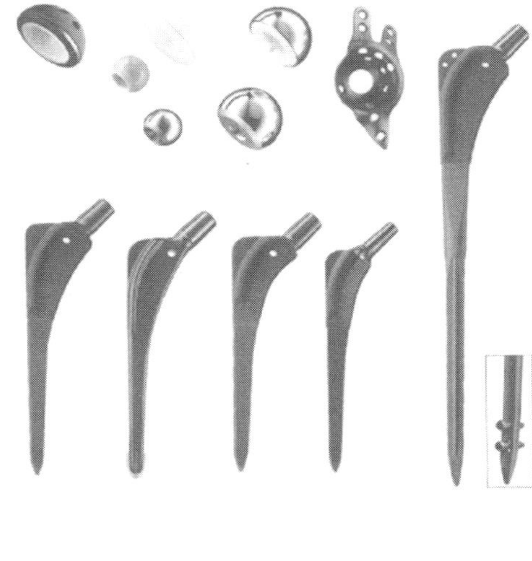

FIG. 5. The Bicontact hip system with stem, cup, and head components for primary, dysplastic, special anatomy, and revision procedures

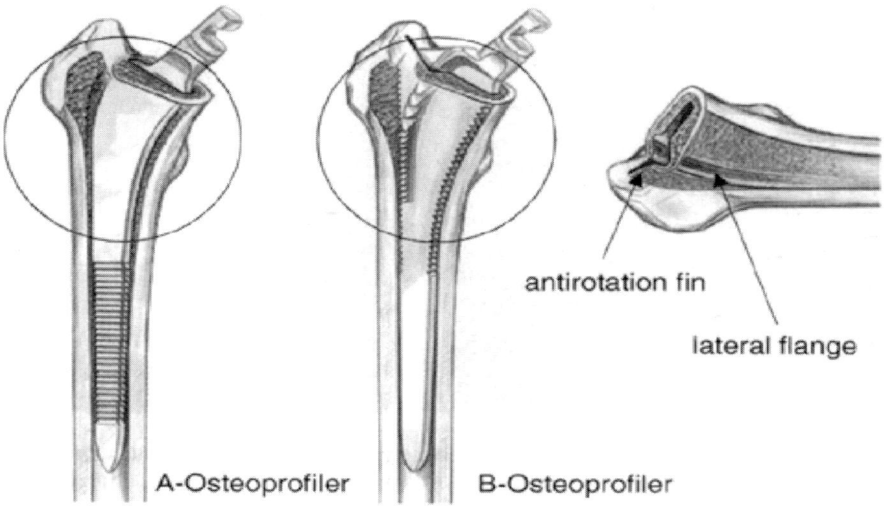

FIG. 6. Bicontact Osteoprofiler system: no rasping, no reaming, no removal of bone. Compression of cancellous bone structures (*A-Osteoprofiler*) and cutting of the proximal Bicontact shape (*B-Osteoprofiler*) for proximal load transfer. With the so-called Osteoprofiler System—reaming or rasping explicitly is not wanted here—no vital living bone is sacrificed in the metaphyseal part of the femur. On the contrary, the cancellous structures present are compressed (condensed) to guarantee optimum stress transmission (stress introduction)

This point, last but not least, has been a learning result of our earlier experiences with numerous revision operations, quite often associated with considerable bone defects (osteolysis) and general periprosthetic bone loss.

Therefore, to pay attention to these facts, we say: "During each primary operation—and also after every revision—a subsequent intervention must be borne in mind." This guiding principle emphasizes the significance of prevention also and precisely in our joint replacement procedures. Load and stress-transfer should occur exclusively in the intertrochanteric region, whereas a distal "press-fit" of the prosthesis stem is avoided for the primary implantation (Fig. 6).

The principle of bone-preserving-implantation techniques is pursued similarly on the acetabular side. The Plasmacup press-fit-anchoring method with expansion fixing at the cortical socket aperture level and a press-fit contact also follows the same principle of bone preservation and bone reconstruction. By this technique, premature protrusion of the socket is avoided.

Thus, the Bicontact system represents a family consisting of various members with a basic generic design [6,7].

Conclusion

Summarising this chapter underlines Judet's saying "experience means learning from failures." This sentence also applies to hip endoprosthetics, where it is precisely from all sorts of failures that a great deal have been learned in the last 46 years. As mentioned earlier, at least 10 to 15 years of results in a uniform group of patients is required to achieve an honest statement on the performance of a procedure. Again: "For every patient, we need an individual decision!" This process involves constant and precise subsequent monitoring of the largest possible patient cohort within the context of a prospective study with the same implant technique (cementless/cemented). Finally, however, we must realize and confess that "Lasting stabilization of endoprostheses still remains an unsolved problem!" For the preoperative evaluation and decision-making process, we have to "*stop and think!*", and strictly follow the algorithm plan for hip replacement, which includes a checklist of the following points:

- Individual patient situation
- Preoperative planning
- Implant design and material
- Technique of implantation (cemented or cementless)
- Postoperative treatment
- Postoperative follow-up and documentation
- Patient consultation in case of problems

Again, to repeat: Because there are still unsolved and open questions in the context of joint replacement, all possibilities for joint-preserving options must be considered and included in the decision-making process, especially in a patient group with a long life expectancy, under the aspect of a temporary and time-gaining procedure (osteotomy, posttraumatic joint reconstruction, etc.). Examples are given in Fig. 7.

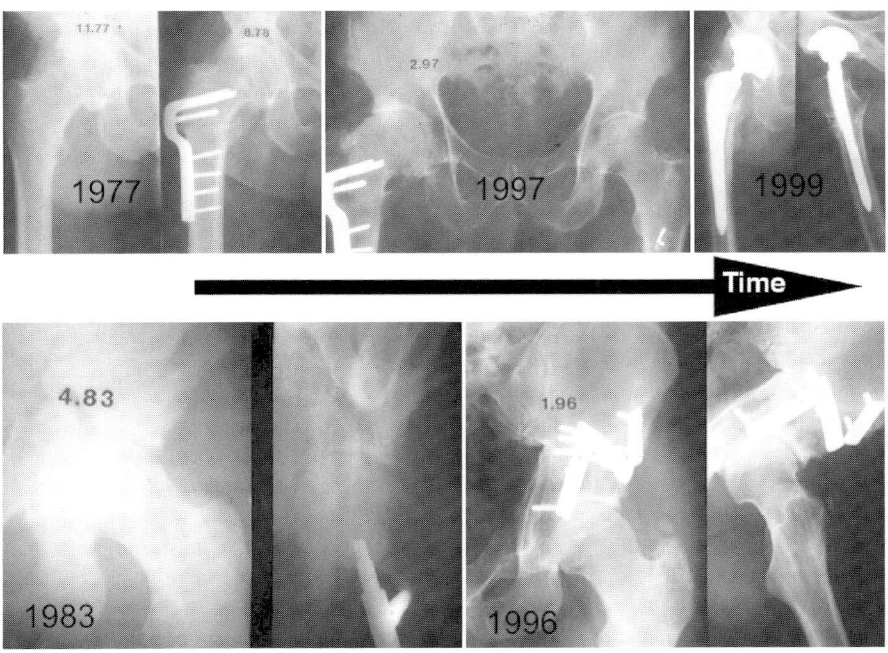

FIG. 7. The indication for joint replacement should be restricted to those situations where joint-conserving treatment cannot help. The aim is to gain time for the patient. Case example 1 (*upper*): osteotomy in 1978 followed by total hip arthroplasty (THA) 20 years later. Case example 2 (*lower*): posttraumatic joint reconstruction in 1983 and situation 13 years later

References

1. Adler CP (1997) Knochenkrankheiten. Diagnostik makroskopischer, histologischer und radiologischer Strukturveränderungen des Skeletts, 2nd Aufl. Springer, Heidelberg
2. Bombelli R (1976) Osteochondritis of the hip: pathogenesis and consequent therapy. Springer-Verlag, Berlin Heidelberg New York
3. Pauwels F (1976) Atlas zur Biomechanik der gesunden und kranken Hüfte. Springer-Verlag, Berlin, Heidelberg, New York
4. Asmuth T, Bachmann J, Eingartner C, et al (1998) Results with the cementless Bicontact stem: multicenter study of 553 cases. In: Weller S, Volkmann R (eds) The Bicontact hip system. Thieme, Stuttgart, pp 63–74
5. Eingartner C, Volkmann R, Winter E, et al (2001) Results of a cementless titanium alloy straight femoral shaft prosthesis after 10 years of follow-up. Int Orthop 25(2): 81–84
6. Song W S, Yoo JJ (2004) Experience with the Bicontact revision stems with distal interlocking. J Arthroplasty 1:27–34
7. Blömer W, Fink U (1997) Biomechanische Aspekte zementfreier Revisionsendoprothesen des Hüftgelenks: eine biomechanische Analyse der Verankerungssituation im Falle von Primär- und Revisionsschäften. In: Schneider E (ed) Unfallchirurg 261:20–41 (special issue)
8. Eingartner C, Heigele T, Dieter J, et al (2003) Long-term results with the Bicontact System: aspects to investigate and to learn from. Int Orthop 27(suppl 1):11–15
9. Flamme C, Wirth CJ, Stukenborg-Colsmann C (2001) Charakteristik der Lernkurve bei der Hüfttotalendoprothese am Beispiel der Bicontact-Prothese. Z Orthop 139:189–193
10. Weller S (2003) 15 years BICONTACT Hip Endoprosthesis System. The past–present–the future. What has been achieved? Int Orthop 27(suppl 1):2–6

Twenty Years of Experience with the Bernese Periacetabular Osteotomy for Residual Acetabular Dysplasia

Reinhold Ganz[1] and Michael Leunig[2]

Summary. Residual acetabular dysplasia is known as the most frequent cause of early osteoarthritis of the hip. The degeneration starts with overload of the rim, leading to a variety of pathologies. This change may cause the femoral head to migrate further out of the socket, resulting in a loss of congruity and generating even higher pressure point loading, which finally leads to rapid destruction of the joint. It is well accepted today that the surgical increase of the load transmission area can slow down this process of destruction and postpone total hip replacement (THR) substantially. Among the different techniques available, reorientation procedures allow for the most physiological correction of the joint mechanics. Our proposition is a reorientation procedure, which was first executed in 1984. Techniques and results have been published on several occasions. Under the name of the Bernese periacetabular osteotomy, the technique has gained popularity, especially in North America. Our 20 years' experience performing this osteotomy through a modified Smith-Peterson approach without dissection of the abductors has clearly shown that confound appreciation of joint mechanics is the key to a successful result. Addressing acetabular retroversion and an insufficient femoral head/neck offset has helped to avoid postosteotomy impingement and significantly improved our results. Today, in our armentarium of surgical techniques to preserve the natural hip joint, the periacetabular osteotomy leads to the most predictable results.

Key words. Hip, Young adults, Dysplasia, Joint preservation, Periacetabular osteotomy

Introduction

Residual acetabular dysplasia is known as the most frequent cause of osteoarthritis of the hip, leading to joint destruction in 25% to 50% of cases by the age of 50 years [1]. In the classic pathomorphology, the degeneration starts early with overload of

[1]Department of Orthopaedic Surgery, Balgrist University Hospital, Forchstr. 340, CH-8008 Zürich, Switzerland
[2]Department of Orthopaedics Surgery, Schulthess Clinic, Lengghalde 2, CH-8008 Zürich, Switzerland

the anterolateral joint, visible by the increased subchondral sclerosis on standard anteroposterior (AP) X-rays [2].

It is well accepted today [3] that surgical increase of the local transmission area and a more even load transmission can slow the process of destruction and postpone total hip replacement substantially. Among the different techniques available, reorientation procedures allow for the most physiological correction of the joint mechanics. We have performed most of the described techniques. Based on limitations with several of the former techniques (Table 1), we defined in 1983 the aspects to be achieved with a new technique as follows: optimal correction including version and medialization of the acetabular fragment; a single approach to avoid repositioning of the patient during the procedure; easy fixation of the fragment allowing for early ambulation; and unlimited access to the joint to treat intracapsular pathologies without the potential risk of avascular necrosis of the acetabular fragment. Finally, the new technique should allow major bilateral correction without narrowing of the birth canal because most of the patients are females of reproductive age.

The new technique, which was tested on 25 cadavers and performed for the first time in March 1984 (Fig. 1), consists of five osteotomy steps beginning with an

Table 1. Characteristics of reorientation procedures

Author(s)	Type of osteotomy	Incisions	Possible intracapsular surgery	Relationship to acetabulum	Perfusion of fragment
Salter [34]	Single	1	—	Distant	++(+)
Sutherland [35]	Double	2	—	Distant	++(+)
Hopf [36]	Double	1(2)	—	Distal intraarticular	(+)
LeCoeur [37]	Triple	3	—	Juxtaarticular	++(+)
Steel [38]	Triple	3	—	Distant	++(+)
Tonnis [39]	Triple	3	—	Juxtaarticular	+++
Carlioz [40]	Triple	3(2)	—	Juxtaarticular	+++
Nishio [41]	Spherical	1	(+)	Close	+(−)
Ninomiya [42]	Spherical	1	(+)	Close	+(−)
Eppright [43]	Spherical	1	(+)	Close	+
Wagner [44]	Spherical	1	(+)	Close	+
Kuznenko [45]	Translation	?	?	?	?
Ganz [5]	Periacetabular	1	++	Juxtaarticular	+++

incomplete cut of the ischium followed by the complete osteotomy of the pubis. For the supra- and retroacetabular chevron-type osteotomy, we abandoned early the detachment of the abductor muscles from the ilium for a complete intrapelvic execution. The last osteotomy is to combine the incomplete cuts (1 and 4 on Fig. 1) and is again performed from the inside of the pelvis [4] (Fig. 2). For the execution, a set of special retractors and osteotomes is needed. Intraoperative fluoroscopy is not necessary, although it is used by most surgeons. Although the execution of the osteotomies becomes easy with time, the precise special orientation of the fragment remains challenging (Fig. 3). For the fixation of the standard correction, 3 × 3.5 mm screws 50 to 80 mm in length are sufficient. Postoperative treatment consists of toe-touch weight-bearing for 6 to 8 weeks. Ninety percent of the hips are consolidated by then for full weight-bearing. Over the following years, several vascular studies have been performed to confirm the intact perfusion of the acetabular fragment [5–8].

The technique and our own results have been published on several occasions [5,9–11]. The procedure has gained popularity, especially in North America [12–19]. Our own experience is based on more than 1500 operated hips over the years.

Possibility of correction				Limiting factors for reorientation	Narrowing of birth canal	Osteotomy crossing growth plate
Anterior cover	Lateral cover	Mediali-sation	Version			
+(+)	+(+)	—	—	Symphysis	—	—
++	++	+	?	Sacrospinal + sacrotubular ligament	—	—
?	?	?	?	Sacrospinal + sacrotubular ligament	?	+
++(+)	++(+)	+	?	Sacrospinal + sacrotubular ligament	?	—
++(+)	++(+)	+	?	Sacrospinal + sacrotubular	?	—
++++	++++	++	?	Periosteum on quadrilateral surface	With large bilateral correction	—
+++	+++	++(+)	?	Sacrospinal ligament	With large bilateral correction	—
+++	+++	(+)	?	Capsule	—	—
+++	+++	(+)	?	Capsule	—	+
+++	+++	(+)	?	Capsule	—	+
+++	+++	++	?	Capsule	—	+
?	?	?	?	?	?	?
++++	++++	++++	+++	Capsule + attached abdominal muscle	—	+

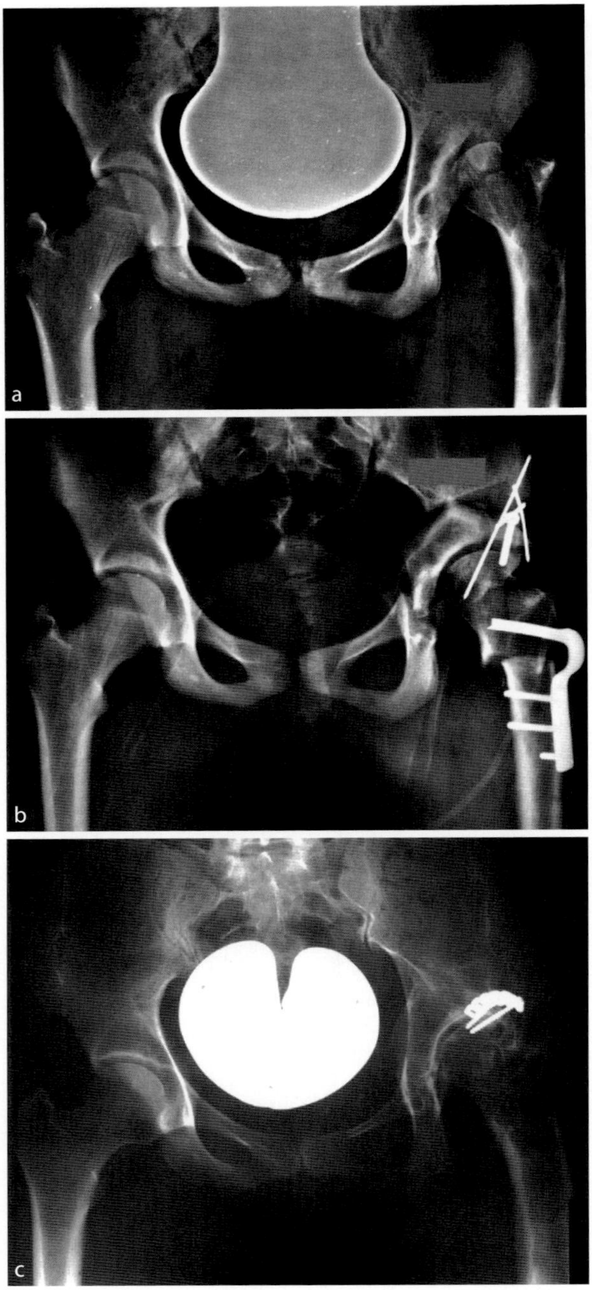

Fig. 1. First case of periacetabular osteotomy (PAO). **a** Anteroposterior (AP) pelvic radiograph of a 13-year-old girl with a proximal femoral focal deficiency (PFFD) of the left side and a functional hip. Previous surgery was a valgus intertrochanteric osteotomy and a femoral shaft lengthening procedure. The acetabulum is very shallow and retroverted; the proximal femur shows a hypoplastic epiphysis on a thick and short femoral neck. **b** Postoperative radiograph after PAO and intertrochanteric revalgization osteotomy. In 1984, the retroversion of the acetabulum was not recognized as part of the pathomorphology and has therefore not been corrected. Eight weeks later, a posterior subluxation was recognized and treated with a posterosuperior shelfplasty using a plate for fixation. **c** The left hip, 21 years after periacetabular surgery, with a reasonably good clinical result (no pain, relative abductor weakness) and a congruent and rather large joint space

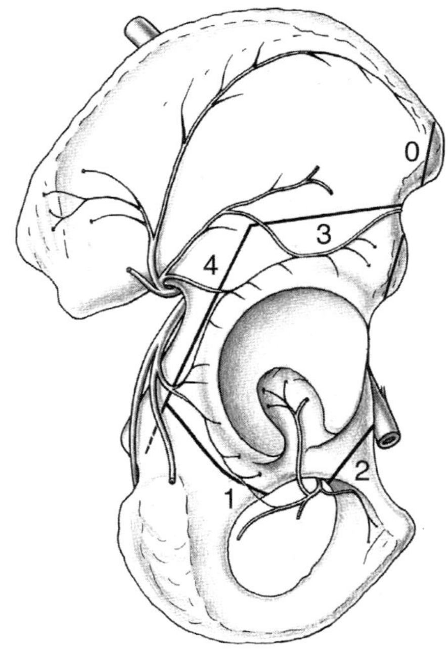

FIG. 2. Schematic drawing of the various osteotomy steps for the periacetabular osteotomy. Osteotomy of the anterosuperior iliac spine (0) is required for a sufficient approach. The first osteotomy is the "blind" partial ischial cut (1), followed by the pubic osteotomy (2); this is followed by the supraacetabular (3) and retroacetabular osteotomy (4), before the controlled fracture is induced

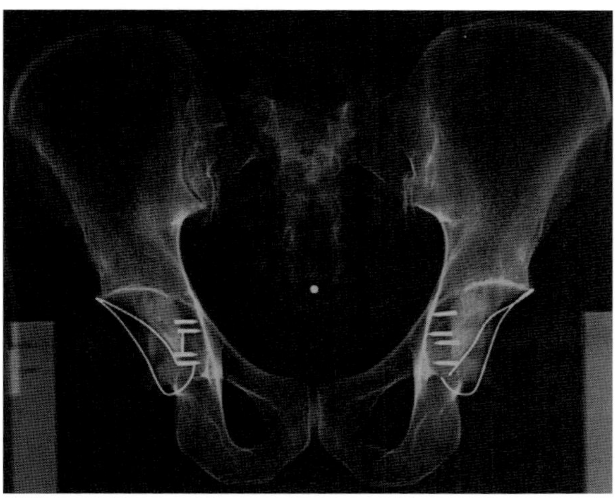

FIG. 3. Orthograde intraoperative AP pelvic radiograph. Orthograde means that the tip of the os coccyx points toward the middle of the symphysis and the distance between the tip of the sacrococcygeal joint and the symphysis ranges between 2 (men) and 4 (women) cm [33]. With such an intraoperative tray, several parameters are controlled: the distance between femoral head and ilioischial line, the inclination of the supraacetabular sclerosis over the femoral head (acetabular index), the anterior and posterior border of the acetabulum, and finally the Menard–Shenton line, which in an ideal condition should be normalized after the periacetabular osteotomy

One of the earlier experiences was the phenomenology of acetabular rim pathologies before the cartilage itself becomes affected. Although it was known that the labrum can become avulsed in hip dysplasia [20], the incidence of such lesions was seen to be much more frequent with radial magnetic resonance (MR) arthrography [21] and potentially accompanied by other rim pathologies as ganglion formation in the labrum, the surrounding tissue, and the periacetabular bone. Rim fractures could be identified as part of a labrum rupture and as such are mostly seen in rather congruent hips [22]. Using MRI, we also could see that some labral ruptures showed the disconnection deep in the acetabular cartilage, indicating a clearly reduced prognosis for a reorientation procedure when compared with a case having avulsion of the labrum alone (Fig. 4).

Our 10 years of results with periacetabular osteotomy (PAO) finally show that cases without labral lesions do better in the long run, indicating that the labrum lesion is a precursor or even the first step of osteoarthritis of a dysplastic hip because it takes part in the load transmission and, when it fails, the head migrates further out of the socket with substantial deterioration of the load transmission and the beginning of rapid joint destruction [22]. The observation that the labrum in acetabular dysplasia is hypertrophic has added a further argument in borderline morphologies where it may be unclear whether the hip suffers from dysplasia or impingement from another pathomorphology such as retroversion [21]. Whether rim pathologies should be treated or left alone while performing a periacetabular osteotomy is the subject of ongoing dis-

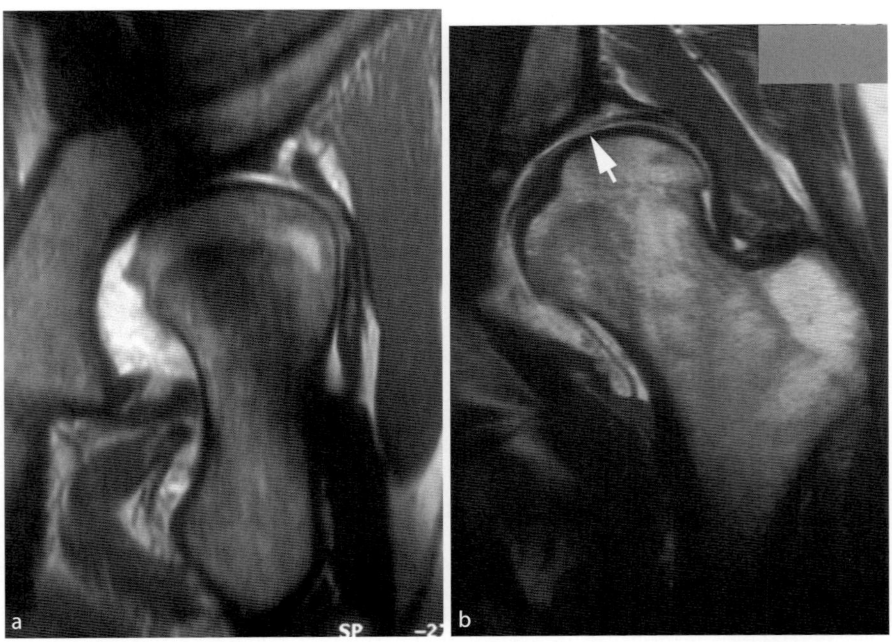

FIG. 4. **a** Magnetic resonance imaging (MRI) shows an avulsion of the labrum from the osseous rim with a substantial gap between the two structures. The femoral head is migrating out of the joint after the labrum as last resistance has failed. **b** Frontal MR image shows that the avulsed labrum comes with a substantial flap of acetabular cartilage (*arrow* indicates level of separation)

cussion. It is a general observation that hips with a small labral avulsion normally become asymptomatic even without an attempt to resect or refix this structure. It may be possible with smaller rim fragments that become unloaded in a similar way after osteotomy and may eventually consolidate. Intraosseous ganglia also can disappear spontaneously after a redirection of the acetabulum. However, as soon as these lesions surpass a certain size, an attempt to treat the lesion is justified or even recommended. This conclusion is especially true for large and floating bucket-handle lesions of a degenerated labrum (Fig. 5) and for large supraacetabular ganglion formation.

We further learned over the years that acetabular dysplasia is not uniform anterolateral insufficiency of coverage of the femoral head but shows a multitude of pure and combined anterior, lateral, and posterior dysplasias. Li and Ganz [23] showed that one of six dysplastic hips were retroverted (Fig. 6). Mast et al. [24] found, with one of three, an even higher number. Although the classic anterolateral dysplasia remains the most common, pure lateral deficiency of coverage is rare and the pure posterior deficiency is an exception, and then is seen in functional hips of proximal

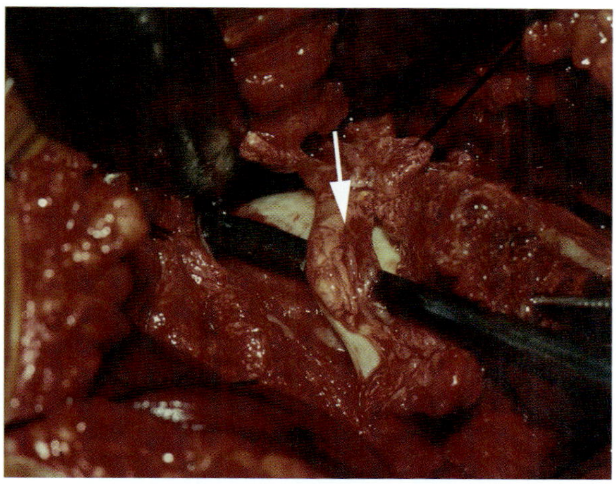

FIG. 5. Intraoperative view of a bucket-handle avulsion of a degenerated labrum (*arrow*)

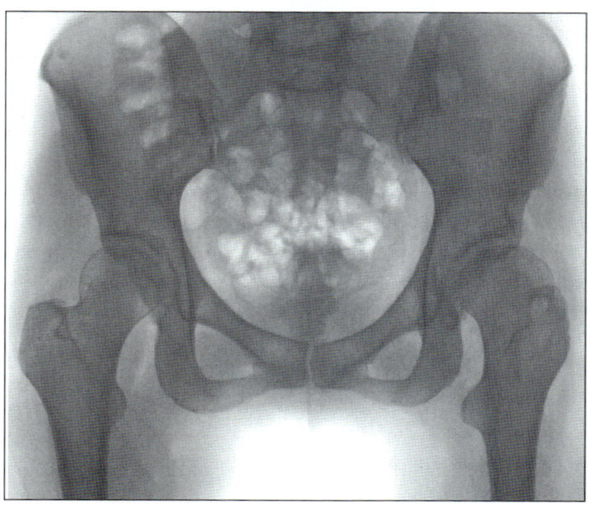

FIG. 6. AP-pelvic radiograph of the dysplastic acetabulum of an Asian woman shows retroversion of the superior one-third of the acetabulum

femoral focal deficiency (PFFD) [25] or posttraumatic dysplasia [26]. One important group of a posterior insufficiency of coverage or anterior overcoverage consists of hips with Salter or triple osteotomies in childhood [27] in which a correct version of the acetabulum was difficult to establish in the presence of an unossified acetabular rim. If a retroverted dysplastic acetabulum is redirected in the same way as an anterolaterally dysplastic acetabulum, the problem of this hip may be increased and further treatment even more difficult. Surgery then becomes necessary (Fig. 7).

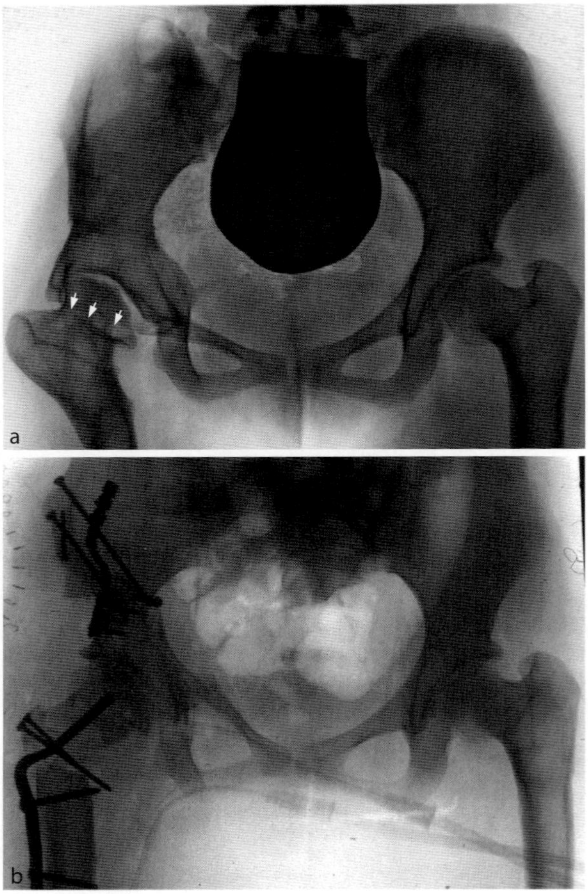

FIG. 7. **a** AP-pelvic radiograph of a 14-year-old girl after three attempts of acetabular redirection and two attempts of proximal femoral osteotomy. The acetabulum is extremely retroverted (*arrows* show the anterior border; the posterior border is hidden behind the inner acetabular wall). On the femoral side the head is deformed, the neck is short, and there is subtrochanteric abduction with medialization of the femoral shaft. The hip showed impingement with 40° flexion, creating severe problems with sitting on a chair. **b** Postoperative radiograph of the pelvis after 40° internal rotation of the acetabulum. To bridge the displacement necessary for such a correction, the plate had to be prebended stepwise. Fixation was then only possible on the inside of the stable ilium and on the outside of the acetabular fragment. On the femoral side, femoral neck lengthening, trochanteric advancement, and subtrochanteric alignment were necessary to regain an anatomical morphology

Our first 75 cases with a minimum of 10 years' follow-up (10–13.8 years) showed good to excellent results in 88% when only hips without signs of osteoarthritis were considered. Taking all hips, the success rate dropped to 73% with good or excellent results [28]. The higher early failure rate was in the group with grade III osteoarthritis [29], an observation that caused us to exclude most of such hips from the indication for a reorientation. A standard AP X-ray, however, may be misleading when the joint space narrowing is rather the result of an anterolateral subluxation and does not represent cartilage loss. Such hips can be an acceptable indication and may lead to a good result for years, helping to postpone an artificial joint for a prosthesis lifetime (Fig. 8). Very early failures were observed also in reoriented hips with a secondary acetabulum.

With our 10-year follow-up study we had unexpectedly found that 30% of the patients had developed impingement symptoms over the years [28]. These symptoms were in most of the patients not severe enough, very severe, or only detectable with the impingement test [30], but in this small group hips were included with perfect corrections of the acetabulum. Further studies showed that the anterolateral head-neck junction in dysplastic hips frequently had no waist, producing a decreased clearance for flexion/internal rotation after correction of the acetabular roof [31].

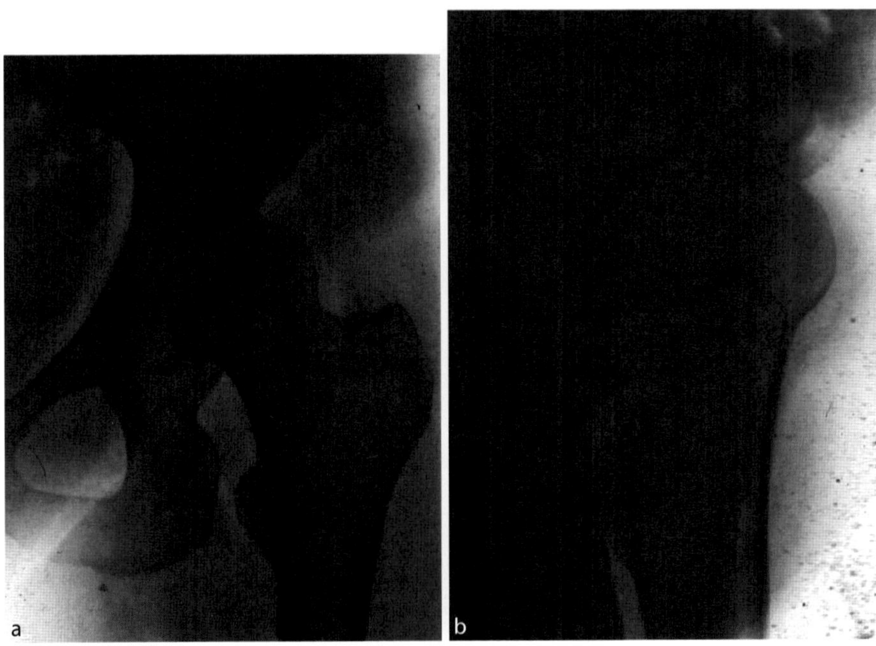

FIG. 8. **a** AP radiograph of the left hip of a 37-year-old woman with subchondral sclerosis and ganglion (cyst) formation and marked joint space narrowing with advanced osteoarthritis. **b** Lateral radiograph of the same day (false profile view) shows fewer secondary signs of arthrosis but anterosuperior migration of the head. **c** Postoperative radiograph of the pelvis immediately after periacetabular osteotomy shows a normal joint space. **d** Ten years later: result with good clinical function. **e** Fifteen years after PAO. The patient has now problems with the left hip and is ready for total hip replacement (THR)

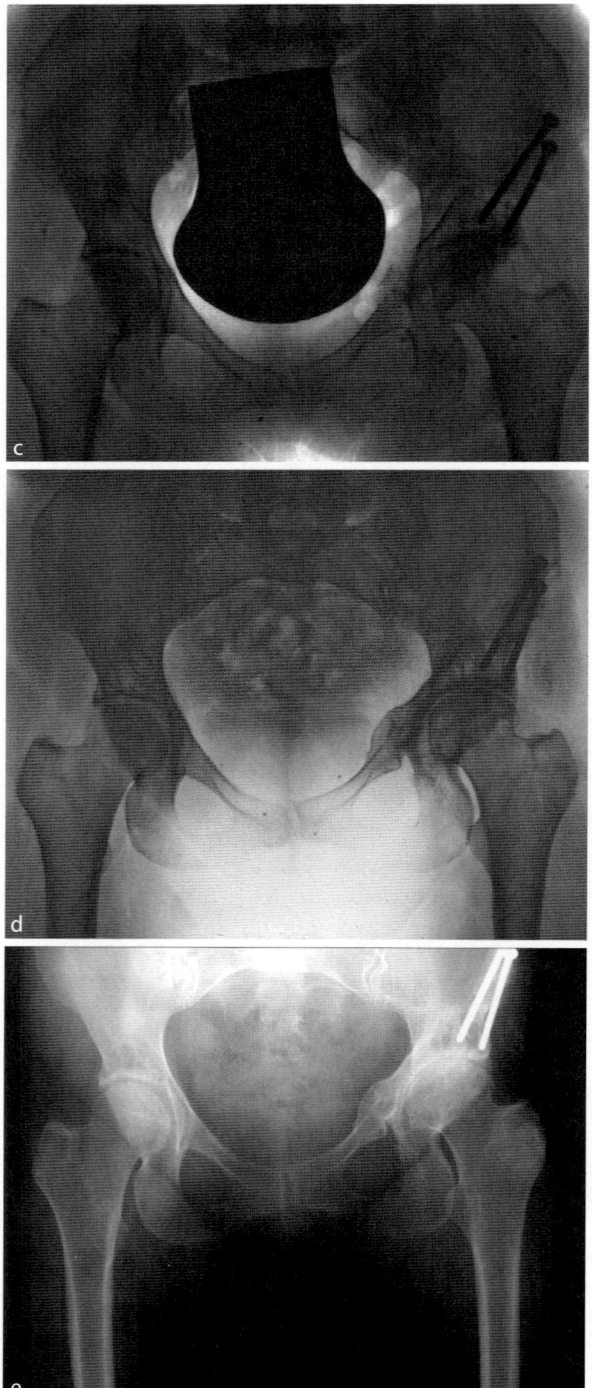

FIG. 8. *Continued*

As an intraoperative consequence we check routinely this motion and perform an anterolateral osteochondroplasty of the head–neck junction in seven of ten hips to improve the offset (Fig. 9). The necessary capsulotomy allows further treatment of any additional intraarticular pathology, which surprisingly often escapes preoperative evaluation. So far, the clinical follow-up of our more recent cases seems to support this additional treatment step.

Retroversion of the acetabulum is not only a phenomenon in residual acetabular dysplasia but is common in nondysplastic hips as well; some of these idiopathic retroversions have a substantial degree. Such hips become symptomatic in early adulthood as a result of impingement of the anterior overcoverage against the head–neck

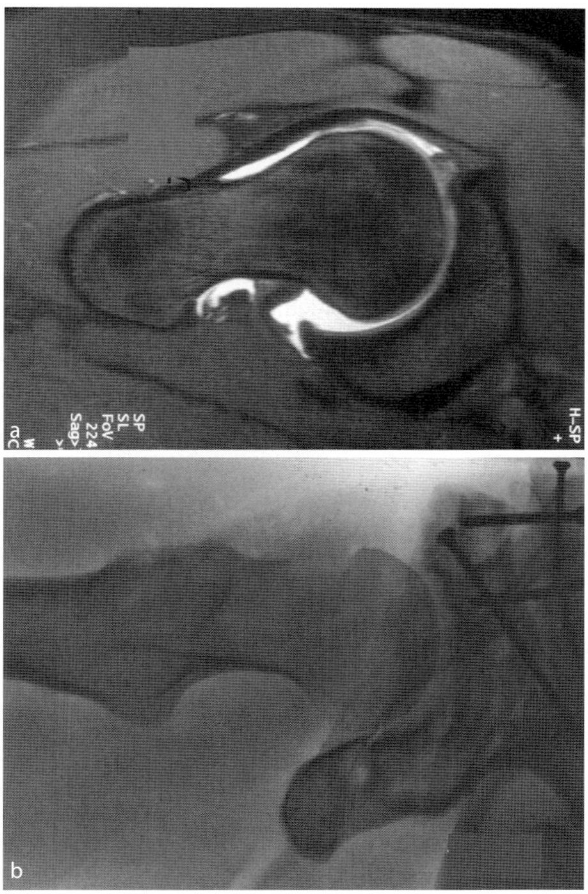

FIG. 9. **a** Coronal MRI section of the symptomatic dysplastic right hip of a 30-year-old woman. The anterior head–neck contour rim is out of sphericity with the risk of impingement after redirection of the acetabulum. **b** The periacetabular osteotomy was executed via an anterior capsulotomy, and the anterior head–neck contour was shaped to avoid impingement and to improve the limited internal rotation in flexion

junction in flexion/internal rotation. Such acetabular morphologies can be treated with a periacetabular osteotomy, reestablishing an anteversion by internal rotation of the acetabular fragment around a vertical axis. The limitation of such a correction is a posterior acetabular rim at or lateral of the center of the femoral head. With such a morphology, rotation of the acetabular fragment would have the risk of posterior impingement [32]. The second limitation is the quality of the acetabular cartilage in the area of anterior overcoverage. Preoperative MRI must show a normal cartilage; otherwise, it is better to trim the anterior overcoverage and refix the labrum. However, one has to take into consideration that some of these hips do not have a reasonable size of acetabular roof to allow complete trimming of the anterior coverage without the risk of producing a dysplasia-like lateral coverage. In general, we prefer to perform the reorientation of the retroverted nondysplastic acetabulum in patients under the age of 20 and do the trimming with refixation of the labrum in older patients with severe retroversion.

Some of the nondysplastic but severely retroverted acetabuli, but also some of the dysplastic acetabuli, show in addition a substantial deformity of the proximal femur, making a surgical step at this level, such as a capsulotomy, necessary.

Because surgery for the acetabular correction and substantial surgery of the proximal femur are hardly possible via a Smith-Peterson approach, we reevaluated the possibility of a posterolateral approach. It is well known that a rotational acetabular osteotomy (RAO) can successfully be performed via a posterolateral approach when the hip joint capsule is left intact. We first studied again the periacetabular blood supply [8]. The fact that the inferior branch of the superior gluteal artery, which runs in a rather mobile periosteal tissue along the distal border of the gluteus minimus and provides the perfusion of the supraacetabular bone together with arcades of the anastomosing supraacetabular artery and branches of the iliolumbar artery [7], can be mobilized and lifted from the bone to be osteotomised offers the possibility of a lateral acetabular reorientation together with a substantial capsulotomy with preserved perfusion of the acetabular fragment [8].

This osteotomy is in its supraacetabular course slightly more proximal to preserve the vessel arcade (Fig. 10). We have successfully performed seven cases so far, all with conditions necessitating a lateral approach (Fig. 11). We will certainly increase the

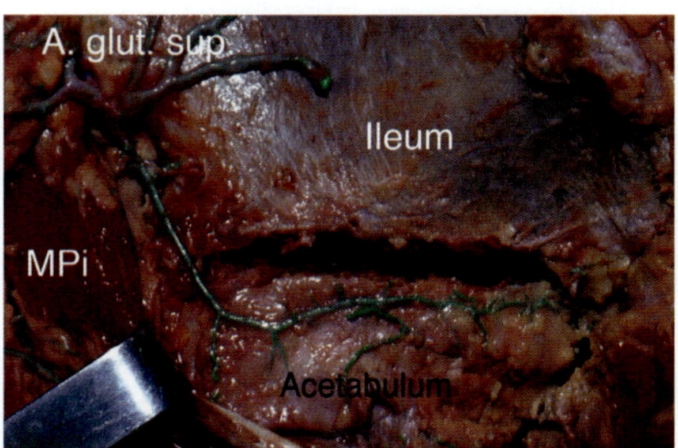

FIG. 10. Anatomical dissection of the lateral iliac wing with the superior gluteal artery (*A. glut. sup*) providing a vascular branch to the superior acetabular rim. The ramus supraacetabularis follows the course of the piriformis muscle (*MPi*) and crosses the line of the osteotomy

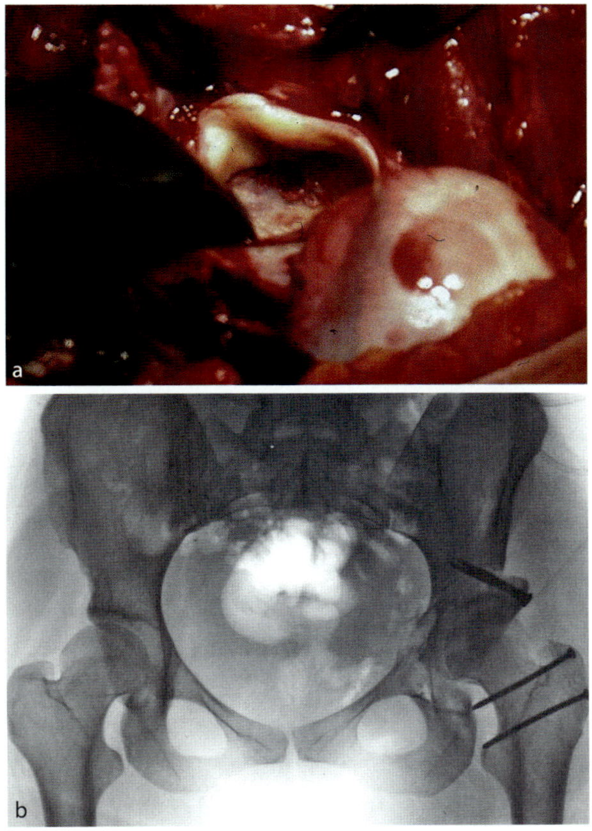

FIG. 11. **a** Intraoperative photograph of a woman who had significant intraarticular pathology and simultaneously an acetabular dysplasia. **b** The periacetabular osteotomy was performed through a transtrochanteric lateral approach

indication with increasing experience; the execution via a Smith-Peterson approach, however, will remain the standard.

In conclusion, in our armamentarium of surgical techniques to preserve the natural hip joint, periacetabular osteotomy is the operation that leads to the most predictable results. The technical execution is demanding, and even more so is orientation of the acetabulum, which must be individualized. The correction must be exact in all parameters, including a normal version of the acetabulum. In addition, one has to consider that the proximal femur may be dysplastic as well, which has to be corrected if possible at the same time.

References

1. Cooperman DR, Wallensten R, Stulberg SD (1983) Acetabular dysplasia in the adult. Clin Orthop 175:79–85
2. Kummer B (1991) The clinical relevance of biomechanical analysis of the hip area. Z Orthop Ihre Grenzgeb 129:285–294
3. Millis MB, Murphy SB, Poss R (1955) Osteotomies about the hip for prevention treatment of osteoarthrosis. J Bone Joint Surg [Am] 77:626–677

4. Leunig M, Siebenrock KA, Ganz R (2001) Rationale of periacetabular osteotomy and background work. Instr Course Lect 50:229–238
5. Ganz R, Klaue K, Vinh TS, et al (1988) A new periacetabular osteotomy for the treatment of hip dysplasias. Technique and preliminary results. Clin Orthop 232:26–36
6. Hempfing A, Leunig M, Notzli HP, et al (2003) Acetabular blood flow during Bernese periacetabular osteotomy: an intraoperative study using laser Doppler flowmetry. J Orthop Res 21:1145–1150
7. Beck M, Leunig M, Ellis T, et al (2003) The acetabular blood supply: implications for periacetabular osteotomies. Surg Radiol Anat 25:361–367
8. Leunig M, Rothenfluh D, Beck M, et al (2004) Surgical dislocation and periacetabular osteotomy through a posterolateral approach: a cadaveric feasibility study and initial clinical experience. Oper Tech Orthop 14:49–57
9. Siebenrock KA, Scholl E, Lottenbach M, et al (1999) Bernese periacetabular osteotomy. Clin Orthop 363:9–20
10. Siebenrock KA, Leunig M, Ganz R (2001) Periacetabular osteotomy: the Bernese experience. Instr Course Lect 50:239–245
11. Leunig M, Ganz R (1988) The Bernese method of periacetabular osteotomy. Orthopade 27:743–750
12. Clohisy JC, Barrett SE, Gordon JE, et al (2005) Periacetabular osteotomy for the treatment of severe acetabular dysplasia. J Bone Joint Surg [Am] 87:254–259
13. Katz DA, Kim YJ, Millis MB (2005) Periacetabular osteotomy in patients with Down's syndrome. J Bone Joint Surg [Br] 87:544–547
14. Matta JM, Stover MD, Siebenrock K (1999) Periacetabular osteotomy through the Smith-Petersen approach. Clin Orthop Relat Res 363:21–32
15. Mayo KA, Trumble SJ, Mast JW (1999) Results of periacetabular osteotomy in patients with previous surgery for hip dysplasia. Clin Orthop Relat Res 363:73–80
16. Murphy S, Deshmukh R (2002) Periacetabular osteotomy: preoperative radiographic predictors of outcome. Clin Orthop Relat Res 405:168–174
17. Sucato DJ (2006) Treatment of late dysplasia with Ganz osteotomy. Orthop Clin N Am 37:161–171
18. Trousdale RT, Cabanela ME (2003) Lessons learned after more than 250 periacetabular osteotomies. Acta Orthop Scand 74:119–126
19. Valenzuela RG, Cabanela ME, Trousdale RT (2003) Sexual activity, pregnancy, and childbirth after periacetabular osteotomy. Clin Orthop Relat Res 418:146–152
20. Dorrell JH, Catterall A (1986) The torn acetabular labrum. J Bone Joint Surg [Br] 68:400–403
21. Leunig M, Podeszwa D, Beck M, et al (2004) Magnetic resonance arthrography of labral disorders in hips with dysplasia and impingement. Clin Orthop 418:74–80
22. Klaue K, Durnin CW, Ganz R (1991) The acetabular rim syndrome. a clinical presentation of dysplasia of the hip. J Bone Joint Surg 73B:423–429
23. Li PL, Ganz R (2003) Morphologic features of congenital acetabular dysplasia: one in six is retroverted. Clin Orthop Relat Res 416:245–253
24. Mast JW, Brunner RL, Zebrack J (2004) Recognizing acetabular version in the radiographic presentation of hip dysplasia. Clin Orthop Relat Res 418:48–53
25. Dora C, Buhler M, Stover MD, et al (2004) Morphologic characteristics of acetabular dysplasia in proximal femoral focal deficiency. J Pediatr Orthop B 13:81–87
26. Dora C, Zurbach J, Hersche O, et al (2000) Pathomorphologic characteristics of posttraumatic acetabular dysplasia. J Orthop Trauma 14:483–489
27. Dora C, Mascard E, Mladenov K, et al (2002) Retroversion of the acetabular dome after Salter and triple pelvic osteotomy for congenital dislocation of the hip. J Pediatr Orthop B 11:34–40
28. Siebenrock KA, Schöll E, Lottenbach M, et al (1999) Periacetabular osteotomy. a minimal follow-up of 10 years. Clin Orthop 363:9–20

29. Trousdale RT, Ekkernkamp A, Ganz R, et al (1995) Periacetabular and intertrochanteric osteotomy for the treatment of osteoarthrosis in dysplastic hips. J Bone Joint Surg [Am] 77:73–85
30. MacDonald SJ, Garbuz D, Ganz R (1997) Clinical evaluation of the symptomatic young adult hip. Semin Arthroplasty 8:3–9
31. Myers SR, Eijer H, Ganz R (1999) Anterior femoroacetabular impingement after periacetabular osteotomy. Clin Orthop 363:93–99
32. Siebenrock KA, Schoeniger R, Ganz R (2003) Anterior femoro-acetabular impingement due to acetabular retroversion. Treatment with periacetabular osteotomy. J Bone Joint Surg [Am] 85:278–286
33. Siebenrock KA, Kalbermatten DF, Ganz R (2003) Effect of pelvic tilt on acetabular retroversion: a study of pelves from cadavers. Clin Orthop 407:241–248
34. Salter RB (1961) Innominate osteotomy in the treatment of congenital dislocation and subluxation of the hip. J Bone Joint Surg [Br] 43:518–539
35. Sutherland DH, Greenfield R (1977) Double innominate osteotomy. J Bone Joint Surg [Am] 59:1082–1091
36. Hopf A (1966) Hüftpfannenverlagerung durch doppelte Beckenosteotomie zur Hüftgelenksdysplasie und Subluxation bei Jugendlichen und Erwachsenen. Z Orthop 101:559–568
37. LeCoeur P (1965) Corrections des défaults d'orientation de l'articulation coxo-femorale par ostéotomie de l'isthme iliaque. Rev Chir Orthop 51:211–212
38. Steel HH (1973) Triple osteotomy of the innominate bone. J Bone Joint Surg [Am] 55:343–350
39. Tonnis D, Behrens K, Tscharani F (1981) A modified technique of the triple pelvic osteotomy: early results. J Pediatr Orthop 1:241–249
40. Carlioz H, Khouri N, Hulin P (1982) Ostéotomie triple juxtacotyloidienne. Rev Chir Orthop Repar Appar Motil 68:497–501
41. Nishio A (1956) Transposition osteotomy of the acetabulum in the treatment of congenital dislocation of the hip. J Jpn Orthop Assoc 30:483
42. Ninomiya S, Tagawa H (1984) Rotational acetabular osteotomy for the dysplastic hip. J Bone Joint Surg [Am] 66:430–436
43. Eppright RH (1975) Dial osteotomy of the acetabulum in the treatment of dysplasia of the hip. J Bone Joint Surg [Am] 57:1171
44. Wagner H (1976) Osteotomies for congenital hip dislocation. In: Proceedings of the 4th open scientific meeting of the Hip Society. Mosby, St. Louis
45. Kuznenko WW, Adiev TM (1977) The translocation of the hip joint in the treatment of secondary arthritis in hip dysplasia in the adult. Orthop Traumatol 6:70

Joint Reconstruction Without Replacement Arthroplasty for Advanced- and Terminal-Stage Osteoarthritis of the Hip in Middle-Aged Patients

Moritoshi Itoman, Naonobu Takahira, Katsufumi Uchiyama, and Sumitaka Takasaki

Summary. In hip osteoarthritis (OA), osteophytes are formed both on the acetabular edge and the margin of the femoral head as a result of biological response, which reflects the natural biological regenerative capacity to heal. We need to try to use these osteophytes more effectively in the treatment of advanced- and terminal-stage osteoarthritis, particularly in middle-aged patients. By improving the biomechanical environment of the hip joint, we can promote biological repair and regeneration of the devastated joint surface. Thus, valgus osteotomy or valgus-flexion osteotomy is a joint regenerative surgery that enhances the regeneration of repair tissues in the articular surface, even for terminal-stage OA. For younger patients, rather than going to total hip replacement immediately, we should first try to resort to means to enhance and capitalize on the capacity of the biological system to heal, repair, and regenerate.

Key words. Osteotomy, Osteoarthritis, Hip joint, Regeneration, Remodeling

Introduction

The recovery of joint function has always proven a great challenge. In the 1860s, improvement of function was attempted with the use of an interposing membrane as a means of preserving the joint. For instance, the JK-membrane used by Dr. Jinnaka was very well known. After Smith-Peterson introduced glass-interposing arthroplasty, he went on to attempt cup arthroplasty, using vitallium. Later, this led to the development of total hip replacement (THR), which culminated in Charnely's introduction of low-friction arthroplasty. On the other hand, McMurray's displacement osteoplasty marked the inception of osteotomy, followed by Pauwels' valgus osteotomy (VO). His method accomplished excellent results with a very good theoretical background [1].

The question of THR versus osteotomy has been a long-debated topic, for the treatment of osteoarthritis (OA) of the hip, in particular. Dr. Terayama stated in 1982 that THR is an excellent surgery, with assured pain relief, good range of motion and

Department of Orthopedic Surgery, Kitasato University School of Medicine, 1-15-1 Kitasato, Sagamihara, Kanagawa 228-8555, Japan

support, and improvement in gait. He dismissed osteotomy as a surgery of the past. Dr. Terayama thus gave up performing osteotomy and introduced an elective strategy for young OA patients whereby the patients could only wait until they were old enough to have THR [2]. On the other hand, Dr. Ueno has performed Pauwels' VO in Japan for a long time with excellent results. He said that osteotomy could have outstanding results if appropriate indication, design, and surgical techniques were employed. He reported that osteotomy was a wonderful method for gaining good pain relief and improvement in gait ability while preserving the joint, a very good demonstration of the artistry of nature. He also said that it did have its disadvantage, which was the need for long and careful aftertreatment [3].

It is certainly true that THR can have extremely good results in the short term, no matter by whom or where the surgery is performed. At a later stage, however, it could have very serious complications, such as aseptic loosening, osteolysis, and infection, and therefore we have doubts about the indication for THR in younger patients. The theoretical background of osteotomy for advanced- and terminal-stage OA was established by Pauwels and was introduced in Japan by Dr. Ueno. Later, Bombelli, who was studying under Pauwels, developed three-dimensional (3-D) valgus-extension osteotomy (VEO), with very good biomechanical theory [4]. When his book was made available in English in 1976, the method was introduced all over the world. However, we had some doubts about the significance of extension in his osteotomy and started to perform valgus-flexion osteotomy (VFO) in 1979 [5].

OA of the hip joint in 1125 patients was treated surgically at Kitasato University Hospital from its foundation up to 2003. Primary THR accounts for 51%, whereas about 40% of cases undergo osteotomy. The breakdown of osteotomy showed that the use of varus osteotomy, or varus combined with some procedures on the acetabular side, or pelvic osteotomy alone, for pre- and initial-stage OA accounts for 48%, and valgus osteotomy alone or valgus plus some procedures, 52%, for advanced- and terminal-stage OA. Thus, more than half of the osteotomy cases were in the advanced or terminal stage.

I present here the artistry of human biology that allows excellent reconstruction of the hip joint, without the use of hip prostheses.

Features of Secondary OA of the Hip

Reviewing the characteristic features of secondary OA caused by developmental dislocation of the hip (DDH) or acetabular dysplasia, we can observe the coexistence of two phases, one being wear and the destructive process on the weight-bearing area, and the other the proliferative and reparative process on the peripheral, non-weight-bearing area. The large capital drop that forms on the posteromedial side seems to come from the biological response of the repair process. Even on the weight-bearing area, abundant buds of reparative tissue, so-called chondroid plugs, that seem to have come from the bone marrow can be observed. Thus, the secondary OA can be characterized by the coexistence of two phases, that is, the destructive phase with the devastation of the biomechanical environment, and the proliferative and reparative phase that occurs as a result of the biological repair process (Figs. 1, 2).

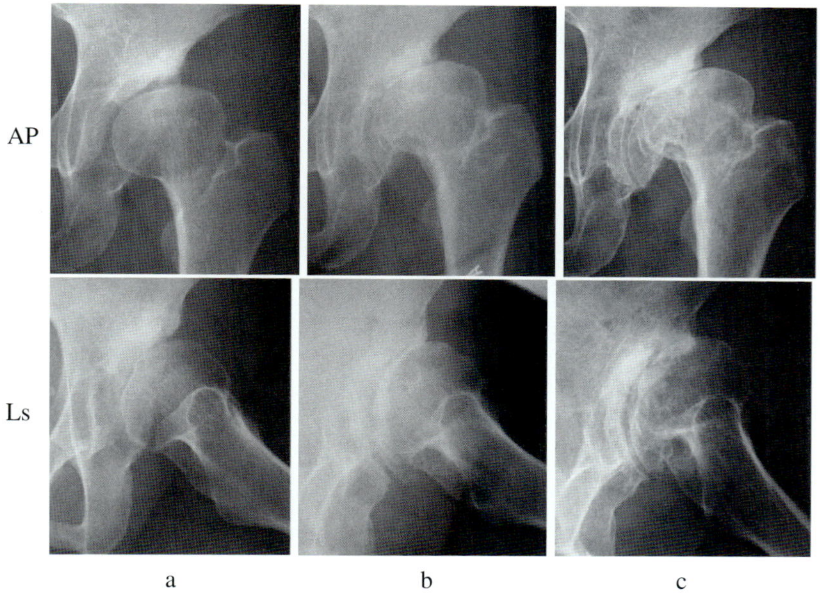

FIG. 1. Natural course of osteoarthritis (OA) of the hip caused by developmental dislocation of the hip (DDH). Radiologic change of the hip of a 45-year-old woman at the first visit. **a** April 1991 (45 years old); **b** April 2001 (55 years old); **c** April 2005 (59 years old). *AP*, anteroposterior; *Ls*, left side

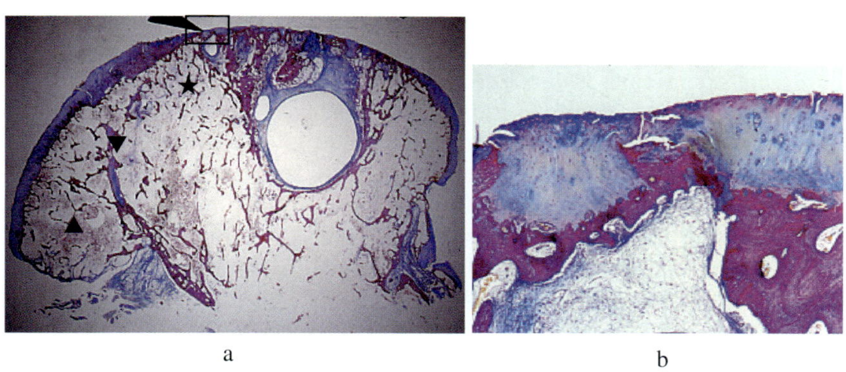

FIG. 2. Histological findings of femoral head harvested from terminal-stage OA. **a** Cross section of the femoral head. ▲, capital drop; ▼, original line of the head. **b** Magnification of chondroid plugs at weight-bearing area (*boxed area* in **a**)

Bombelli used the big capital drop and double floor, formed on the posteromedial side. With applying strong valgus beyond so-called congruency, he destroyed the mechanical environment, and then reduced the anterior quarter of the femoral head, which protruded laterally as a result of the excessive valgus orientation, back into the acetabulum by extension in his VEO [4]. However, if we look closely, we can see that there are cases where the size of the medial capital drop tends to be relatively small.

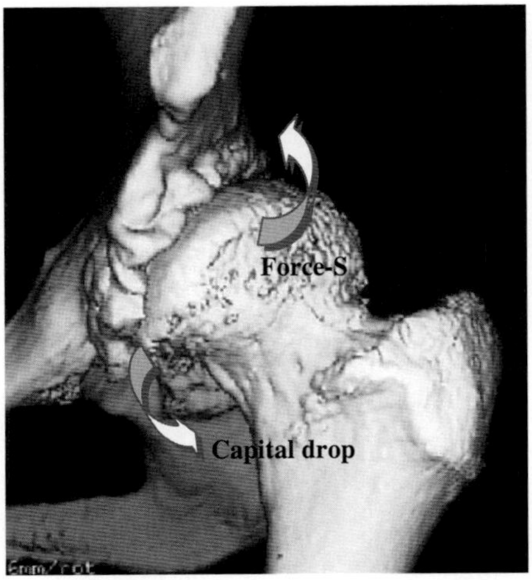

FIG. 3. Three-dimensional (3-D) computed tomography (CT) findings. The three-dimensional relationship of the capital drop and force S presents an S-curve

There is a corresponding double floor. Three-dimensional computed tomography (3-D CT) shows that the capital drop, in fact, is bigger on the posterior side in most cases. The capital drop is formed in the posteromedial-inferior direction, which is in agreement with the direction of slippage of the femoral head in slipped capital femoral epiphysis. Conversely, the force-S that pushes out the femoral head laterally has a three-dimensional S-curve, going into the anterolateral-superior direction (Fig. 3) [5,6]. The old weight-bearing surface gradually displaces into an anterolateral-superior direction, thereby losing its original function; this has led us to change our procedure from extension to flexion osteotomy [5,6].

The weight-bearing surface is subjected to gradual wear and loss, and the old weight-bearing surface of the femoral head deviates into the anterolateral-superior direction, losing its function. Despite all that, there seems to be some budding of reparative tissues in this environment (see Fig. 2). In the marginal non-weight-bearing area, bony and cartilaginous tissues are regenerated and proliferated in the posteromedial-inferior direction. Assuming that the capital drop and the double floor are serving to form a new joint, then surgery will be needed to induce the natural healing capacity and to promote the regeneration of reparative tissues. This realization led us to combine flexion with valgus osteotomy [5,7,8].

Indication and Preoperative Planning of Valgus-Flexion Osteotomy

The indication of VFO includes the following:

1. Patients under the age of 60.
2. Extension/flexion range of motion (ROM) should be at least 40° or more, preferably 60° or more.
3. Adduction of 15° or more.

4. Lateral-type OA in the advanced and terminal stage.
5. Femoral head having a mushroom shape.
6. Hinge adduction must be observed in dynamic radiogram; with adduction, the lateral joint space must open wide in the shape of a wedge (Fig. 4) [7,9].
7. Acetabular head index (AHI) must be 60% or greater. If the AHI is less than 60% with inadequate formation of the roof osteophyte, it should be combined with Chiari's pelvic osteotomy for valgus [10–13].

Preoperative planning using tracing paper is extremely important. Most OA patients have adduction contracture, which must be first corrected. The osteotomy line is drawn at the lesser trochanter level; the tracing for the femur will then be brought into adduction position. With adequate adduction, the lateral joint space is opened. The head will be fixed before the osteotomy. If the distal fragment is adapted to the proximal osteotomy line, there is a risk of causing genu valgum, and therefore the distal fragment must be moved laterally [5,9,12]. The increased length that results from the transposition will be resected to shorten that to the correct length.

The patient's preoperative radiologic image, the final drawing, and images immediately after VFO and at 10-year follow-up are shown in Fig. 5. If the osteotomy is performed exactly as planned, there is a substantial widening of the lateral joint space. Ten years later, very good remodeling of the trabeculae was seen. The patient had an operation on the contralateral side 2 years after the index surgery and had enjoyed very good results at 8 years.

I am always asked the question of why flexion rather than extension, or how I determine the flexion angle. We always look at motion with a fluoroscope to decide whether to use flexion or extension [9]. As shown on Fig. 6, when the patient is in valgus-flexion position, there is substantial widening of the lateral joint space. In Bombelli's (valgus-extension) position, on the other hand, widening of the joint space is not enough when comparing it with that in valgus-flexion. For this patient, we decided to perform VFO with 35° of valgus and 20° of flexion.

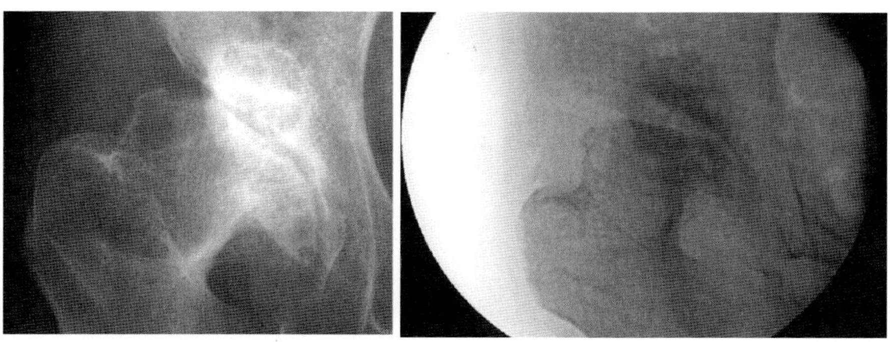

a b

FIG. 4. Hinge adduction must be observed with passive adduction under anesthesia before surgery; the lateral joint space must open wide in the shape of a wedge. **a** Preoperative anteroposterior (AP) radiogram in neutral position. **b** Radiogram in position of passive adduction under anesthesia

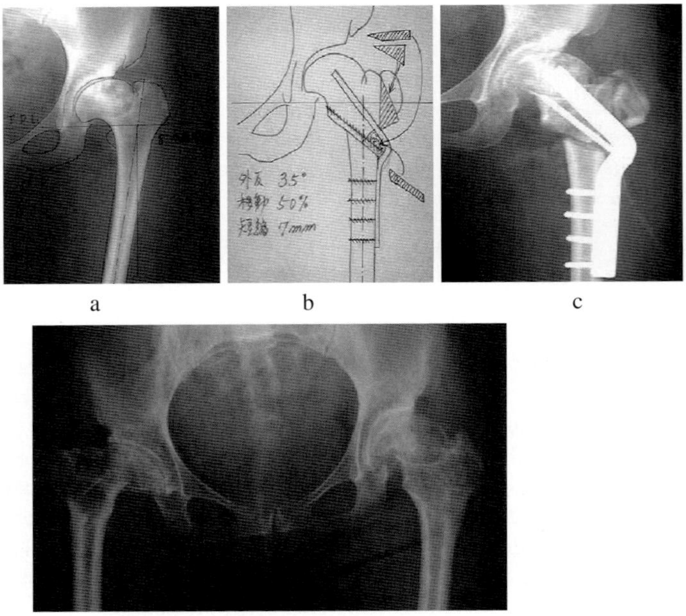

a b c

d

FIG. 5. Preoperative planning and results of valgus-flexion osteotomy (VFO) for 34-year-old woman at surgery. **a** Preoperative AP radiogram with 8° adduction contracture. **b** Preoperative planning on tracing paper. **c** Immediately postoperative radiogram showed osteotomy was performed accurately following preoperative planning. **d** Left hip, 10 years after VFO. For the right hip, the same procedure was indicated 2 years after index osteotomy

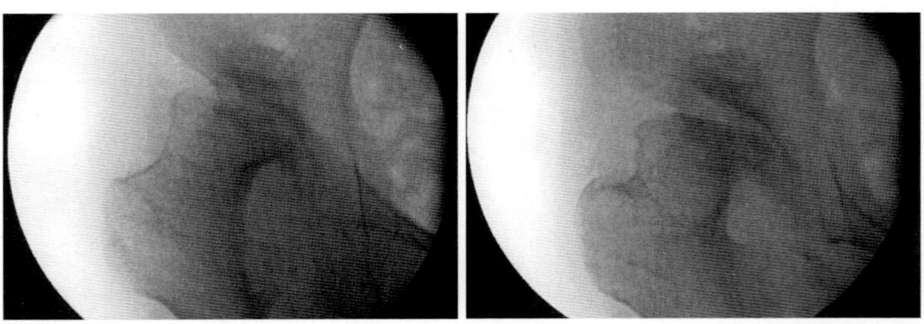

a b

FIG. 6. How to decide whether to perform flexion or extension using dynamic fluoroscopic examination under anesthesia. **a** Valgus-extension (Bombelli) position. **b** Valgus-flexion position. Substantial widening of lateral joint space is shown

Clinical and Radiologic Results

For 229 hips in advanced- and terminal-stage OA, we have performed either VFO or VEO, mainly valgus-flexion. For 82 hips, Chiari's pelvic osteotomy was combined.

Our postoperative rehabilitation program is the following:

1. On day 2, patients start passive and active ROM exercise and use of wheelchair.
2. At week 2, one-third partial weight-bearing starts.
3. At week 6, two-thirds partial weight-bearing starts and the patient is discharged from the hospital.
4. At 3 to 4 months, full weight-bearing starts, when bone union is expected. The follow-up period is 3 to 24 years, an average of 14.5 years.

The evaluation of the clinical results includes the hip scoring system by the Japanese Orthopaedic Association (JOA Hip Score) for clinical outcome, our assessment method of radiologic findings, and cumulative survivorship. Of the 229 hips, 2 were excluded due to technical failure because these 2 patients had to convert to THR less than 2 years after osteotomy.

Clinical results are presented on Fig. 7. At 1 year postoperative, the score became 76, up from 51, and at 5 years, it goes up further, to almost 80 points. Then, particularly among the patients with severe joint contracture, the score started to decline gradually, and at final follow-up, the score dropped down to 73. Compared to the preoperative hip score, it was still significantly better.

The results of radiologic evaluation are shown in Fig. 8. We looked at the degree of joint space widening, degree of improvement in bone cysts and osteosclerosis, and the degree of trabecular remodeling. If the parameters nearly normalized, they were assessed as "good." If there was no widening of the joint space, or if there was residual or worsening of bone cysts or osteosclerosis, or if there is no improvement or worsening of the trabecular structure, the results were considered "poor" [6]. Preoperatively, all cases were "poor" because they are mostly in their terminal stage. At 5 years after osteotomy, all cases had improvements, with "good" or "fair," but after 10 years, we started to see "poor" cases again.

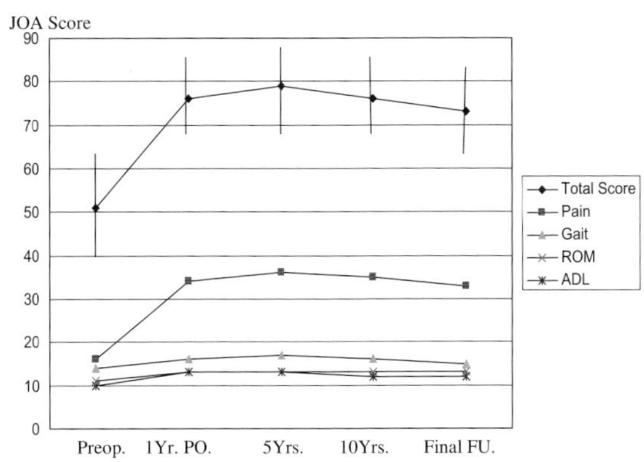

FIG. 7. Clinical results of VFO

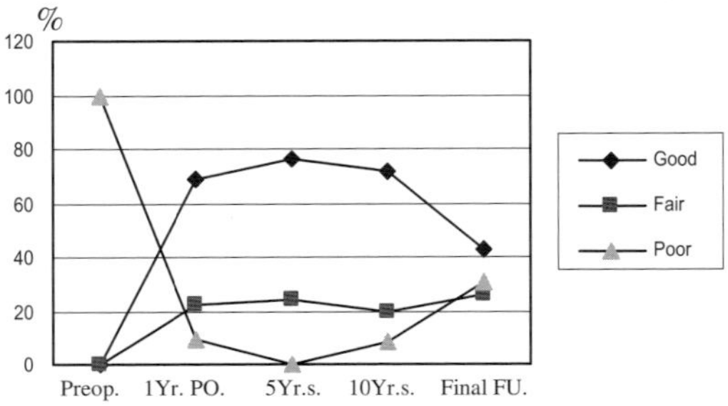

FIG. 8. Radiologic results of VFO

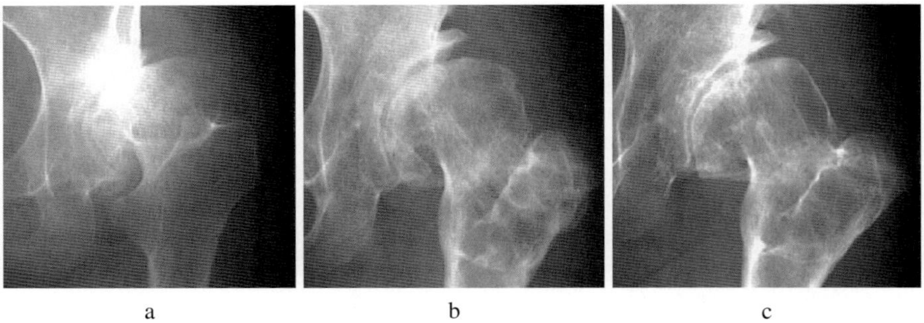

FIG. 9. Postoperative radiologic remodeling course of 45-year-old woman. **a** Preoperative radiogram. **b** At 2 years after VFO, good remodeling had occurred at the joint line and resorption of the anterolateral part of the head had started. **c** At 15 years after VFO, the anterolateral part of the femoral head had completely resorbed, and joint remodeling was excellent

Case 1 was a 45-year-old woman with dysplastic OA. At 18 years after VFO, a very good remodeling had been achieved with widening of the joint space and near normalization of the trabecular structure. She had a very significant lateral protrusion of the head (Fig. 9a); this part did not function for weight-bearing. After VFO, gradual resorption of the anterolateral part of the head that is not functioning had occurred. With VFO, the old femoral head is further pushed out anterolaterally and loses its function. It is then resorbed and disappears (Fig. 9c).

Case 2 was a 52-year-old woman who was treated by VFO. The inclined weight-bearing surface showed significant osteosclerosis and cyst formation on the preoperative radiogram (Fig. 10a). Osteotomy was performed with 35° valgus and 20° flexion. At 19 years later, the roof osteophyte gradually grew and matured to a horizontal direction, widening the weight-bearing surface (Fig. 10c).

I present the characteristic radiographic change during the initial stage after VFO. For the patient presented on Fig. 11, osteotomy was performed with 30° valgus and 20° flexion. The X-ray finding taken at 3 months after VFO showed hinge adduction between capital drop and double floor and remarkable bone atrophy in the previous weight-bearing area (Fig. 11b). In general, marked bone atrophy occurs within 3 to 6 months postoperatively, which disappears almost completely within 1 year. The

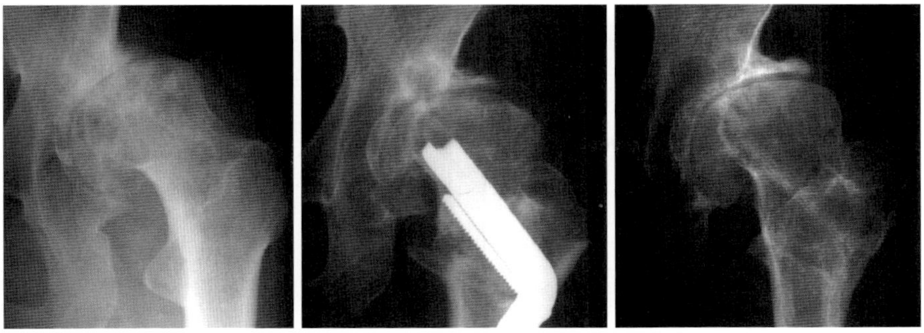

a b c

FIG. 10. A 52-year-old woman with terminal-stage OA. **a** Preoperative radiogram presented terminal-stage OA with severe adduction contracture. **b** At 2 years after VFO. **c** At 19 years after VFO, it is clear that remodeling of the joint line and trabecular structure has occurred. In addition, the weight-bearing area has widened by a horizontally grown roof osteophyte, making a stable joint

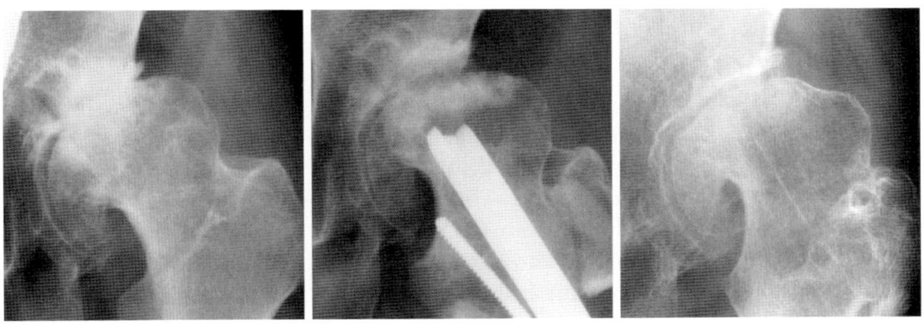

a b c

FIG. 11. Appearance of marked bone atrophy of the previous weight-bearing area during 3–6 months after surgery is a characteristic finding in patients who have a favorable postoperative course. **a** Preoperative radiogram of the hip joint of a 50-year-old woman. **b** At 3 months after VFO, remarkable atrophy of the old weight-bearing area of both the acetabulum and the femoral head is seen. **c** At 20 years after VFO, joint remodeling and good function were still maintained

femoral head line returns, with widening of the joint space and remodeling of the trabecular structure. If a roof osteophyte is initially present, it further grows and eventually reaches maturation [11].

Survivorship analysis was conducted taking either the time of conversion to THR or the time when the JOA hip score was less than 50 as the endpoint. It is clear that at 15 years, 59% for VFO alone, and 58% for VO plus Chiari's pelvic osteotomy, are seen, the latter group being somewhat inferior (Fig. 12) [11].

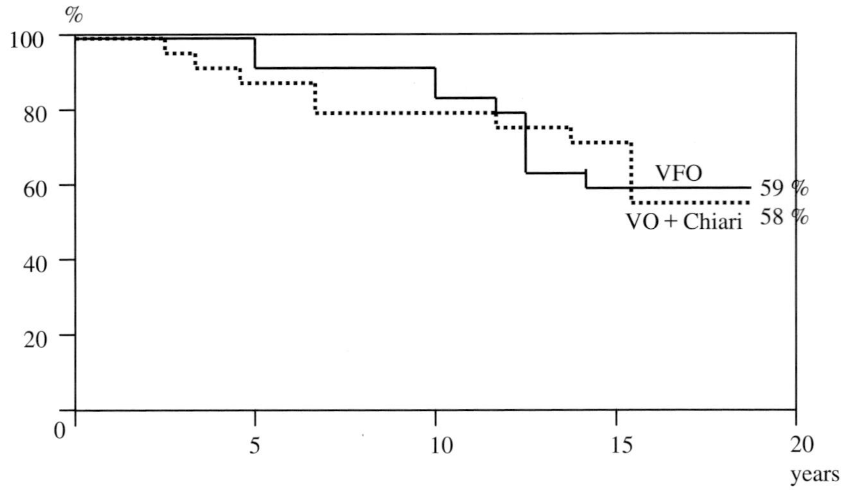

FIG. 12. Results of survivorship analysis based on the Kaplan–Meier method. *VO*, valgus osteotomy

Complications of VFO

The complications of the operation included 4 cases of intraoperative fracture; 2 were a highly comminuted head fracture and they were excluded from the analysis. The other 2 cases had uneventful healing. There were 3 cases of transient sciatic nerve paresis in Chiari combination. Seven cases had superficial infection and 3 cases delayed healing and non-union. The latter cases were successfully treated by additional procedures such as implant exchange with bone graft. There were 12 cases of deep vein thrombosis, but no pulmonary embolism.

Contributing Factors on Clinical and Radiologic Results

As for the factors contributing to clinical results, Maistrelli et al. showed in 1990 that age and body weight are relevant factors, associated with clinically poor results ($P < 0.05$) [14]. Our series showed that the results are very poor when the range of motion of the joint was less than 40°. Age and body weight were not contributing factors of the outcome [6].

Radiologic changes after VFO were studied by Dr. Uchiyama. Cysts disappeared in about 3 months to 1 year; osteosclerosis began to disappear somewhat later than the disappearance of cysts; for the growth of roof osteophyte, only 1 of 6 cases without an initial presence of roof osteophytes showed new growth. If roof osteophytes were present at the beginning, and if the initial size was about 6–10 mm, good growth and maturation were observed in more than half the cases. In cases where roof osteophytes are absent, we cannot expect new growth. Dr. Uchiyama also studied factors contributing to the radiologic results. He said that preoperative AHI must be 60% for

TABLE 1. Contributing factors to radiologic results of valgus-flexion osteotomy (VFO)

	Good 19 (63.3%)	Fair 10 (33.3%)	Poor 1 (3.3%)
Preoperative AHI (%)	71.0 ± 11	69.0 ± 10	61
Postoperative AHI (%)	73.0 ± 13	69.0 ± 10	54
Length of RO (mm)	8.5 ± 4.5	8.0 ± 6.3	0
Width of postoperative joint space	2.9 ± 1.4	1.9 ± 0.6	1

AHI, acetabular head index; RO, roof osteophyte
Data are mean ± SD
Source: From Uchiyama et al. [11]

the surgery. However, successful cases had preoperative AHI of 70%–73%; AHI immediately postoperative was 73%, the length of the roof osteophyte was 8.5 mm, and the widening of the joint gap was about 3 mm. If these parameters were less, the results tended to be poor. Other factors, such as age, body mass index (BMI), Sharp's angle, or the size of the capital drop, were not directly associated with the results (Table 1) [11].

Discussion of the Biological and Biomechanical Mechanism of VFO

Now I turn to a discussion of the biological and biomechanical mechanism of VFO.

The basic idea is that biological effects can be introduced with the improvement of the biomechanical environment in the diseased hip joints. To ascertain the biological effect, we performed histological evaluation of 15 joints with good postoperative remodeling of the articular surface. At the time of implant removal, 1 to 3 years after osteotomy, histological specimens were taken from the patients with their consent. Under arthroscopic control, biopsy specimens were harvested, through the blade channel, from the area where there was no joint cartilage before the index surgery [15,16]. The arthrogram showed some radiolucent lines, above and below the contrast medium, which area was harvested (Fig. 13) [15,17].

I present one very conspicuous case in our histological findings. The tissue is very well stained by Safranin-O; the superficial layer has formed a relatively smooth articular surface. Unlike normal cartilage, however, the feature is that the fibrous structure is relatively coarse. Looking at the superficial layer, there are spindle-shaped cells within the fibrous structure that run in parallel to the articular surface (Fig. 14a). The middle layer has relatively round cells with bright cytoplasm, conceivably cartilaginous cells, within the meshlike network of the fibrous structure (Fig. 14b). In the deep layer, within the fibrous structure, which runs completely perpendicular to the weight-bearing surface and stains strongly with Safranin O, bright round cartilaginous cells are observed. Another point to note is that the deepest part of the reparative tissue maintains communication with the bone marrow, and no tidemarks or subchondral bone plate are found (Fig. 14c). The tissue, therefore, most likely has originated in the bone marrow. If S-100 protein is used to stain the tissue, most cells stain positive, substantiating the finding that they are indeed chondrocytes (Fig. 14d). On the basis

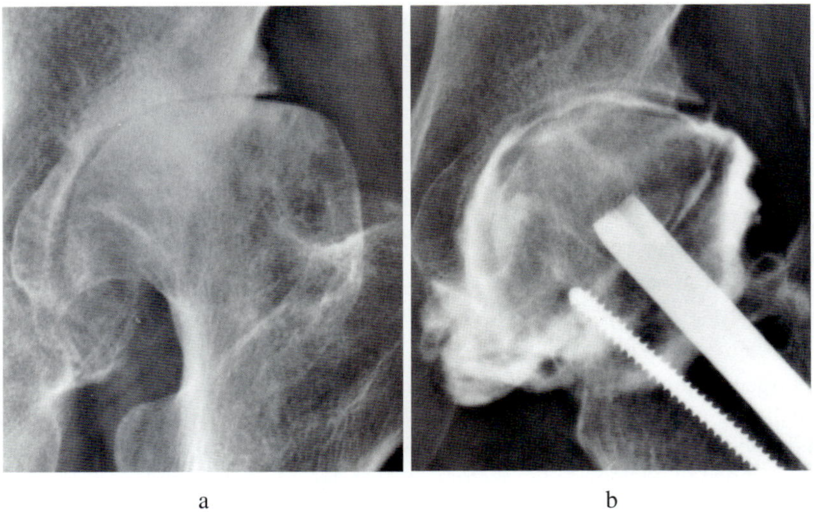

FIG. 13. A 58-year-old woman treated by VFO. **a** Preoperative radiogram showed terminal-stage OA. **b** Arthrogram findings, 1 year after surgery

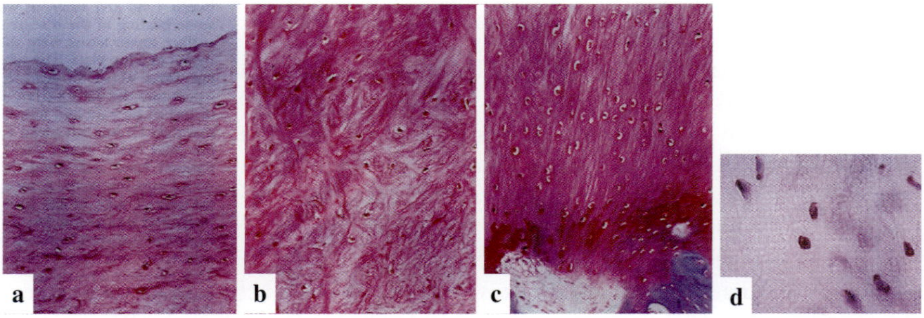

FIG. 14. Histological findings of surface repair tissue harvested from the femoral head of the patient presented on Fig. 13. **a** Superficial layer; **b** middle layer; **c** deep layer (Safranin-O stain, ×95). **d** S-100 protein-positive cells. (From Itoman et al. [15])

of these findings, we can conclude that undifferentiated cells derived from the bone marrow have been differentiated into chondrocytes, which then produced the cartilaginous reparative matrix.

Tissue engineering has recently become a popular topic. Regeneration of cartilage means cellular proliferation and matrix production. Valgus-flexion osteotomy recruits undifferentiated mesenchymal cells from the bone marrow, which in turn will differentiate, proliferate, and produce cartilage matrix. It is a joint-regenerating procedure, in the true sense of the word.

It is believed that such a biological response is triggered by the improvement of biomechanical environment. To prove this, a number of parameters were studied, using Frankel's free-body technique. The center of rotation of the head is plotted as the center of a circle by a digitizer, by taking 5 points on the weight-bearing surface, and its position within a coordinate was calculated by computer. I wish to call particular attention to the resultant force (RF), which is the sum of force applied to the hip joint and the average pressure acting on the unit area of the femoral head (Pu). As a result of measurement and calculation, it was determined that RF was about 243 preoperatively, which decreased to about 70.9% postoperatively. As a result of the increased area of the weight-bearing surface with an extended roof osteophyte and medialization of the center of rotation, the average surface pressure (Pu) was reduced to about 44.2% of preoperative level (Table 2) [5,8]. Such an improvement in the mechanical weight-bearing environment seems to bring about the biological response. Despite the improvement, however, the levels of RF and Pu would never match those of ten cases of normal control women.

To present what I mean, the force applied on the hip joint (RF) has a counterforce of RF'. RF' is composed of P, which is perpendicular to the articular surface, and S, which is parallel to the articular surface. S is a force, directed lateral to the joint, that pushes out the femoral head laterally, in the dysplastic OA, which has an inclined acetabular weight-bearing surface. When the articular surface becomes more horizontal after VFO with horizontal growth of the roof osteophyte, RF' is now composed of P, which is still perpendicular to the articular surface, and Q, which is a force that pushes in the femoral head medially, a stabilizing force, instead of S. With this, the weight-bearing environment for a stable joint is now available. Hip joint score was improved from 51 to 92; the average surface pressure was significantly improved from 0.78 to 0.26, which means that a very good condition is being maintained (Fig. 15) [5,8].

Coming back to the old discussion about the reparative and regenerative capacity of articular cartilage, the literature shows that there is no repair of damage and defect localized in the cartilage in situ, in other words, there is no intrinsic repair of cartilage. Damage and defect that extends to subchondral bone, however, can be repaired by tissue derived from the bone marrow or capsular or synovial tissue around the cartilage. That is to say that an extrinsic pathway for repair is believed to be present.

Table 2. Change in biomechanical environment by VFO

	Preoperative	Postoperative (%)[a]	Control[b]
c/b	0.24	0.31 (127.5)	0.34
M (kg)	200.9	142.4 (70.9)	101.7
RF (kg)	242.9	182.9 (75.3)	138.9
θ (degrees)	70.6	71.3	75.6
Pu (kg/cm²)	52.0	23.0 (44.2)	18

c/b, lever arm ratio; M, body weight; RF, resultant force; θ, inclination of abductor muscle; Pu, average pressure acting on the unit area of the femoral head

[a] Percentage of preoperative value

[b] Normal control group: 10 cases of same-age women

From Itoman [8]

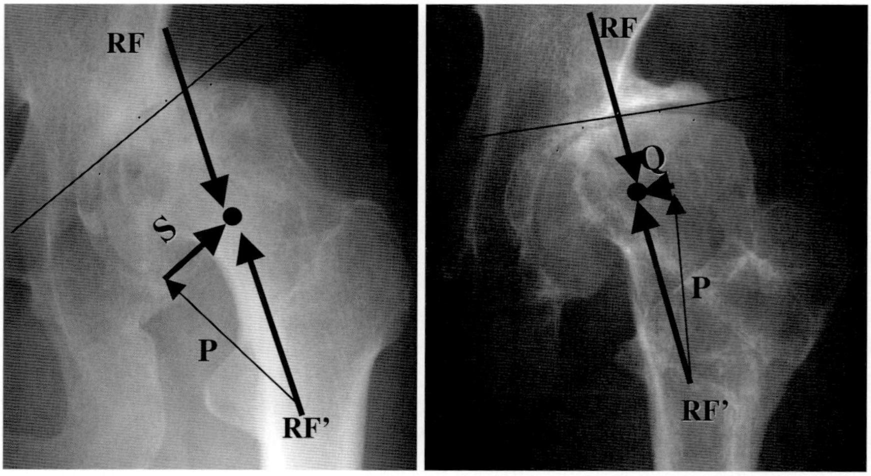

a b

Fig. 15. The 52-year-old woman with terminal-stage OA presented on Fig. 10 shows remarkable improvement in biomechanical environment. **a** Preoperative radiogram. **b** Radiogram taken 5 years after VFO. *RF*, resultant force; *S*, force-S; *P*, force-P; *Q*, force-Q

As we consider the mechanism of joint regeneration in our VFO, there is a remodeling process in which bone structure is reconstructed under an improved mechanical environment, and at the same time, the expanded joint gap harbors interposing reparative tissues. That is the biological reparative process, triggered in response to the changes in the dynamic biomechanical environment. The chondroid plug in the weight-bearing surface, which is highly capable of regeneration, continues to become worn under the very harsh weight-bearing conditions of OA and loses its regenerative ability. However, with VFO, when the environment is improved, the chondroid plug will spread on the articular surface, proliferate overall, and form the cartilage matrix [15,18]. That is the mechanism of the joint regeneration process in VFO.

The basic principle of OA treatment for the pre- and initial stage of OA, where the cartilage is still intact, is to enlarge the weight-bearing area and to improve congruency and the mechanical environment, thereby preventing the destruction of cartilage and preventing the progression of OA. In the case of advanced- and terminal-stage OA, when there is no longer cartilage in the weight-bearing surface, then the congruency should be destroyed first to improve the mechanical condition and to assist the formation of repair tissue and promote the repair of the articular surface. It is in fact a process of joint regeneration. The question is whether the cartilage would simply disappear, or whether chondroid plug-producing bone marrow would appear in the articular surface. This was our turning point. This is where we would have to completely change our way of thinking. If we wanted to treat all cases the same way, with enlarged weight-bearing area and improved congruency, as was the case in pre- and initial-stage OA, there is a limit to what we could accomplish.

Significance of VFO for Advanced- and Terminal-Stage OA in Middle-Aged Patients

Dr. Takatori presented the effectiveness of rotational acetabular osteotomy (RAO). His chart shows the change in JOA score in relay-type treatment [19]. For example, what happens if RAO is performed at the age of 35, as opposed to doing nothing at that age and THR at the age of 45? If a patient did nothing until 45, she would have progression of OA and require THR at 45. She would need a revision surgery in the first half of her sixties. Assuming that she enjoys an average life span, she would require a second revision. However, if the patient had an RAO at the age of 35, her first THR would be around the age of 60, and the second THR around 75, and she would only require a single revision surgery in her lifetime. So Dr. Takatori emphasized that it would be better to have RAO first.

Now the next question is what happens if the patient was not treated by RAO and had VFO at the age of 45, instead of THR. The average course of VFO shows that the patient would require her first THR around the age of 60, and her second THR, or revision, at the age of around 75. Even if the patient is not indicated for RAO because of the advanced or terminal stage of OA, it is questionable whether she should have THR for her first surgery. The question here, however, is the difference of the clinical result that can be expected from THR versus VFO at the age of 45. It is true that osteotomy would only result in a score of up to 80. The gap in results cannot be filled no matter what you do (Fig. 16) [13]. Thus, it is all up to the surgeon to decide whether one would be willing to accept this, or whether one would prefer multiple revisions.

Before summarizing this paper, I present a very interesting case. In 1977, a 64-year-old patient came to me. She had very severe pain and I recommended THR (Fig. 17a). While plans were being made, an nonsteroidal antiinflammatory drug (NSAID) was given on a pro re nata (PRN) basis, and I instructed her to start using crutches. In the meantime, the pain was relieved. Five years later, almost all orthopedic surgeons must think that THR was definitely necessary with this condition (Fig. 17b). However, this was only a radiologic finding, and she was no longer complaining of much pain.

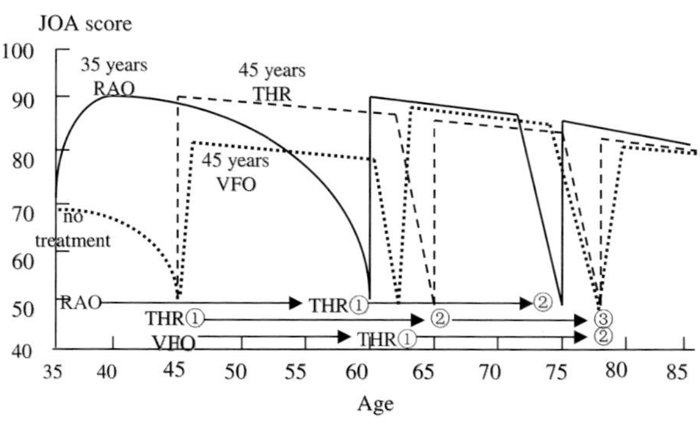

Fig. 16. Estimated curve of Japanese Orthopedic Association (JOA) hip score based on Takatori's relay-type treatment algorithm for OA of the hip. *RAO*, rotational acetabular osteotomy; *THR*, total hip arthroplasty. (Modified from Takahira et al. [13])

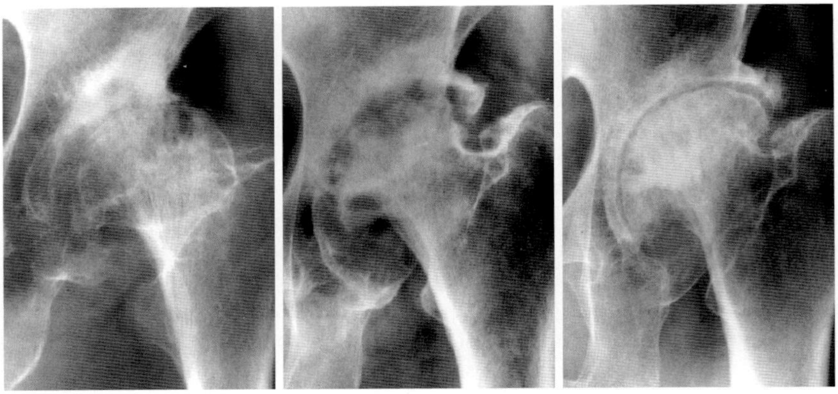

a b c

Fig. 17. Radiologic natural course of severe OA of the hip joint. **a** A 64-year-old woman at her first visit to my outpatient clinic. **b** Five years later, severe destruction of the joint has occurred. On the other hand, marked development of roof and floor osteophytes can be seen. **c** Fourteen years later, excellent remodeling of the entire hip joint has been completed

This is not simple destruction. The formation of a fine set of roof osteophyte and floor osteophyte can be seen on the radiogram. After 5 more years, her hip joint had good function without any pain. Four more years, and the patient is now 78 (Fig. 17c). Joint space is very wide, the roof osteophyte has matured, and the joint was reconstructed and regenerated into a nice spherical joint.

Osteoarthritis is characterized by the coexistence of wear and a destructive phase and the proliferative, reparative, and regenerative phase. The biological system has an innate capacity to repair. It seems, at the present time, that not only the patients but we, the orthopedic surgeons, hurry too much. It may be that we are nipping the natural reparative capacity in the bud by rushing too much. So, we do not actively recommend an operation on our part until the patient asks for surgery. Only when the patient asks for surgery do we then would provide information about the type of operation that can be offered. I believe that is the call of orthopedic surgeons.

As Dr. Sugioka said in his lecture, hospital administrators need to improve financial status by ensuring a shorter length of stay. On other hand, however, in my day-to-day practice, I strongly feel that osteoarthritis cases should not be dealt with in the same manner as rheumatoid arthritis and other destructive joint diseases.

Conclusion

I have tried to describe the principles of treatment of OA of younger patients and to share our results and experience with joint preservation surgery in advanced and terminal cases, emphasizing the significance of osteotomy.

Osteophytes are formed on the acetabular edge and margin of the femoral head as a result of biological response to the biomechanical environment of the joint, reflecting the natural biological regenerative capacity to heal. We need to try to more effectively use these osteophytes. By improving the biomechanical environment of the hip joint, we need to promote biological repair and regeneration of the devastated joint surface. Thus, it is not too much to say that VO or VFO is a joint regenerative surgery that enhances the regeneration of repair tissues in the joint surface even for terminal-stage OA. For younger patients, rather than going to THR straightaway, we should first try to resort to means to enhance and capitalize on the capacity of the biological system to heal, repair, and regenerate.

References

1. Pauwels F (1976) Biomechanics of the normal and diseased hip. Springer-Verlag, Berlin, Heidelberg, New York
2. Terayama K (1982) Natural process and waiting strategy for treatment of osteoarthritis of the hip (in Japanese). Seikei-Saigai-Geka 25:1–4
3. Ueno R (1982) After reading [Natural process and waiting strategy for treatment of osteoarthritis of the hip] (in Japanese). Seikei-Saigai-Geka 25:193–195
4. Bombelli R (1976) Osteoarthritis of the hip. Springer-Verlag, Berlin, Heidelberg, New York
5. Itoman M, Yamamoto M (1984) From valgus-extension osteotomy to valgus-flexion osteotomy as a treatment of advanced coxarthrosis (in Japanese). Seikei-Saigai-Geka 27:863–870
6. Itoman M, Yonemoto K, Sekiguchi M, et al (1992) Valgus-flexion osteotomy for middle-aged patients with advanced osteoarthritis of the hip: a clinical and radiological evaluations. J Jpn Assoc Orthop 66:195–204
7. Itoman M, Yamamoto M, Sasamoto N, et al (1986) Valgus-osteotomy for treatment of advanced coxarthrosis in the young adult. Seikei-Geka to Saigai-Geka 35:549–553
8. Itoman M (1988) Valgus-flexion osteotomy for severely advanced osteoarthritis of the hip joint in middle aged patients. Int Coll Surg Thailand 30:21–23
9. Takahira N, Itoman M (2006) Valgus-flexion osteotomy for advanced and terminal stage osteoarthritis of the hip (in Japanese). MB Orthop 19:48–53
10. Sekiguchi M, Itoman M, Izumi T, et al (1998) Middle-term results of combined valgus and Chisir pelvic osteotomies for advanced osteoarthritis of the hip (in Japanese). Hip Joint 24:116–120
11. Uchiyama K, Takahira N, Komiya K, et al (2004) The results of combined valgus and Chiari pelvic osteotomies for osteoarthritis of the hip (in Japanese). Hip Joint 30: 364–369
12. Itoman M, Sekiguchi M, Kai H, et al (1993) Valgus-flexion osteotomy for severely advanced osteoarthritis of the hip joint (in Japanese). J Musculoskel System 6: 747–752
13. Takahira N, Uchiyama K, Takasaki S, et al (2005) Valgus osteotomy combined with Chiari pelvic ostetotomy for the treatment of advanced osteoarthritis in patients less than 50 years old (in Japanese). J East Jpn Orthop Traumatol 17:132–137
14. Maistrelli GL, Gerundini M, Fusco U, et al (1990) Valgus-extension osteotomy for osteoarthritis of the hip. J Bone Joint Surg 72B:653–657
15. Itoman M, Yamamoto M, Yonemoto K, et al (1992) Histological examination of surface repair tissue after successful osteotomy for osteoarthritis of the hip joint. Int Orthop 16:118–121
16. Itoman M, Yonemoto K, Yamamoto M, et al (1991) Trochanteric valgus-flexion osteotomy for subluxated coxarthrosis: radiological and histological studies on joint remodeling (in Japanese). Hip Joint 17:235–239

17. Yonemoto K, Itoman M, Ueta S, et al (1990) Radiological study of the valgus osteotomy of the proximal femur in the subluxated osteoarthritis of the hip (in Japanese). Hip Joint 16:57–62
18. Tamai A, Masuhara K, Oneda Y, et al (1985) Intertrochanteric osteotomy and its combined arthroplasty for osteoarthritis of the hip: an arthroscopic and histological study on the regenerated articular surface of the postoperative joints (in Japanese). Hip Joint 11:217–223
19. Takatori Y (2003) Probability and surgery for osteoarthritis of the hip joint (in Japanese). Seikeigeka 54:1335–1339

Part IV
Total Hip Arthroplasty: Special Cases and Techniques

Minimally Invasive Hip Replacement: Separating Fact from Fiction

Claire F. Young and Robert B. Bourne

Summary. Total hip arthroplasty is one of the most successful procedures introduced in the twentieth century. Hip surgery performed through a small incision has been widely promoted [1]. Although minimally invasive surgery (MIS) total hip replacement has been greeted with enthusiasm by those wishing to embrace the technique; others have voiced concern or even scepticism. Those extolling the virtue of the minimally invasive approach tout the potential benefits, such as reduced soft tissue trauma, reduced postoperative pain, and quicker rehabilitation. Sceptics of minimally invasive hip arthroplasty are concerned by increased operative difficulty, reduced visualization of the operative landmarks, the increased risk of complications, and the obvious downside of a learning curve associated with the introduction of new techniques. The question remains "Are minimally invasive hip arthroplasties safe and as efficacious as conventional hip replacements?" To date, there has been widespread marketing both to surgeons and to the public about the proposed merits of MIS techniques, but few objective data have been published on this topic. This chapter reviews the technique and published literature to delineate the advantages and pitfalls of performing minimally invasive total hip arthroplasty surgery.

Key words. Minimally invasive surgery, Total hip arthroplasty

Introduction

Less-invasive surgery has become a trend in every surgical discipline. Examples are laparoscopic cholecystectomy which has largely replaced open cholecystectomy in general surgery, minimally invasive robotic heart surgery where stenotomy is not necessary, and in orthopaedics where arthroscopic meniscal surgery has made open menisectomy obsolete. Not surprisingly, interest in less-invasive total hip replacement has emerged.

What are the driving forces to lead surgeons to try less-invasive hip arthroplasty surgery? First, patients come to surgeons requesting it, often having researched the technique with the aid of the Internet or learned of the procedure through the popular

Department of Orthopaedics, London Health Sciences Centre–University Campus, 339 Windermere Road, London, Ontario, N6A 5A5, Canada

TABLE 1. Advantages and disadvantages for various different minimally invasive surgery (MIS) total hip arthroplasty techniques

	Advantages	Disadvantages
Two incision	Intranervous	Fluoroscopy required
Anterior	Intranervous	Femur difficult
Direct lateral	Small incision	?MIS
Posterior	Less invasive	?Dislocation

press. These patients believe that there will be less pain and quicker recovery. Proponents of the procedure allege that patients who undergo total hip arthroplasty surgery via a minimally (less) invasive technique have significantly earlier ambulation, less need of walking aids, a more favourable and earlier discharge from hospital, decreased transfusion requirements, and better functional recovery.

Less-invasive total hip arthroplasty surgery originated with the work of Heuter, Judet, and Keggi [2]. In recent years it has been rediscovered and popularized by Sculco, Berger, and Dorr [3–5].

Minimally invasive total hip arthroplasty involves a smaller skin incision, usually between half to one quarter the length of a conventional skin incision for this surgery, and attempts to minimize the extent of associated soft tissue trauma. Berger defines MIS as surgery where "muscles and tendons are not cut" [6]. Recent developments to aid successful MIS surgery have been the introduction of specialized instrumentation, computer-assisted surgery, the utilisation of fluoroscopic guidance, and specific MIS implants.

The success of conventional total hip arthroplasty surgery has relied on adequate exposure to allow visualization of both the acetabulum and proximal femur. This exposure enabled correct orientation of the implanted prostheses based on visualized anatomical landmarks. One of the concerns with minimally invasive techniques are that with a small incision the surgeon would have poor visualization and this could lead to malposition of the prostheses, neurovascular injury, and poor implant fixation, therefore compromising the short- and long-term results of a procedure which has become one of the most successful advances in surgical technology of the twentieth century.

Minimally invasive total hip arthroplasty has generated a lot of controversy within the orthopaedic community and a great deal of publicity in the popular press. In a randomized controlled trial involving 219 patients, Ogonda et al. [7] reported the results of minimally invasive hip arthroplasty performed through a posterior surgical approach by a very experienced arthroplasty surgeon. Randomization was to either undergo total hip arthroplasty through a standard 16-cm incision or a short incision of less than 10 cm. The authors concluded that minimally invasive total hip arthroplasty performed through a single-incision posterior approach by a high-volume surgeon, with extensive experience in less-invasive approaches, was safe and reproducible. The study however showed no significant benefit between the groups in terms of the severity of post-operative pain, the use of post-operative analgesic medications, the need for blood transfusion, length of hospital stay, or early functional recovery.

Minimally/less-invasive total hip replacement is an umbrella term used to encompass what is actually a "family" of operations. Each of which have advantages and disad-

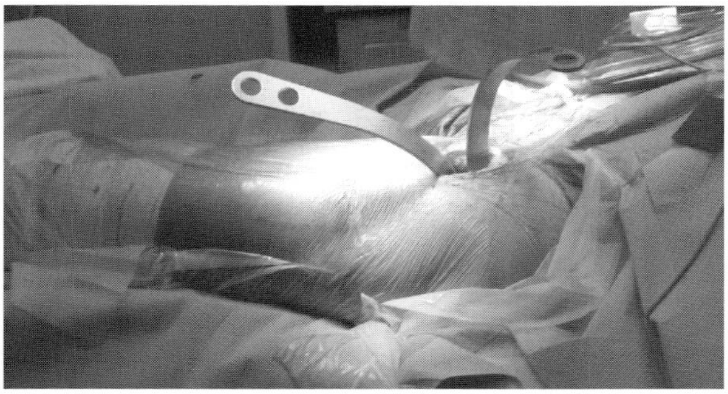

FIG. 1. Intraoperative photograph shows position of specialized retractors during minimally invasive surgery (MIS) anterior approach

vantage (Table 1). This family of less-invasive hip approaches includes anterior, anterolateral, direct lateral, posterior, and two-incision surgical approaches.

Anterior Approach Technique

A modified Smith–Peterson approach is used for a MIS anterior technique. This approach requires the femoral head to be removed, often piecemeal. It gives excellent visualization of the acetabulum, allowing acetabular preparation and implant insertion with relative ease. Surgery via this approach has many disadvantages. First, there is a very steep learning curve as it utilizes a less-common approach for arthoplasty surgery. Second, in this approach access to the femoral canal for implantation of the femoral stem is difficult, prompting many surgeons to use a radiolucent fracture table, fluoroscopy, and specialized implants (Fig. 1). Third, occasionally the surgeon needs to make a second incision. No level-one data have been published on the anterior MIS approach to total hip replacement.

Two-Incision Approach Technique

The two-incision technique was developed by Mears and popularized by Berger [1,4]. This approach utilizes a modified anterior Smith–Peterson incision, which is approximately 4–6 cm, directly over the femoral neck for preparation and implantation of the acetabular component. A separate posterior incision, 3–4 cm in length, in line with the femoral canal is required for the femoral canal preparation and stem implantation (Figs. 2, 3). The procedure is aided by fluoroscopy for placement of the skin incisions, guidance of instrument use and for verification of prosthesis positioning. Customized instrumentation and illuminated retractors aid successful surgery. Specially developed, non-hemispherical acetabular reamers have been found to be helpful to prepare the acetabulum, and a cup inserter with dogleg handle helps avoid both soft tissue and bone impingement. Newly designed femoral canal reamers are also required for proximal canal preparation. Fully porous coated distally fixed stems are advocated for this approach. A rigorous critical pathway for early rehabilitation was devised. Post-operative pain regimens for these patients included surgery per-

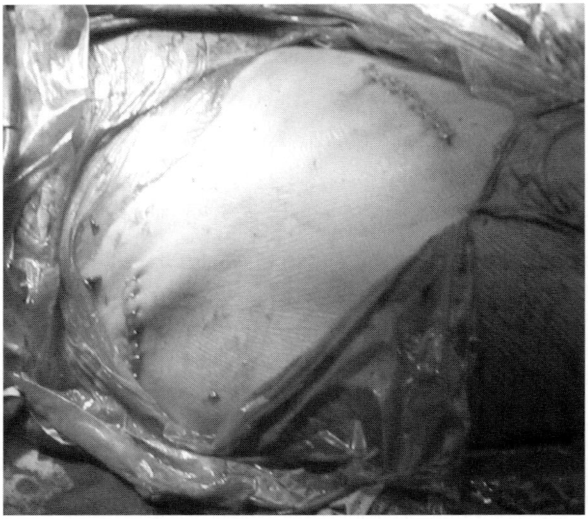

FIG. 2. Intraoperative image at completion of surgery for which two-incision MIS approach technique shows an anterior Smith–Peterson incision for acetabular implantation and a separate posterior incision for femoral component implantation

formed under regional anaesthesia, a combination of non-narcotic analgesic medications, and the utilisation of portable local anaesthetic infusion pumps [8]. Patients selected for this surgical approach all receive accelerated physical therapy with immediate weight-bearing and physiotherapy within the first 24h.

Berger, one of the early enthusiastic proponents of the two-incision technique, reported on his, single-surgeon, results of the first 100 total hip arthroplasties performed using this approach [4]. After the first 12 cases performed, he initiated an outpatient protocol in which 85% of patients were discharged home (not to other care facilities) on the day of surgery and the remaining 15% the day following surgery. One intraoperative proximal femoral fracture was reported for the first 100 cases. There were no dislocations and no hospital readmissions. Radiographic analysis of component positioning for the first 30 cases showed 91% of femoral stems in neutral alignment (a range of neutral to 3° valgus). The average abduction angle for the acetabular component was 45° (range, 36°–54°). Berger concluded that the two-incision technique was safe and facilitated a rapid patient recovery. Mears' results were similar in a highly selected patient population, with 90% of patients discharged home within 24h of surgery [1].

Concerns regarding the two-incision technique are based on several factors. First, there is a high reported complication rate. Mears reported a 2.8% proximal femoral fracture rate (which is three times higher than that in conventional surgery) [1]. Furthermore, it has been claimed that this technique avoids muscle or tendon damage; however, a cadaveric study conducted and reported by Mardones et al. revealed that the muscle damage to the gluteus medius and minimus muscles was substantially greater using the two-incision technique than with a miniposterior approach [9]. Damage was also noted to the external rotators. In addition, even those surgeons who advocate the benefits of this technique admit that there is a learning curve and that appropriate training is required [1].

The evolution of this two-incision technique is still in its infancy. The early experience of a group of 159 surgeons who had completed a designated training programme was followed. A learning curve over the first ten cases for the surgeons showed a significant decrease in mean operative and fluoroscopic screening time; however, key complications (fractures, dislocations, and nerve deficits) were not reduced over the first ten cases [10].

Berger admits that the technique is technically challenging, and states that surgery via this approach should only be attempted after proper hands-on training, which should include cadaveric workshops as an essential component of that training process. The hope is that this training will lead to a decreased complication rate and assure success when the two-incision approach is performed on patients [11].

The many surgeons who oppose the two-incision technique remain sceptical and claim that promotion of this form of minimally invasive hip arthroplasty is being commercially driven and has been marketed without appropriate evidence-based evaluation. Although there are reports from those who have developed the technique on the early clinical results, it will be several years before the mid- or long-term results are available on these patients [1,11].

In conclusion, two-incision minimally invasive total hip arthroplasty surgery is technically challenging and requires specialized training before use on patients. It is interesting to note that of those surgeons who train for the procedure, 90% gravitate to using another approach for total hip surgery.

Anterolateral Approach Technique

The anterolateral or direct lateral approach is well known to surgeons. It has also been utilised for MIS surgery. A shorter skin incision is made and similar muscle dissection down to the joint is performed.

Wenz et al. compared two groups of patients: 124 patients following MIS and 62 patients after conventional direct lateral approach total hip arthroplasty [12]. They wanted to assess the accuracy and reproducibility of implantation, determine if obesity influenced the outcome and technique, and compare operative and postoperative outcomes. They found that the advantages of MIS were that the patients had a decreased transfusion requirement, had a better functional recovery, ambulated significantly earlier, required significantly less transfer assistance, and required significantly less skilled nursing care after discharge. There was no difference in the accuracy of implant positioning, and obesity did not adversely alter patients' operative approach or outcome.

Posterior Approach Technique

This "mini-incision" posterior approach is the most commonly used less-invasive surgical technique for total hip replacement. The less-invasive posterior approach involves a 10-cm oblique incision which, unlike the two-incision approach, is nonproprietary (Figs. 4, 5). The gluteus maximus tendon is split in line with its fibres,

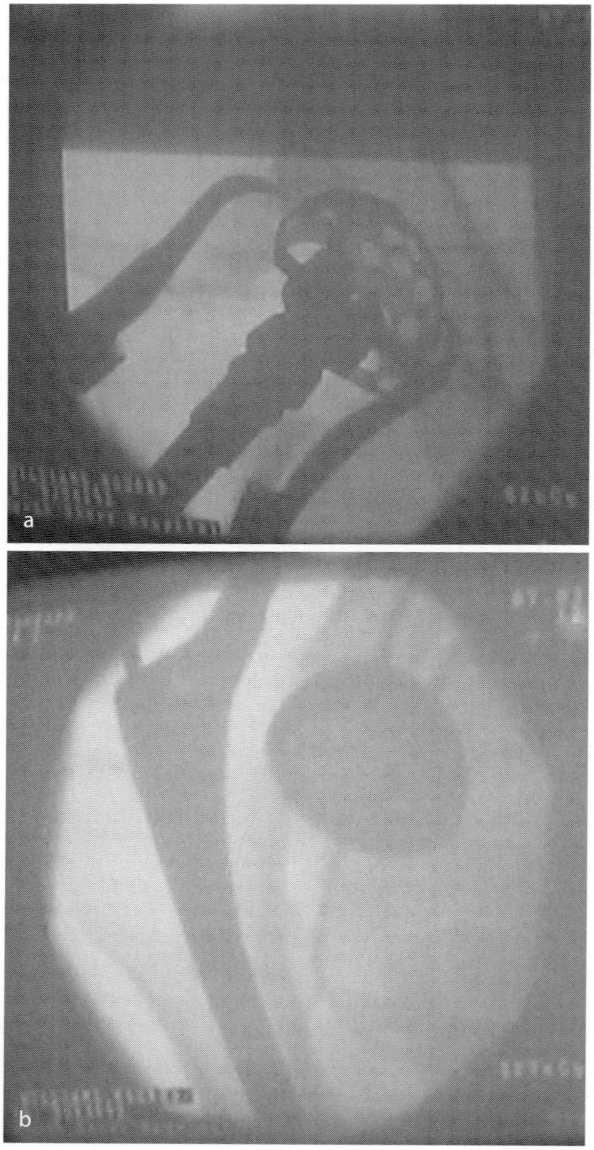

Fig. 3. Intraoperative fluoroscopic images during two-incision MIS approach. **a** Acetabular reaming during two-incision MIS approach. **b** Femoral stem implantation

and the short external rotators and capsule are elevated off the back of the femur in a single flap. Cemented or cementless prostheses can be implanted through this approach implant malpositioning hip. Acetabular socket retroversion (or varus positioning of the femoral stem) are more common with this approach (Figs. 5, 6).

Waldman et al. outlined their early experience with the first 32 total hip arthroplasties in which they used this approach [13]. Mean hospital stay was 3 days with 87% of patients discharged to their own home, the remaining 13% to a rehabilitation facility. There were no reported complications with a mean follow-up of 7 months.

Results of computer navigation in association with a mini-incision posterior approach technique were reported by DiGioia et al. [14], who compared 33 patients following surgery through a standard incision (mean length, 20.2 cm) to a matched group after surgery through a mini-incision (mean, 11.7 cm). All surgery was performed with the aid of computer navigation. He found that the mini-incision group had less limp and better stair-climbing at 3 months, and less limp and improved stair-climbing and distance walked at 6 months.

Sculco et al. reported the results of patients who had undergone MIS total hip arthroplasty through a posterolateral approach with a minimum follow-up of 1-year [15]. This report included a randomized trial in which 22 patients with a mean incision length of 8 cm were compared to 24 patients with a standard 15-cm incision. They found reduced blood loss and faster recovery in the MIS group. Complications encountered were 4 dislocations, 1 femoral fracture, 2 neuropraxias, and 2 wound haematomas. All components were in an acceptable position.

Conclusion

The evidence to date in support of minimally invasive total hip arthroplasty is not convincing. The published data, with the exception of the Ogonda et al. paper already mentioned [7], involve small population groups who have only undergone short-term follow-up. Most studies employ poor methodology with a lack of control groups.

Current practice of this technique requires careful patient selection, a body mass index less than 30, and a routine uncomplicated total hip arthroplasty. Intraoperative soft tissue balancing is important to prevent dislocation, as is the use of larger femoral heads (32 or 36 mm), lipped acetabular liners, and cross-linked polyethylene.

The interest in minimally invasive total hip replacement is growing and will continue to grow. It has sparked a reevaluation of all aspects of hip replacement surgery: reduction and management of postoperative pain, minimization of blood loss, reduction in length of hospital stay, promotion of earlier rehabilitation, and improved cosmesis.

Most surgeons recognize that the potential for complications increases with the limited exposure that is afforded by MIS techniques [16,17]. Advocates of less-invasive procedures suggest that the marriage of the technologies of MIS and computer-assisted surgery may be the future. This is a reasonable hypothesis, but computer navigation adds an additional complexity and cost to the operative procedure.

Careful review of component positioning following minimally/less-invasive techniques shows greater acetabular cup retroversion and femoral stem placement in

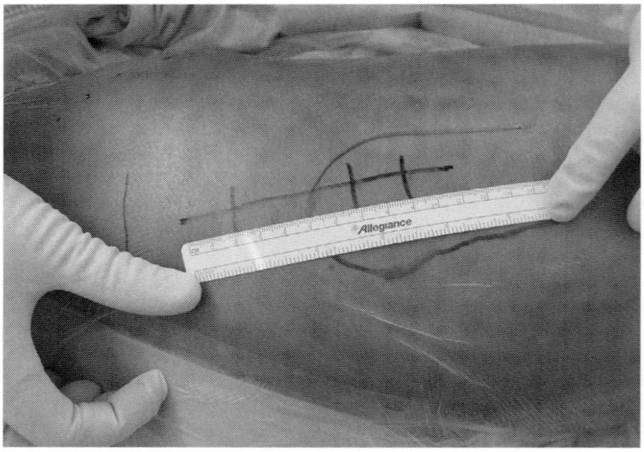

FIG. 4. Preoperative skin marking for MIS direct lateral approach

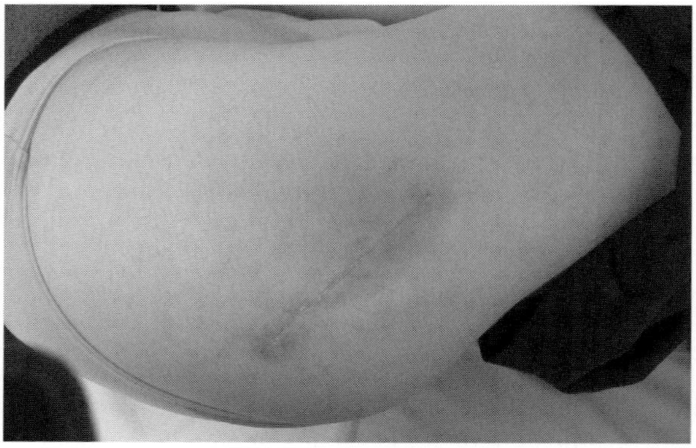

FIG. 5. Clinical photograph of right hip scar following MIS posterior approach

varus (Figs. 5, 6). Several authors have reported increased implant malposition when a minimally invasive technique was undertaken. Woolson et al. reported a higher percentage of acetabular cup malposition and poor fit and fill of femoral components inserted without cement in a series of 135 primary unilateral total hip replacements [18].

The National Institute of Clinical Excellence (NICE) is an independent British organization responsible for providing national guidance on promotion of good health and prevention and treatment of ill health. It has published guidance on minimally invasive hip arthroplasty, which recommends that "there is insufficient evidence on the safety and efficacy of the two-incision technique for it to be performed without special arrangement for consent, audit or research" [19]. Guidance on single mini-incision hip replacement recommends that "there may be benefits to this procedure but it should only be used in appropriately selected patients by clinicians with adequate training in the technique" [20].

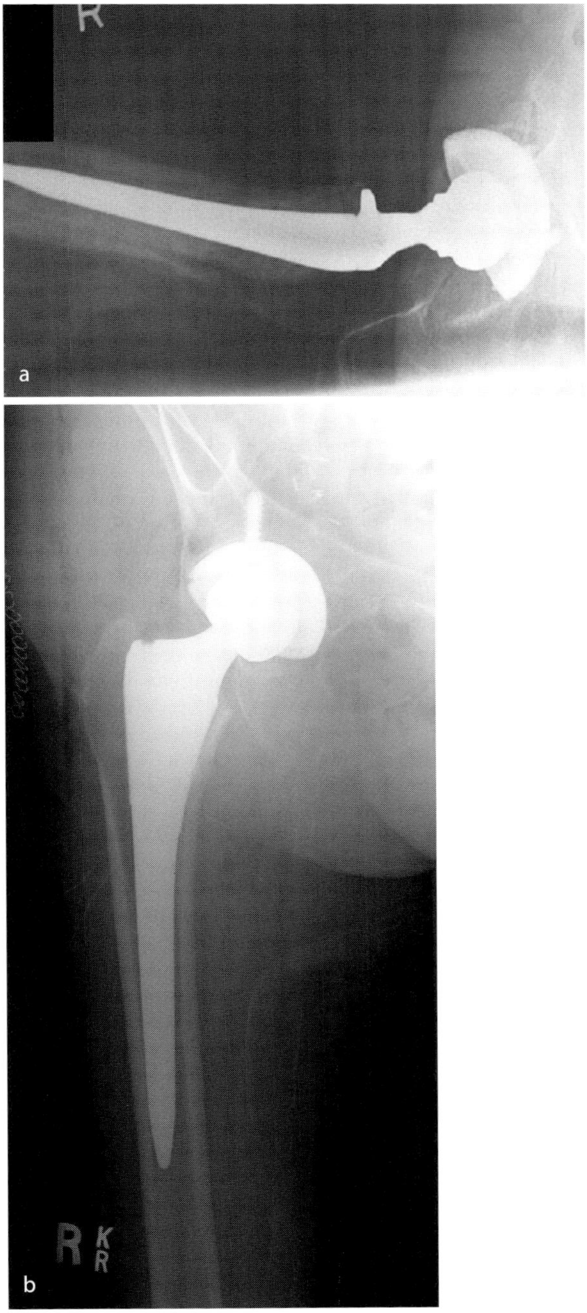

Fig. 6. Component malposition following MIS surgery. **a** Postoperative radiograph shows retroverted acetabular cup. **b** Postoperative radiograph shows varus femoral stem

Despite its purported popularity among surgeons, a minimally invasive approach for total hip arthroplasty surgery is performed by less than 10% of surgeons in Canada [21]. The initial enthusiasm for minimally invasive total hip arthroplasty seems to be waning due to less-precise component positioning and the greater risk of complications associated with this technique.

References

1. Berry DJ, Berger RA, Callaghan JJ, et al (2003) Minimally invasive total hip arthroplasty. Development, early results, and a critical analysis. J Bone Joint Surg [Am] 85A(11):2235–2246
2. Light TR, Keggi KJ (1980) Anterior approach to hip rthroplasty. Clin Orthop Relat Res 152:255–260
3. Wright JM, Crockett HC, Delgado S, et al (2004) Mini-incision for total hip arthroplasty: a prospective, controlled investigation with 5-year follow-up evaluation. J Arthroplasty 19(5):538–545
4. Berger RA (2003) Total hip arthroplasty using the minimally invasive two-incision approach. Clin Orthop Relat Res 417:232–241
5. Inaba Y, Dorr LD, Wan Z, et al (2005) Operative and patient care techniques for posterior mini-incision total hip arthroplasty. Clin Orthop Relat Res 441:104–114
6. Berger RA (2004) Minimally invasive THR using two incisions. Orthopedics 27(4): 382–383
7. Ogonda L, Wilson R, Archbold P, et al (2005) A minimal-incision technique in total hip arthroplasty does not improve early postoperative outcomes. A prospective, randomized, controlled trial. J Bone Joint Surg Am 87A(4):701–710
8. Berger RA (2004) The technique of minimally invasive total hip arthroplasty using the two-incision approach. Instr Course Lect 53:149–155
9. Mardones R, Pagnano MW, Nemanich JP, et al (2005) The Frank Stinchfield Award: muscle damage after total hip arthroplasty done with the two-incision and mini-posterior techniques. Clin Orthop Relat Res 441:63–67
10. Archibeck MJ, White RE Jr (2004) Learning curve for the two-incision total hip replacement. Clin Orthop Relat Res 429:232–238
11. Berger RA, Duwelius PJ (2004) The two-incision minimally invasive total hip arthroplasty: technique and results. Orthop Clin N Am 35(2):163–172
12. Wenz JF, Gurkan I, Jibodh SR (2002) Mini-incision total hip arthroplasty: a comparative assessment of perioperative outcomes. Orthopedics 25(10):1031–1043
13. Waldman BJ (2002) Minimally invasive total hip replacement and perioperative management: early experience. J South Orthop Assoc 11(4):213–217
14. DiGioia AM III, Plakseychuk AY, Levison TJ, et al (2003) Mini-incision technique for total hip arthroplasty with navigation. J Arthroplasty 18(2):123–128
15. Sculco TP, Jordan LC (2004) The mini-incision approach to total hip arthroplasty. Instr Course Lect 53:141–147
16. Fehring TK, Mason JB (2005) Catastrophic complications of minimally invasive hip surgery. A series of three cases. J Bone Joint Surg [Am] 87A(4):711–714
17. Bal BS, Haltom D, Aleto T, et al (2005) Early complications of primary total hip replacement performed with a two-incision minimally invasive technique. J Bone Joint Surg [Am] 87A(11):2432–2438
18. Woolson ST, Mow CS, Syquia JF, et al (2004) Comparison of primary total hip replacements performed with a standard incision or a mini-incision. J Bone Joint Surg [Am] 86A(7):1353–1358

19. Minimally Invasive Two-Incision Surgery for Total Hip Replacement (2005) National Institute for Clinical Excellence Interventional Procedure Guidance 112, London. www.nice.org.uk
20. Single Mini-Incision Hip Replacement (2006) National Institute for Health and Clinical Excellence Interventional Procedure Guidance 152, London. www.nice.org.uk
21. Canadian Joint Replacement Registry 2005 Report (2005) Canadian Institute for Health Information, Ottawa. www.cihi.ca

Hip Resurfacing: Indications, Results, and Prevention of Complications

Harlan C. Amstutz[1], Michel J. Le Duff[1], and Frederick J. Dorey[2]

Summary. The purpose of the present study was to review the indications and assess the clinical results of a current metal-on-metal hip resurfacing design in a population of patients treated for secondary osteoarthritis (OA) in which 208 patients (238 hips) underwent metal-on-metal hybrid hip resurfacing with a diagnosis of nonprimary OA. The patients were young (average age, 41.4 years), and 62% were male. The study group presented greater risk factors [Surface Arthroplasty Risk Index (SARI) score] for resurfacing than a control group of patients operated for primary OA. The average follow-up was 5.6 years. All clinical scores showed significant improvements postoperatively ($P < 0.001$). Kaplan–Maier survivorship at 4 years was 95%, using any revision as endpoint. In comparison with primary OA patients, the study group had slightly inferior results, explained by the difference in risk factors. However, improvements in the surgical technique suggest that these risk factors can be overcome because early failures pertained to the stage of development of the surgical technique. Specific training programs for resurfacing are needed to minimize the learning curve of surgeons newly undertaking this procedure.

Historical Review

The history of hip resurfacing has previously been described in the literature [1–3], and the recent success of the procedure came after a long evolution driven by the need to find a viable conservative prosthetic solution for young and active patients with end-stage arthritis. The origin of hip resurfacing is commonly attributed to Smith-Petersen [4], who was followed by subsequent designs referred to as "double cups" in which the joint bearing was replaced by two adjacent congruent surfaces sliding against each other. The popularity of the concept led to the development of numerous designs worldwide [5–13].

[1]Joint Replacement Institute at Orthopaedic Hospital, 2400 South Flower Street, Los Angeles, CA 90007, USA
[2]Los Angeles Children's Hospital, Los Angeles, CA, USA

The poor mid- and long-term performance of these early resurfacing designs nearly led to the demise of the concept itself when, in fact, technological factors such as the lack of adequate component fixation and particularly the metal-on-polyethylene bearing materials were causing rapid failure rates [14,15]. However, the resurfacing concept was kept alive in a few centers because of the results of hemiresurfacing fixed with acrylic, in which aseptic loosening of the device has not been observed in 25 years of experience in the senior author's series [16,17]. This observation originated the idea that a low-wear metal-on-metal (MOM) bearing material was the likely key to the success of total resurfacing.

The need to accommodate a femoral head of a large diameter led to the choice of cobalt-chromium-molybdenum, which combined low wear and strength with a reduced thickness, for the acetabular component, so that the procedure became bone conserving for the acetabulum as well as for the femoral head and neck. Currently, only metallic devices can be manufactured with thin-walled one-piece cementless sockets and excellent wear properties, especially for large femoral heads [18,19], making MOM the bearing of choice for resurfacing.

Introduction

Hip resurfacing with MOM bearings is the fastest growing procedure in the world and is playing a major role in the treatment of osteoarthritis (OA), especially for young patients [20–24]. However, most of the results published to date relate to resurfacing in a population essentially composed of patients treated for idiopathic or "primary" OA. In Asia, primary OA is extremely rare [25,26], and hip arthroplasty essentially applies to degenerative changes secondary to developmental dysplasia of the hip (DDH), osteonecrosis (ON), posttrauma (PT), slipped capital femoral epiphysis (SCFE), Legg–Calve–Perthes (LCP) disease, and inflammatory diseases (rheumatoid arthritis, etc.). Kobayashi et al. have reported the effects of theses differences on the long-term clinical and survivorship results of primary Charnley total hip arthroplasties [27].

The purpose of the present study was to review the indications and assess the clinical results of a current metal-on-metal hip resurfacing design in a population of patients treated for nonprimary OA.

Materials and Methods

From a series of more than 950 hips treated with metal-on-metal hybrid resurfacing (Conserve Plus; Wright Medical Technology, Arlington, TN, USA), 208 patients (238 hips) underwent the procedure between November 1996 and June 2005 for a diagnosis other than primary OA.

The degeneration of the articular cartilage was secondary to DDH in 82 hips (34.5%), ON in 70 (29.4%), PT in 35 (14.7%), LCP disease in 20 (8.4%), SCFE in 13 (5.5%), inflammatory joint disease in 15 (6.3%), pigmented villonodular synovitis in 2 (0.8%), and melorheostosis in 1 (0.4%). There were 129 males (62%) and 79 females (38%). The average age of the patients at the time of surgery was 41.4 years (range, 14–63). Forty-six hips (19.3%) had undergone a prior operation before resurfacing, including 13 osteotomies, 12 core decompressions, 14 pinnings of the femoral head, 2 hemiresurfacings, and 5 other procedures.

All the procedures reported here were performed by the senior author. The surgical technique employed in this series has been described in detail in previous publications [28–30], and the effects of the modifications made from the initial surgical technique have been evaluated [31].

The patients were evaluated preoperatively, immediately after surgery, at 3 to 4 months, at 1 year, and then at yearly intervals. Radiographic data consisting of a low anteroposterior pelvis view, a modified table down-lateral, and a Johnson lateral view [32] were collected at each visit. The radiographic analysis was similar to that reported in our previous publications [21]. Two patients were lost to follow-up, leaving 236 hips for review.

The clinical outcome of the surgeries was evaluated pre- and postoperatively using the University of California at Los Angeles (UCLA) hip scoring system [33] and the Short-Form 12 questionnaire (SF-12) [34]. The Harris hip score [35] was calculated postoperatively as an overall assessment of success comparable to other studies. The Surface Arthroplasty Risk Index (SARI) [22] was calculated for each hip to evaluate the suitability of the group to be treated with a resurfacing procedure.

A statistical analysis was performed using Kaplan–Maier survivorship curves and log-rank tests for comparison of survivorship data. Paired Student's t tests were used for comparison of preoperative to postoperative clinical scores, and two-sample equal-variance t tests were used for comparisons of clinical scores with other groups of patients.

Results

Clinical Results

At a mean follow-up of 5.6 years (range, 1.0–9.5), all clinical scores improved significantly, although they did not quite reach the average scores of primary OA patients, except for the physical component of the SF-12 survey (Table 1). SARI scores were high on average for the study group (3.2 vs 2.3 for the primary OA patients, $P = 0.001$), and this difference was explained by a greater percentage of previous surgeries (19.3% vs 0.2%), a lower body weight (78.2 kg vs 85.1 kg, $P = 0.001$), and a greater percentage of hips with cystic defects larger than 1 cm in the study group (55.0% vs 30.9%).

Radiographic Results

Seven hips (2.9%) from the study group presented substantial metaphyseal stem radiolucencies [21] at the last radiographic follow-up. Only one of these was associated with clinical symptoms of loosening in a patient who was lost to follow-up. The others were all pain free despite an average follow-up time of 4.6 years (range, 2.0–7.0) since the appearance of the radiolucency (Fig. 1).

A narrowing of the femoral neck of 10% or more at the junction with the femoral component was observed in ten hips, but no definite association could be made with femoral component failure.

TABLE 1. Clinical scores of the study group (pre- and postoperative) and in comparison with patients operated for primary osteoarthritis (OA)

	Study group, preoperative	*P*	Study group, postoperative	*P*	Primary OA, postoperative
UCLA hip scores					
Pain	3.3	0.001	9.3	0.008	9.5
Walking	5.9	0.001	9.5	0.002	9.7
Function	5.4	0.001	9.3	0.014	9.6
Activity	4.4	0.001	7.2	0.001	7.7
SF-12					
Physical	31.6	0.001	50.6	0.718	50.9
Mental	46.1	0.001	51.2	0.001	54.2
HHS	—	—	91.8	0.023	93.5

UCLA, University of California at Los Angeles; SF-12, Short-Form 12 questionnaire; HHS, Harris hip score

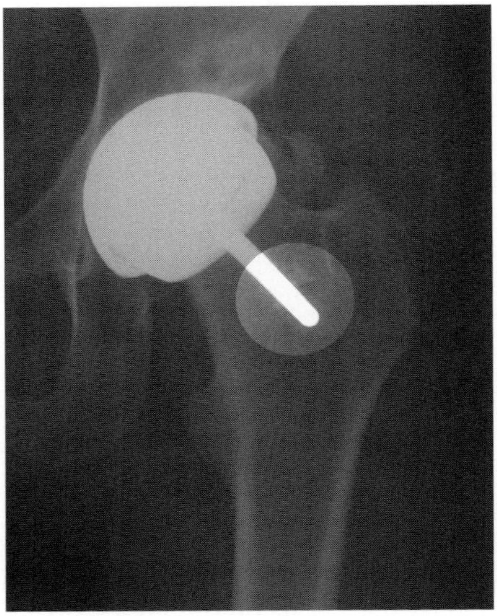

FIG. 1. Seven-year-postoperative radiograph of a 40 year-old woman who underwent metal-on-metal resurfacing for developmental dysplasia of the hip (DDH). The region of interest highlights a radiolucency, which has been visible around the metaphyseal stem for more than 6 years, indicating imperfect initial fixation with first-generation cementing technique (cyst size was 2 cm). The patient has no clinical symptoms, indicating a degree of stability commensurate at this time with her activity level of 7 and her weight of 67 kg

Complications

There were a total of 14 complications (overall rate, 5.9%) that did not require conversion to a total hip replacement (THR) in this series. Four were dislocations (1.7%), from which 3 resolved with closed reduction and 1 necessitated acetabular component reorientation. There were 4 femoral nerve palsies (1.7%), which all fully recovered without any specific treatment. There was also 1 femoral vein clot (0.4%) followed by extracapsular bleeding secondary to the use of heparin. One hematogenous sepsis happened 10 days after surgery and was treated with soft tissue debridement and antibiotics. One of 5 patients operated through a lateral transtrochanteric approach developed a trochanteric bursitis, which resolved with the removal of wires used in the reattachment of the greater trochanter.

A component size mismatch that occurred early in the series before prepackaging of the components was resolved with replacement of the acetabular shell with a 2-mm-thicker custom component of the appropriate inner diameter. One hip required a reexploration to remove residual bone cement trapped in the joint after hip reduction. Finally, one hip needed acetabular reconstruction after the acetabular shell protruded through the acetabular wall. The patient was heavy, had poor bone quality, and had undergone simultaneous bilateral resurfacing (the event occurred on the first hip operated). In addition, the wall had presumably been further weakened by overreaming.

Conversions to THR

Thirteen hips were converted to a THR in this series. The reasons for revision included 2 for fracture of the femoral neck, 9 (in 8 patients) for femoral component loosening, 1 for late hematogenous sepsis, and 1 for recurrent subluxation secondary to ischial–trochanteric impingement. The femoral neck fractures occurred at 2 and 5 months after surgery (both with a diagnosis of DDH in patients with poor bone quality) [36], and the loosening of the femoral component occurred at an average of 53.4 months (range, 23–100) after resurfacing.

Taking any revision as endpoint, the Kaplan–Maier survivorship of the study group at 4 years was 95.0% (95% confidence interval, 90.1–97.5). In comparison, the hips operated for primary OA had a slightly superior 4-year survivorship with 96.6% (95% confidence interval, 93.4–98.3; log-rank test, $P = 0.056$). However utilizing second-generation technique [31], there has been only 1 loosening and 2 radiolucencies in the most recent 138 hips, and none when the stem was cemented in despite the presence of large cystic defects.

Discussion

The clinical and radiographic results of this very young series of challenging cases are certainly encouraging, even though they did not quite match the performance of resurfacing in primary OA patients performed with first-generation bone preparation and cementing techniques. The difference in survivorship results is accountable to this group presenting greater risk factors, and patient selection should play an important role in the success of the procedure with secondary OA patients. However, changes in the initial surgical technique [31] resulted in a significant improvement in the initial stability and durability of the prosthesis by eliminating the cases of early femoral component loosening. These latter results suggest that a successful resurfacing is possible even with the most challenging cases, and certainly the midterm follow-up review of this series of patients confirms this statement (Fig. 2). However, longer-term follow-up will be important, and we advise patients who have risk factors to avoid impact sporting activities.

The challenge of resurfacing nonprimary OA patients varies with the etiology of each case. Patients with DDH mainly present anatomical challenges (shallow acetabulum, greater femoral anteversion and neck–shaft angle, lower offset, and leg length inequalities). Our experience with resurfacing is limited to Crowe class I and II DDH,

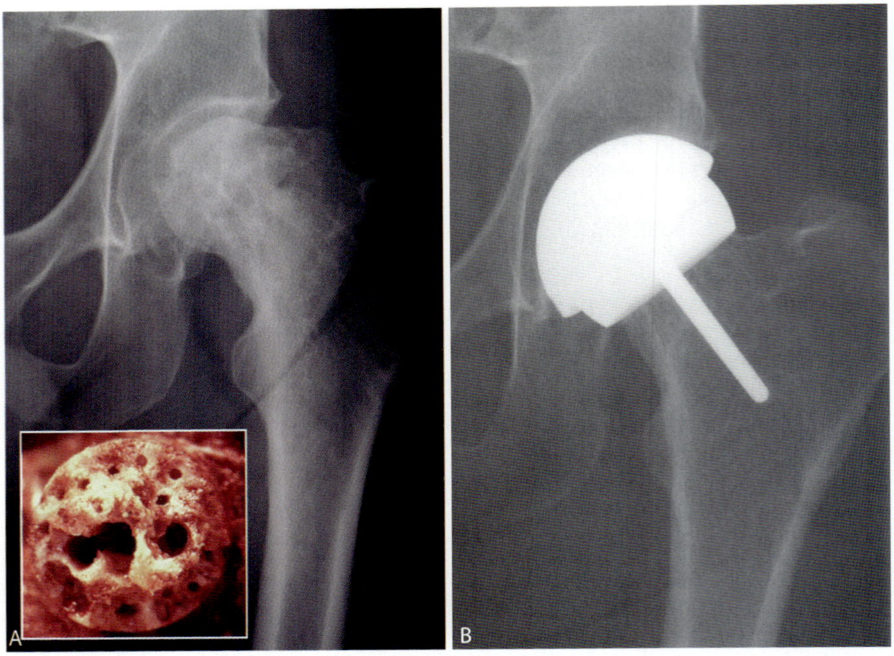

FIG. 2. **A** Anteroposterior radiograph of a 47-year-old man with posttraumatic osteonecrosis consecutive to a bicycling accident. The femoral neck fracture was pinned, and the tracks are visible both on the radiograph and in the intraoperative photograph (*insert*). Note the extensive defects in the femoral head before reconstruction. The additional area for fixation due to the pin tracks may have enhanced the initial fixation. **B** Nine years after metal-on-metal resurfacing, the patient has resumed a very active lifestyle (including ski racing), and his UCLA hip scores are 10 for pain, walking, and function, and 9 for activity

and the results for this etiology were characterized by perfect acetabular initial and enduring component stability, despite incomplete lateral acetabular coverage of the socket (up to 10%–20%), without the need for a special component with adjunct side bar and screw fixation. The rough surface with small porous beads (75–150 μm) provides excellent initial stability when a 1-mm-interference anteroposterior fit is obtained between the anterior and posterior columns. Femoral component durability has been more of a challenge because of failure to provide intimate fixation with good-quality bone, but this problem now appears to be solved with the second-generation surgical technique and cementing of the stem in patients with risk factors.

The technical difficulty of resurfacing patients with LCP disease or SCFE is also related to the anatomical characteristics of these hips. The femoral head is generally flattened, the neck–shaft angle is lower than average, the neck is wide and short, and range of motion is consequently reduced (Fig. 3). Notching of the thicker medial cortex of the femoral neck was sometimes necessary to fit the femoral component when the head–neck ratio approached 1 and the standard-thickness sockets were utilized. However, no femoral neck fractures have been recorded in our series with

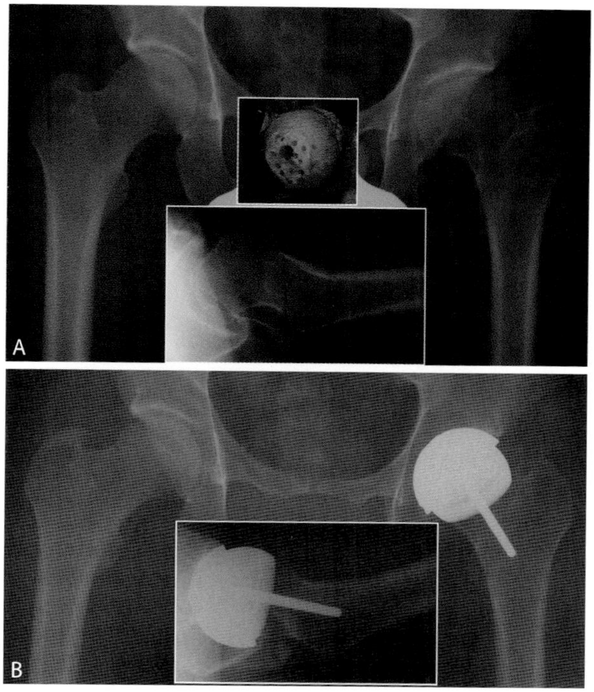

FIG. 3. **A** Anteroposterior radiograph of a 32-year-old man with osteoarthritis (OA) of the left hip secondary to Legg–Calve–Perthes (LCP) disease. *Inserts* show the Johnson lateral radiograph and the femoral head (*above*) after preparation. Note the flattening of the head, cystic defects, incongruity with the acetabulum, wide neck with low head–neck ratio, and increased anteversion, which are typical features of LCP with secondary OA. **B** At 2 years after metal-on-metal Conserve Plus resurfacing using the 3.5-mm acetabular shell. This component allows a gain of 3 mm in femoral head diameter without any extra reaming on the acetabular side as compared to the standard 5-mm shell. There was no need to notch the neck to conserve acetabular bone stock. The component was positioned in a slight posterior-to-anterior position

this etiology [37]. Notching has not been necessary in more-recent cases utilizing the thin (3.5-mm) shells. In DDH, LCP, and SCFE, 1 mm of leg equalization is generally possible when necessary. Leg lengthening should only be performed by bringing the socket to a more anatomical location and not by leaving the femoral component proud.

Patients with osteonecrosis of the hip present challenges of a different nature. The femoral head often presents with extensive yellowish, friable necrotic bone, which must be completely removed down to the underlying white hard reparative bone to ensure proper component fixation. The residual defects are often large, and these should not be grafted, and the stem should be cemented to maximize the fixation area. Our results highlight that the etiology of osteonecrosis itself does not constitute a contraindication for resurfacing and that the risk factors for the procedure are similar to that of primary OA [16].

Etiologies other than primary OA do not present challenges only to hip resurfacing: numerous reports have shown inferior results when treated with total hip arthroplasty (THA) [38–42] because poor bone quality and hip anatomy also affect conventional reconstructions [43]. In that respect, a prosthetic solution that preserves bone stock on both the acetabular and the femoral sides is particularly indicated for a population of young patients likely to undergo revision surgery within their lifetime. From this perspective, hip resurfacing not only conserves bone at surgery but also preserves bone mineral density of the proximal femur [44–46], another advantage over conventional hip replacement where proximal femoral stress shielding [47,48] can frequently be observed with a decrease in bone mineral density [49–51].

Finally, for hip resurfacing to take its place in the array of conservative solutions for young and active patients, specific training for new surgeons needs to be made available because the procedure is technically more difficult than a conventional THR. Our experience has led to a significant reduction of the complication rate, and minimizing this learning curve for other surgeons is essential for the future success of the procedure, in particular with the most challenging cases.

References

1. Grigoris P, Roberts P, Panousis K, et al (2005) The evolution of hip resurfacing arthroplasty. Orthop Clin N Am 36(2):125–134
2. Amstutz HC, Grigoris P, Dorey FJ (1998) Evolution and future of surface replacement of the hip. J Orthop Sci 3(3):169–186
3. Amstutz HC, Le Duff MJ (2006) Background of metal-on-metal resurfacing. Proc Inst Mech Eng [H] 220(2):85–94
4. Smith-Petersen MN (1948) Evolution of mould arthroplasty of the hip joint. J Bone Joint Surg 30 B:59–75
5. Charnley JC (1961) Arthroplasty of the hip: a new operation. Lancet 1:1129
6. Muller ME, Boitzy A (1968) Artificial hip joints made from PROTOSOL. Bull Assoc Study Probl Intern Fixation 1, pp 1–5
7. Gerard Y (1978) Hip arthroplasty by matching cups. Clin Orthop 134:25–35
8. Nishio A, Eguchi M, Kaibara N (1978) Socket and cup surface replacement of the hip. Clin Orthop 134:53–58
9. Tanaka S (1978) Surface replacement of the hip joint. Clin Orthop 134:75–79
10. Trentani C, Vaccarino F (1978) The Paltrinieri–Trentani hip joint resurface arthroplasty. Clin Orthop 134:36–40
11. Amstutz HC, Graff-Radford A, Gruen TA, et al (1978) THARIES surface replacements: a review of the first 100 cases. Clin Orthop 134:87–101
12. Wagner H (1978) Surface replacement arthroplasty of the hip. Clin Orthop 134: 102–130
13. Townley CO (1982) Hemi and total articular replacement arthroplasty of the hip with the fixed femoral cup. Orthop Clin N Am 13(4):809–894
14. Charnley JC (1963) Tissue reactions to polytetrafluoroethylene. Lancet 2:1379
15. Kabo JM, Gebhard JS, Loren G, et al (1993) In vivo wear of polyethylene acetabular components. J Bone Joint Surg 75B(2):254–258
16. Beaulé PE, Amstutz HC, Le Duff MJ, et al (2004) Surface arthroplasty for osteonecrosis of the hip: hemiresurfacing versus metal-on-metal hybrid resurfacing. J Arthroplasty 19(12):54–58
17. Beaulé PE, Schmalzried TP, Campbell P, et al (2001) Duration of symptoms and outcome of hemiresurfacing for hip osteonecrosis. Clin Orthop 385:104–117

18. Smith SL, Dowson D, Goldsmith AA (2001) The effect of femoral head diameter upon lubrication and wear of metal-on-metal total hip replacements. Proc Inst Mech Eng [H] 215(2):161–170
19. Rieker CB, Schon R, Konrad R, et al (2005) Influence of the clearance on in-vitro tribology of large diameter metal-on-metal articulations pertaining to resurfacing hip implants. Orthop Clin N Am 36(2):135–142
20. Back DL, Dalziel R, Young D, et al (2005) Early results of primary Birmingham hip resurfacings. An independent prospective study of the first 230 hips. J Bone Joint Surg 87B(3):324–329
21. Amstutz HC, Beaule PE, Dorey FJ, et al (2004) Metal-on-metal hybrid surface arthroplasty: two to six year follow-up. J Bone Joint Surg 86A:28–39
22. Beaulé PE, Dorey FJ, Le Duff MJ, et al (2004) Risk factors affecting early outcome of metal on metal surface arthroplasty of the hip in patients 40 years old and younger. Clin Orthop 418:87–93
23. Beaulé PE, Le Duff MJ, Campbell PA, et al (2004) Metal-on-metal surface arthroplasty with a cemented femoral component: a 7–10 year follow-up study. J Arthroplasty 19(12):17–22
24. Daniel J, Pynsent PB, McMinn DJW (2004) Metal-on-metal resurfacing of the hip in patients under the age of 55 years with osteoarthritis. J Bone Joint Surg 86B:177–188
25. Nakamura S, Ninomiya S, Nakamura T (1989) Primary osteoarthritis of the hip joint in Japan. Clin Orthop 241:190–196
26. Hoaglund FT, Yau AC, Wong WL (1973) Osteoarthritis of the hip and other joints in southern Chinese in Hong Kong. J Bone Joint Surg 55A(3):545–557
27. Kobayashi S, Eftekhar NS, Terayama K, et al (2001) Primary Charnley total hip arthroplasty: a comparison of American and Japanese cohorts followed for 10–20 years. J Arthroplasty 16(3):340–350
28. Amstutz HC, Beaulé PE, Le Duff MJ (2001) Hybrid metal on metal surface arthroplasty of the hip. Oper Tech Orthop 11(4):1–10
29. Beaulé PE, Amstutz HC (2002) Surface arthroplasty of the hip revisited: current indications and surgical technique. In: Singha R (ed) Hip replacement: current trends and controversies. Dekker, New York, pp 261–297
30. Amstutz HC, Beaule PE, Dorey FJ, et al (2006) Metal-on-metal hybrid surface arthroplasty: two to six-year follow-up study—surgical technique. J Bone Joint Surg [Am] Vol 88-A, Suppl 1 part 2, pp 234–249
31. Amstutz HC, Le Duff MJ, Campbell PA, et al (2006) The effects of technique changes on aseptic loosening of the femoral component in hip resurfacing. Results of 600 Conserve Plus with a 3–9 year follow-up. J Arthroplasty (in press)
32. Laage H, Barnett JC, Brady JM, et al (1953) Horizontal lateral roentgenography of the hip in children; a preliminary report. J Bone Joint Surg 35A(2):387–398
33. Amstutz HC, Thomas BJ, Jinnah R, et al (1984) Treatment of primary osteoarthritis of the hip. A comparison of total joint and surface replacement arthroplasty. J Bone Joint Surg 66A(2):228–241
34. Ware JE, Kosinski M, Keller SD (1998) SF-12: How to score the SF-12 Physical and Mental Health Summary Scales, 3rd edn. Quality Metric, Lincoln, RI
35. Harris WH (1969) Traumatic arthritis of the hip after dislocation and acetabular fractures: treatment by mold arthroplasty. An end-result study using a new method of result evaluation. J Bone Joint Surg 51A(4):737–755
36. Amstutz HC, Campbell PA, Le Duff MJ (2004) Incidence and prevention of neck fractures after surface arthroplasty. J Bone Joint Surg 86A(9):1874–1877
37. Amstutz HC, Su EP, Le Duff MJ (2005) Surface arthroplasty in young patients with hip arthritis secondary to childhood disorders. Orthop Clin N Am 36(2):223–230
38. Brinker M, Rosenberg A, Kull L, et al (1994) Primary total hip arthroplasty using noncemented porous-coated femoral components in patients with osteonecrosis of the femoral head. J Arthroplasty 9(5):457–468

39. Ortiguera CJ, Pulliam IT, Cabanela ME (1999) Total hip arthroplasty for osteonecrosis. Matched-pair analysis of 188 hips with long-term follow-up. J Arthroplasty 14(1): 21–28
40. Radl R, Hungerford M, Materna W, et al (2005) Higher failure rate and stem migration of an uncemented femoral component in patients with femoral head osteonecrosis than in patients with osteoarthrosis. Acta Orthop Scand 76(1):49–55
41. Lehtimaki MY, Lehto MU, Kautiainen H, et al (2001) Charnley total hip arthroplasty in ankylosing spondylitis: survivorship analysis of 76 patients followed for 8–28 years. Acta Orthop Scand 72(3):233–236
42. Lehtimaki MY, Kautiainen H, Lehto UK, et al (1999) Charnley low-friction arthroplasty in rheumatoid patients: a survival study up to 20 years. J Arthroplasty 14(6): 657–661
43. Kobayashi S, Saito N, Horiuchi H, et al (2000) Poor bone quality or hip structure as risk factors affecting survival of total-hip arthroplasty. Lancet 355(9214):1499–1504
44. Kishida Y, Sugano N, Nishii T, et al (2004) Preservation of the bone mineral density of the femur after surface replacement of the hip. J Bone Joint Surg 86B(3):185–189
45. Amstutz HC, Ebramzadeh E, Sarkany A, et al (2004) Preservation of bone mineral density of the proximal femur following hemisurface arthroplasty. Orthopaedics 27(12):1266–1271
46. Harty JA, Devitt B, Harty LC, et al (2005) Dual energy X-ray absorptiometry analysis of peri-prosthetic stress shielding in the Birmingham resurfacing hip replacement. Arch Orthop Trauma Surg 125(10):693–695
47. Kronick JL, Barba ML, Paprosky WG (1997) Extensively coated femoral components in young patients. Clin Orthop 344:263–274
48. McLaughlin JR, Lee KR (2000) Total hip arthroplasty in young patients: 8- to 13-year results using an uncemented stem. Clin Orthop 373:153–163
49. Marchetti ME, Steinberg GG, Greene JM, et al (1996) A prospective study of proximal femur bone mass following cemented and uncemented hip arthroplasty. J Bone Miner Res 11(7):1033–1039
50. McCarthy CK, Steinberg GG, Agrsen M, et al (1991) Quantifying bone loss from proximal femur after total hip arthroplasty. J Bone Joint Surg 73B(5):774–778
51. Kilgus DJ, Shimaoka EE, Tipton JS, et al (1993) Dual-energy X-ray absorptiometry measurement of bone mineral density around porous-coated cementless femoral implants. Methods and preliminary results. J Bone Joint Surg 75B(2):279–287

Current Trends in Total Hip Arthroplasty in Europe and Experiences with the Bicontact Hip System

HARTMUTH KIEFER

Summary. Many aspects of hip implant design and materials have been developed in different European countries, where more than 600 000 hip replacement procedures were performed in 2005. The leading cemented implant designs come from Europe and are today used worldwide as a gold standard in total hip arthroplasty. For cementless hip stem designs, the straight and tapered stem design developments contributed to the increasing success of cementless hip arthroplasty for younger patients. New implant concepts, such as hip resurfacing and shorter cementless hip stems, are today mostly used in Europe and may also influence the future of hip arthroplasty. However, long-term experience with standard cemented and tapered cementless stem implants in combination with advanced press-fit cups and wear couples set high standards of clinical success. These standards must be matched by all new implants and developing trends in primary hip joint replacement.

Key words. Total hip arthroplasty, Europe, Tapered hip stem, Cementless

Introduction

This overview and review of current total hip arthroplasty (THA) trends attempts to summarize the dedicated development steps of hip implant design in Europe, the resulting current trends for THA treatment, and long-term experience with the flat and tapered cementless Bicontact hip stem.

Hip Replacement in Europe

Of a population of 610 million in Europe, 380 million live in countries within the European Union. More than 600 000 hip replacement procedures were performed in 2005. Table 1 shows the number of hip replacements in 2005 in selected European countries and regions.

Department of Orthopaedic and Trauma Surgery, Lukas Hospital, Hindenburgstraße 56, D-32257 Buende, Germany

TABLE 1. Hip replacement procedures in selected European countries and regions

Country	Population	Hip replacements in 2005
Germany	82 million	180000
France	59 million	100000
England	60 million	90000
Italy	58 million	70000
Austria and Switzerland	15 million	32000
Spain	40 million	30000
Benelux	27 million	40000
Scandinavia	24 million	35000

Hip replacement in Europe was mainly influenced by the initial cemented hip design developments in England in the 1960s by Charnley [1], the beginning of cementless hip replacement in France by Judet [2] and Lord [3] in the 1970s, and the subsequent development of straight and tapered stem designs in Switzerland, Austria, and Germany by Müller in 1984 [4], Zweymüller in 1980 [5], Spotorno in 1983 [6], and Weller [7]. The Scandinavian countries contributed excellent hip register data surveillance in Sweden from 1979 onwards [8]. Later, other Scandinavian countries also started hip registers—Norway in 1987 [9], Finland in 1993 [10], and Denmark in 1995 [11]. The results from the Scandinavian hip registers supported the use of several leading cemented stem designs, as cementless hip stems were not used to the same extent.

Many European cementless acetabular implant designs of the 1970s and 1980s were developed as screw cup designs, either conical or spherical in shape [12]. These screw cup sockets where mostly used in Europe until the introduction of cementless press-fit cup designs, which became more popular at the end of the 1980s. The use of ceramic modular heads was introduced in Europe when these materials were implanted from the mid-1970s by Boutin [13] in France and Mittelmeier and Heisel [14] in Germany. The 28-mm modular metal-on-metal THA was introduced by Weber [15] at the end of the 1980s and was followed by the third generation of ceramic-on-ceramic THA in the mid-1990s [16].

Current Hip Stem Designs and Developments

Contemporary cementless hip stems were introduced in Europe in the mid-1980s. The leading European designs were flat and tapered, and bone preparation was similar to the basic principle of the cemented Müller straight stem, which was invented in Switzerland. A comparable cementless tapered hip stem design was also developed in the United States [17]. However, most U.S. hip designs of that period were rounded distally, more filling, porous coated [18], hydroxyapatite coated [19], or anatomical [20,21], and bone preparation was mostly based on an initial distal reaming procedure.

The flat stem cross section seems to be the key to success for cementless European hip stem designs. This basic design feature leads to a high rotational implant stability.

Disadvantages of flat stem designs were the limited rotational stem positioning and the increased risk of femoral fracture during broaching of the femoral canal.

Secondary proximal load transfer with high primary stability is today a proven biomechanical principle for cementless hip stems. Compared with more distally anchoring implants, proximal load transfer requires an extended range of implant sizes, and the depth of stem insertion might sometimes be limited.

Preservation of muscle and bone during THA intervention seems to be the most important aspect in the current trend of discussions in total hip replacement, even if implant positioning is more difficult with smaller incisions and minimized surgical approaches. In an effort to find dedicated implant solutions for younger and more active patients, contemporary resurfacing implants are becoming popular in Europe. Based on the experience of McMinn et al. [22], the metal-on-metal technology has been used since the early 1990s. Potential disadvantages of surface replacement are femoral head fractures as a result of implant malpositioning and specific aspects of and contraindications for metal-on-metal joint articulation.

The concept of cementless proximal implant fixation is also aimed at the treatment of younger patients. Various shorter hip stem designs are currently in clinical evaluation. At present, most of these implants are being used in Germany. Short hip stem designs also have possible disadvantages, as implant positioning is more difficult than with straight standard stems. Varus alignment can cause unexpected periprosthetic bone remodeling and implant loosening. Apart from the reported experience of Morrey et al. [23], no clinical data or experience are yet available for cementless shorter hip stem designs.

The introduction of navigation technology supports implant positioning for the acetabular component and recently also for the femoral implant [24]. Hip navigation has followed the developments of knee navigation and is also useful in less invasive hip surgery procedures. However, THA navigation is much easier in supine patient positioning, and more information is needed for optimal alignment for individual patient anatomy conditions.

Most of the current trends and developments in hip replacement mentioned here have taken place in European countries, with most of these procedures being introduced in Germany. The German health system allow surgeons to use all commercially available and CE-approved implants for hip replacement. However, most patients are treated with well-documented cemented or cementless hip implants with which much experience has already been gained; new implant technologies are often used without experience or long-term data, and there is no German hip register as in Scandinavia.

Experiences with the Bicontact Hip Stem

As a tapered hip stem implant for which long-term experience exists, the Bicontact hip system (B. Braun Aesculap, Tuttlingen, Germany) was developed by Weller et al. [25] and first implanted in 1987 in Tübingen, Germany. The aspect of bone preservation was one of the most important challenges in the development of the Bicontact implant during 1985 and 1986. At this time, experiences with other European flat and straight stems were promising. The original Bicontact implant was designed according to these principles and remains unchanged to this day.

Special attention was focused on the preservation of bone during femoral canal preparation. The Bicontact instrumentation was designed with so-called osteoprofilers. The A-osteoprofiler is used first to compress cancellous bone in the proximal femur instead of removing bone. The B-osteoprofilers were designed to cut the proximal Bicontact stem shape into the femoral bone. Final bone preparation with the B-osteoprofilers ensures the proximal load transfer of the Bicontact hip stem.

Proximal bone contact was additionally supported by the principles of proximal load transfer; this could be confirmed by analysis of the proximal bone–implant interfaces in the Gruen zones 1 and 7 [26]. Only 0.5% of radiolucent lines in these zones were found in the Bicontact multicenter study of 553 implantations in four German institutions [27]. The titanium microporous stem coating supports the periprosthetic bone apposition in the proximal load transfer area [28].

The first 500 Bicontact implantations in Tübingen were followed up in two prospective follow-up series, cemented and cementless [29]. Early follow-up series confirmed the very low incidence of postoperative thigh pain in the cementless Bicontact implantations with comparable results to the cemented stems of similar, uncoated design.

The cementless Bicontact stem series in particular formed the subject of continuous follow-up work [30–32]. The latest follow-up of this series with 250 implantations was recently published by Eingartner et al. [33] with stem survival rates of 96.6% at 14 years. Special aspects of the proximal load transfer could be found in cases where screw-type sockets implanted in the first Bicontact series of 1987–1989 had loosened. Even where there was severe polyethylene wear and acetabular osteolysis, the proximally coated Bicontact stem was somehow sealed against polyethylene wear particles. This remarkable feature of the titanium plasmaspray coating is the subject of further investigations.

Primary and secondary Bicontact implant stability was analysed by Eingartner et al. [34] using an X-ray analysis of stem migration with the EBRA-FCA software [35]. In a group of 71 cases, the mean axial stem subsidence was 0.2 mm at 3 and 6 months, 0.3 mm at 1 year, and 0.5 mm at 10 years.

Periprosthetic bone remodeling in the proximal coated Bicontact stem area was investigated by dual-energy X-ray absorptiometry (DEXA) [36]. The relative values of the proximal bone mineral density declined by 20% at 6 months but did not change in the subsequent follow-up periods.

Bicontact was introduced into Japan in 1994 [37] and into Korea in 1996 [38] with specific hip stem types designed for the special requirements of the smaller femoral canal dimensions. For this reason, the Bicontact standard stem range was extended with an SD series for dysplastic femoral canal conditions and the Bicontact N series for narrow femoral canal conditions in secondary osteoarthritis.

Conclusion

European hip stem design concepts have influenced the successful development of total hip arthroplasty in the cemented and cementless techniques. Straight tapered hip stems offer reliable biomechanical concepts for cementless fixation. Even if different biomechanical concepts can lead to successful implant designs, we use the favourable characteristics of the proximal bone preservation hip implant concept in our institution.

Not all current trends in hip arthroplasty are based on experience and sufficient clinical data. Implantation for hip arthroplasties in younger patients should not lead us to an uncritical use of less-experienced methods and implants. However, innovation in medicine must also be studied with new technologies that seem to be promising for the benefit of our patients.

References

1. Wroblewski BM, Fleming PA, Siney PD (1999) Charnley low-frictional torque arthroplasty of the hip. 20-to-30 year results. J Bone Joint Surg [Br] 81(3):427–430
2. Bettin D, Greitemann B, Polster J, et al (1995) Long term results of uncemented Judet hip endoprostheses. Int Orthop 19(3):144–150
3. Keisu KS, Mathiesen EB, Lindgren JU (2001) The uncemented fully textured Lord hip prosthesis: a 10- to 15-year followup study. Clin Orthop 382:133–142
4. Müller ME (1992) Lessons of 30 years of total hip arthroplasty. Clin Orthop Relat Res 274:12–21
5. Swanson TV (2005) The tapered press fit total hip arthroplasty: a European alternative. J Arthroplasty 20(4 suppl 2):63–67
6. Romagnoli S (2002) Press-fit hip arthroplasty: a European alternative. J Arthroplasty 17(4 suppl 1):108–112
7. Weller S, Rupf G, Ungethum M, et al (1988) The Bicontact Hip System (in German). Med Orthop Tech 108:222–227
8. Malchau H, Garellick G, Eisler T, et al (2005) Presidential guest address. The Swedish Hip Registry: increasing the sensitivity by patient outcome data. Clin Orthop Relat Res 441:19–29
9. Espehaug B, Furnes O, Havelin LI, et al (2006) Registration completeness in the Norwegian Arthroplasty Register. Acta Orthop 77(1):49–56
10. Eskelinen A, Remes V, Helenius I, et al (2006) Uncemented total hip arthroplasty for primary osteoarthritis in young patients: a mid- to long-term follow-up study from the Finnish Arthroplasty Register. Acta Orthop 77(1):57–70
11. Pedersen AB, Johnsen SP, Overgaard S, et al (2006) Total hip arthroplasty in Denmark: incidence of primary operations and revisions during 1996–2002 and estimated future demands. Acta Orthop 76(2):182–189
12. Effenberger H, Imhof M, Richolt J, et al (2004) Cement-free hip cups. Current status (in German). Orthopade 33(6):733–750
13. Boutin P (2000) Total hip arthroplasty using a ceramic prosthesis. Pierre Boutin (1924–1989). Clin Orthop Relat Res 379:3–11
14. Mittelmeier H, Heisel J (1992) Sixteen-years' experience with ceramic hip prostheses. Clin Orthop Relat Res 282:64–72
15. Weber BG (1996) Experience with the Metasul total hip bearing system. Clin Orthop Relat Res 329(suppl):S69–S77
16. Willmann G (1998) Ceramics for total hip replacement: what a surgeon should know. Orthopedics 21(2):173–177
17. McLaughlin JR, Lee KR (2000) Total hip arthroplasty in young patients. 8- to 13-year results using an uncemented stem. Clin Orthop Relat Res 373:153–163
18. Engh CA Jr, Young AM, Engh CA Sr, et al (2003) Clinical consequences of stress shielding after porous-coated total hip arthroplasty. Clin Orthop Relat Res 417: 157–163

19. D'Antonio JA, Capello WN, Manley MT, et al (2001) Hydroxyapatite femoral stems for total hip arthroplasty: 10- to 13-year followup. Clin Orthop Relat Res 393: 101–111
20. Kawamura H, Dunbar MJ, Murray P, et al (2001) The porous coated anatomic total hip replacement. A ten to fourteen-year follow-up study of a cementless total hip arthroplasty. J Bone Joint Surg [Am] 83(9):1333–1338
21. Archibeck MJ, Berger RA, Jacobs JJ, et al (2001) Second-generation cementless total hip arthroplasty. Eight to eleven-year results. J Bone Joint Surg [Am] 83(11): 1666–1673
22. Daniel J, Pynsent PB, McMinn DJ (2004) Metal-on-metal resurfacing of the hip in patients under the age of 55 years with osteoarthritis. J Bone Joint Surg [Br] 86(2):177–184
23. Morrey BF, Adams RA, Kessler M (2000) A conservative femoral replacement for total hip arthroplasty. A prospective study. J Bone Joint Surg [Br] 82(7):952–958
24. Kiefer H, Othman A (2005) Orthopilot total hip arthroplasty workflow and surgery. Orthopedics 28(10 suppl):s1221–s1226
25. Weller S, Braun A, Gekeler J, et al (1998) The Bicontact hip implant system. Thieme, Stuttgart
26. Gruen TA, McNeice GM, Amstutz HC (1979) Modes of failure of cemented stem-type femoral components: a radiographic analysis of loosening. Clin Orthop Relat Res 141:17–27
27. Asmuth T, Bachmann J, Eingartner C, et al (1998) Results with the cementless Bicontact stem: multicenter study of 553 cases. In: Weller S, Volkmann R (eds) The Bicontact hip system. Thieme, Stuttgart, pp 63–74
28. Weller S, Braun A, Gellrich JC, Gross U (1999) Importance of prosthesis design and surface structure for primary and secondary stability of uncemented hip joint prostheses. In: Learmonth ID (ed) Interfaces in total hip arthroplasty. Springer, London, pp 81–101
29. Volkmann R, Eingartner C, Winter E, et al (1998) Mid term results in 500 titanium alloy straight femoral shaft prostheses—cemented and cementless technique. Eur J Orthop Surg Traumatol 8:133–139
30. Eingartner C, Volkmann R, Winter E, et al (2000) Results of an uncemented straight femoral shaft prosthesis after 9 years of follow-up. J Arthroplasty 15(4):440–447
31. Eingartner C, Volkmann R, Winter E, et al (2001) Results of a cemented titanium alloy straight femoral shaft prosthesis after 10 years of follow-up. Int Orthop 25:81–84
32. Eingartner C, Heigele T, Dieter J, et al (2003) Long term results with the BiCONTACT System: aspects to investigate and to learn from. Int Orthop 27(suppl 1):S11–S15
33. Eingartner C, Heigele T, Volkmann R, et al (2006) Long-term results of an uncemented straight femoral shaft prosthesis. Hip Int 6:23–32
34. Eingartner C, Ilchmann T, Dieter J, et al (2005) Subsidence pattern of a cementless straight titanium femoral stem: a radiographic study with EBRA-FCA. Hip Int 15:85–91
35. Biedermann R, Krismer M, Stöckl B, et al (1999) Accuracy of EBRA-FCA in the measurement of migration of femoral components of total hip replacement. Einzel-Bild-Röntgen-Analyse femoral component analysis. J Bone Joint Surg [Br] 81:266–272
36. Reiter A, Gellrich JC, Bachmann J, et al (2003) Changes of periprosthetic bone mineral density in cementless bicontact stem implantation; influence of different para-meters. A prospective 4-year follow-up (in German). Z Orthop Ihre Grenzgeb 141(3): 283–288
37. Braun A, Hieda H, Domae Y (2005) Hip joint symposium 2004. Bicontact 10 years summit conference, Japan. B. Braun Aesculap, Tokyo
38. Yoo JJ, Kim YM, Yoon KS, et al (2005) Follow-up study alumina-on-alumina total hip arthroplasty. A five-year minimum. J Bone Joint Surg [Am] 87:530–535

Crowe Type IV Developmental Hip Dysplasia: Treatment with Total Hip Arthroplasty. Surgical Technique and 25-Year Follow-up Study

Luc Kerboull, Moussa Hamadouche, and Marcel Kerboull

Summary. A consecutive series of 118 total hip arthroplasties was performed for Crowe type IV developmental hip dysplasia in 89 patients. The mean age of the patients was 52 years. All procedures were carried out through a transtrochanteric approach by the same surgeon. In all cases, the acetabular component was placed at the level of the true acetabulum. The mean lengthening of the operated limb was 3.8 cm. The average follow-up of the whole series was 16.9 years. At the last follow-up evaluation, 41 patients (48 hips) had died and 7 patients (9 hips) were lost to follow-up. Forty patients (61 hips) were still alive at a mean follow-up of 22 years. At the time of last follow-up, the mean Merle d'Aubigné hip score was 17 compared with 10.6 preoperatively. The survival rate, with revision for any reason as the endpoint, was 75% at 25-year follow-up.

Key words. Hip arthroplasty, Congenital dislocation, Long term

Introduction

In complete congenital dislocation of the hip, the femoral head is located entirely outside the original acetabulum, whether or not the hip has been treated during childhood. In this condition, the femoral head articulates with the iliac wing, superiorly to the true acetabulum or superiorly and posteriorly. The true acetabulum is usually small, porotic, triangularly shaped, and filled with fatty and fibrous tissue. The anterior wall is thin, whereas the posterior ischial wall is thick. The femur also is dysplastic, with a narrow medullary canal, a small head, and an anteverted neck, but of normal length. This distorted anatomy may have been worsened by surgical procedures, especially femoral valgus osteotomy.

Subsequent additional anatomical abnormalities include an elongated capsule, extending from the rim of the true acetabulum to the femoral head. The course of the nerve and arteries is altered, but they are not actually shortened. The periarticular muscles are not contracted substantially; some, such as the external rotators, are elongated. Their courses frequently are altered, however.

Marcel Kerboull Institute, 39 Rue Buffon, 75005 Paris, France

The abnormal location of the hip in association with the frequent asymmetry of the dislocation accounts for several anatomical and physiological changes, including leg length discrepancy, pelvic tilt, structural changes in the lumbosacral spine, and malalignment of the ipsilateral knee. Total hip arthroplasty (THA), performed for developmental dysplasia of the hip, aims at providing the patient with a pain-free, stable, and mobile hip, while equalizing leg length and decreasing low back and knee pain through the improvement of static body balance.

At our institution, the senior author (M.K) started performing THA for Crowe type IV dislocated hips in 1970 despite Charnley and Feagin's [1] strong advice "not to attempt the operational reconstruction of nonreduced congenital dislocated hips." This chapter reports on the long-term clinical and radiologic outcome of THA performed for Crowe type IV dislocated hips [2]. These hips correspond to type III or IV of Eftekhar [3] or total dislocation of Hartofilakidis et al. [4] and Harris et al. [5].

Materials and Methods

A total of 89 patients (8 men and 81 women) had 119 Crowe type IV developmental hip dysplasias. Of the 119 complete dislocations, 30 were bilateral, and 59 were unilateral with the contralateral hip being in a low dislocation or subluxation situation (15 hips), dysplastic (23 hips), or normal (21 hips). This group of patients underwent 118 consecutive THAs performed between 1970 and 1986. All the procedures were carried out by the senior author (M.K.). The mean age of the patients at the time of the index THA was 52 years (range, 29–78 years). For 34 of the 118 dislocated hips, THA was the first procedure; the remaining 84 hips underwent various surgical procedures before THA, including attempted open reduction (11 hips), shelf procedure (32 hips), femoral osteotomy (23 hips), Girdlestone (8 hips), arthrodesis (1 hip), and cup or acrylic arthroplasty (9 hips). In no instance, however, was the femoral head replaced into the true acetabulum. The indication for THA was pain in the dislocated hip, associated with stiffness and limitation in activity, for 78 of the 89 patients. In the remaining 11 patients (12.4%), lower back or ipsilateral knee pain was the primary complaint.

Preoperatively, a thorough assessment of the patients was performed, including evaluation of the dislocated and contralateral hip and the state of the knees and lumbosacral spine. Pelvic tilt, fixed deformities, lumbosacral residual motion, leg shortening, true and apparent leg length discrepancy, knee malalignment, and skeletal disorders resulting from previous operations were noted. Several radiographs were obtained during the assessment. Anteroposterior and lateral radiographs of the lumbosacral spine in a standing position were obtained routinely, with a long-standing view of the lower part of the body with anteroposterior and lateral radiographs of the pelvis and upper part of the femur.

The prostheses used in this series were original Charnley (Thackray, Leeds, England) for 10 patients and Charnley–Kerboull (MK1; Benoist Gierard, Howmedica, Herouville Saint Clair, France) for 79 patients. Both components were cemented with CMW type 1 (Thackray). Before the operation, preoperative planning was done to determine the suitable components, the level of neck section with respect to the desirable lengthening of the operated limb, and sometimes the need for an alignment femoral osteotomy.

The surgical technique has been described in detail elsewhere [6]. The THA was carried out with the patient in a lateral decubitus position, through a transtrochanteric approach. Joint capsule, scar fibrous tissue, shelf, and osteophytes were removed carefully and completely. The dissection of the inferior part of the elongated capsule led to the true acetabulum, which was exposed properly by a hooked retractor inserted beneath the inferior margin. The acetabulum then was prepared to obtain a hemispherical bone cavity with the use of curved gouges. No reaming of the cavity was performed because of the inherent fragility of the acetabular walls. A socket, 37 to 42 mm in outside diameter, was cemented into the acetabular cavity. In 81 of the 118 procedures, a bone autograft obtained from the femoral head and neck was used to enlarge and reinforce the roof on the undeveloped original acetabulum. The femoral component was implanted at the level of the lesser trochanter except in 5 hips, in which it had to be placed below. In this series, a femoral osteotomy was performed in 21 hips. In 19 of them, the osteotomy was performed to align an angulated femur that had been osteotomized previously, whereas in 2 hips the osteotomy was performed to shorten the femur. Although reduction was usually tight, muscle releases or tenotomies were not performed. Reduction was achieved by pressure directed inferiorly on the femoral neck, with the limb held in adduction, the hip flexed slightly, and the knee flexed at 90° to relax the sciatic nerve. Reattachment of the greater trochanter was carried out routinely using three or four wires. Postoperative treatment included anticoagulation therapy and systemic antibiotics. Passive motion exercises of the operated joint were undertaken immediately postoperatively. Patients were free to walk with two supports after 3–7 days. Full weight-bearing usually was allowed after 6 weeks.

Clinical and radiologic evaluation was performed every year for the first 5 postoperative years and every 2–3 years thereafter. Hip functional results were rated according to the d'Aubigné grading system [7] and the Harris hip score [8]. The hip score was classified into six categories: excellent, 18 points; very good, 17 points; good, 16 points; fair, 15 points; poor, 14 points; and bad, ≤13 points. Radiologic analysis was performed on serial anteroposterior radiographs of the pelvis. On the pelvic side, the position of the socket relative to the horizontal and vertical teardrop lines according to De Lee and Charnley [9] were noted. Linear wear was measured according to the technique described by Livermore et al. [10]. On the femoral side, parameters investigated included the evolution of radiolucent lines in the seven zones of the femur and stem subsidence. Loosening was defined according to the criteria of Johnston et al. [11] as definite, probable, and possible. A long-standing radiograph of the lower part of the body was performed 1 year postoperatively to assess the result of the THA pelvic tilt, leg lengthening, and residual length discrepancy. Finally, correction of the lordosis and lateral curvature of the spine were evaluated on anteroposterior and lateral radiographs of the lumbar spine.

A survivorship analysis was performed to determine the overall success of the THA. Failure was defined as an implant that had been revised or that was radiologically loosened at the time of follow-up. The survival curve was derived from the cumulative survival rate over time, as calculated from the actuarial life table.

At the last follow-up evaluation, 41 patients (48 hips) had died and 7 patients (9 hips) were lost to follow-up. The follow-up of 48 patients ranged from 1 to 10 years for 14 and 10 to 27 years for the remaining 34. Forty patients (61 hips) were still alive with a mean follow-up of 22 years (range, 18–32 years). The average follow-up of the whole series was 16.9 years (range, 1–32 years).

Results

Complications were as follows. One intraoperative fracture of the femur was treated with cerclage wires and healed with no further complication. One peroneal nerve palsy recovered completely less than 1 week after the procedure. Two nonunions of the greater trochanter required revision to unite. One patient experienced a dislocation 2 weeks after THA. An open reduction had to be performed, and no further episode was observed.

Heterotopic ossifications were observed in four hips and were classified according to Brooker et al. grading [12]: Brooker II in two hips, Brooker III in one hip, and Brooker IV in one hip. The two latter hips had to be revised to perform heterotopic bone removal. No case of infection was recorded in this series.

At the last follow-up examination, clinical results according to the d'Aubigné [7] grading system were rated as excellent in 56 of the 118 hips (47.5%), very good or good in 33 hips (28%), pretty good in 11 (9.3%), and poor in 18 hips (15.2%). The mean functional d'Aubigné hip score improved from 10.6 preoperatively to 17 at the latest follow-up. The mean Harris hip score [8] improved from 32 preoperatively to 86 at the latest follow-up. Of the 118 hips, 10 had a persistent instability and a positive Trendelenburg sign. In the 19 hips in which a femoral alignment osteotomy was performed in conjunction with the THA (Fig. 1), the results were rated as good or excellent in 16 hips (82%). The mean functional hip score in this group of patients was 16.9.

One femoral and 22 acetabular definite loosenings occurred in this series. Twenty-one of them were revised 6–21 years postoperatively. Two additional hips were revised for heterotopic bone formation. In this respect, of the 118 hips, 23 hips were revised

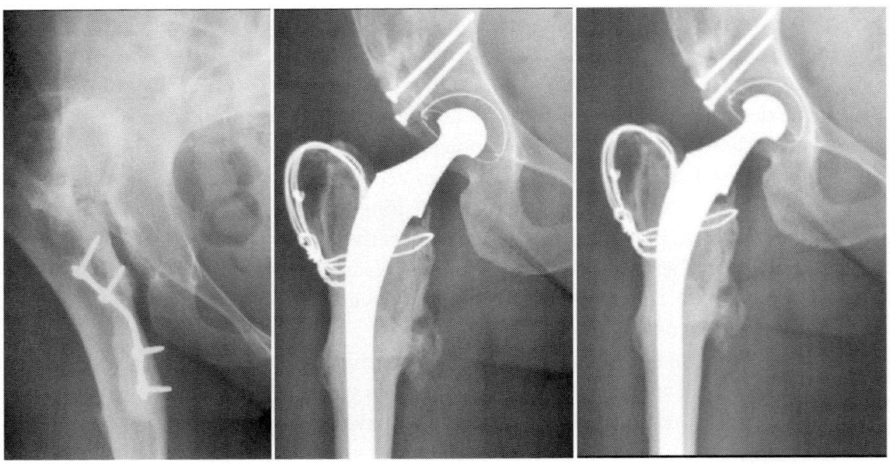

FIG. 1. This 41-year-old woman had in her childhood a previous abduction osteotomy for the treatment of a total hip dislocation. A total hip replacement was performed with an alignment femoral osteotomy and acetabular augmentation. *Right:* X-rays 18 years postoperative show only mild wear of the cup without any change of the fixation of the implants

at a mean of 15 years follow-up (19.5%). The survivorship analysis, with radiologic loosening as the endpoint, yielded a 99% cumulative survival rate at 20 and 25 years, respectively, for the femoral component and, for the acetabular component, 87% at 20 years and 79% at 25 years. The survival rate of the THA with revision for any reason as the endpoint was 78% at 20 years and 75% at 25-year follow-up.

The average preoperative limb shortening measured 4.8 cm (range, 3–8 cm). Full correction was possible in 63 of the 118 hips and within 1 cm in 42 hips. The mean lengthening of the operated limb was 3.8 cm (range, 2–7 cm). The mean leg length discrepancy measured 2.6 cm preoperatively versus 0.4 cm after THA. Fifty-nine patients had no residual discrepancy after THA, whereas leg length discrepancy was 1–3 cm in the remaining 30 patients. The leg length discrepancy decreased in 69 patients, remained unchanged in 14 patients who had no preoperative discrepancy, and increased in 3 patients. In 2 patients, the preoperative leg length discrepancy was so significant that a diaphyseal shortening of the longer femur was performed to obtain equality (Fig. 2).

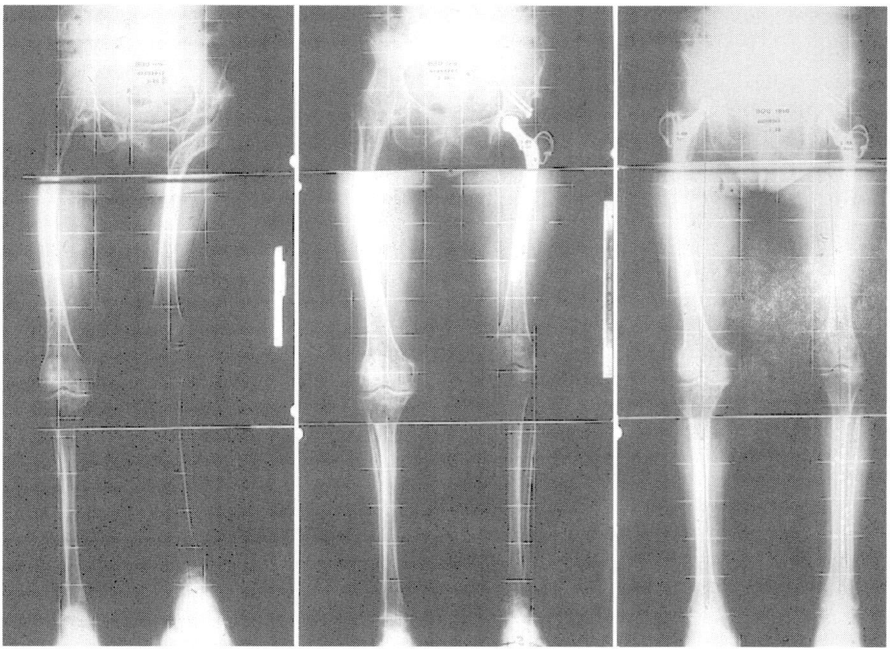

Fig. 2. A 75-year-old woman with a high dislocation of the left hip associated with a major diaphyseal femoral angulation and an apparent valgus of the knee of 20°. On the right side, there is an ankylosed hip associated with an arthritic varus deformity of the knee. Lateral pelvic tilt and leg length discrepancy are noted. The main complaint was low back and knee pain. After bilateral total hip arthroplasty (THA) combined with a femoral alignment osteotomy on the left side and femoral shortening on the right side, leg length discrepancy and pelvic tilt and malalignment of the knee have decreased greatly. Low back pain has been relieved completely, and function of the knees has been improved greatly

The reconstruction of the hip at the level of the true acetabulum resulted in a medialization of the hip, which could increase a valgus deformity, usually by 5°–10°, which is often not enough to relieve knee pain completely. The correction of an abduction position of the femur owing to a stiff hip or a femoral angulation improves the function of the ipsilateral knee. Of the 18 painful knees before THA, symptoms were improved greatly in 10, whereas 8 required an osteotomy or a total knee arthroplasty.

Lateral pelvic tilt was corrected in more than 50% of the cases, at least partially, as also were lordosis and lateral curve of the lumbar spine. Low back pain was reduced in 40 patients, but 4 patients required a laminectomy for treatment of a lumbar canal stenosis.

Discussion

Most authors have recommended the use of a transtrochanteric approach to perform a THA on a dislocated hip. Some have favored the so-called trochanteric slide, however, to reduce the risk of trochanteric nonunion [13–15]. In the senior author's experience, no major difficulties were encountered during trochanteric reattachment. We believe that careful trochanteric reattachment can prevent most of the these problems, as in the current series only 2 nonunions of 118 procedures (1.7%) occurred. Different approaches have been described in these complex situations, including a subtrochanteric osteotomy [16], a Smith-Petersen approach [17], and an extended iliofemoral approach [18]. These exposures required tendon and soft tissue release, however, which may increase the risk of muscle weakness and subsequent hip instability.

Generally, it is believed that the best location to place the socket is the level of the true acetabulum for mechanical and anatomical reasons. A small acetabular component, 37–42 mm outside diameter, combined with a 22.2-mm head and associated with a bone autograft obtained from the patient's femoral head and neck to achieve satisfactory acetabular superior and posterior coverage is, in our opinion, the best approach. Some authors [19–21] have recommended performing a deliberate and controlled fracture of the medial wall to place the prosthetic acetabular component within the available iliac bone to avoid the use of a bone graft. The early results of this acetabuloplasty were promising but did not provide, in the longer term, better results than those that have been obtained with bulk autograft bone. Some long-term studies have reported high rates of failure of the acetabular component related to bone graft resorption [22,23], although this complication did not occur in other reports [23–26]. In the current series, neither resorption of the graft nor acetabular loosening occurred in the absence of polyethylene wear and periacetabular osteolysis. We believe that graft resorption occurs primarily in association with osteolysis induced by polyethylene wear debris particles. The fate of uncemented sockets in the long term in the case of periacetabular osteolysis is debatable [27].

Muscle releases associated with tenotomies have been advocated to expose the true acetabulum properly or reduce the hip. We do not agree with this opinion. Great attention was always paid to retaining all the periarticular muscles. Bringing down the hip to the level of the true acetabulum and limb lengthening to 7 cm always was possible, provided that the entire articular capsule, scar tissue, osteophytes, and, when present, a shelf were removed. Retention of all the periarticular muscles results in better hip function, however, and protects the nerves and vessels against excessive elongation. This retention might be the reason for only 1 transient peroneal nerve palsy occurring in the current series, despite the fact that 30 limbs were lengthened more than 4 cm. The risk of nerve palsy increases in the case of high dislocation with a lengthening superior to 4 cm, and it has been recommended that limb lengthening be limited to 4 cm or even 2 cm. We believe that limb lengthening greater than 4 cm can be safe, provided that tension in the sciatic nerve is assessed intraoperatively and reduction of the hip is performed with the limb in adduction, the hip slightly flexed, and the knee flexed by 90°. This position should be maintained for 5–8 days postoperatively.

Bringing down the hip to the level of the dysplastic true acetabulum, which is located lower than a normal acetabulum, requires shortening of the femur. Some have advocated the use of a diaphyseal resection, so as not to exceed 4 cm in lengthening. It also has been proposed to correct excessive antetorsion at the site of the osteotomy. We prefer to resect the neck at the level of the lesser trochanter, retaining the insertion of the psoas tendon, because we believe it is easier. In the current series, this approach almost always was enough to reduce the hip and to avoid any difficulty related to excessive femoral antetorsion. A small femoral component with a straight stem was required but not a custom-made implant. Shortening of the femur was carried out not because reduction of the hip was impossible, but because the contralateral femur below a normal hip had been shortened during adolescence to equalize leg length.

The results of the current series, previously reported [28], remain in the very long term satisfactory and durable, with a survival rate free of loosening at 25 years of 99% for the femoral component and 79% for the acetabular component. Comparison with other reported series is difficult because of the inclusion of dysplastic, subluxated, and dislocated hips in most of the series. We found in the literature only two series of Crowe type IV dislocated hips. Hartofilakidis et al. [29] reported on 84 hips at a mean of 7.1 years follow-up with a 13% failure rate at 6.4 years. Numair et al. [30] reported on the results of 46 Charnley THAs at a mean of 9.9 years follow-up with a revision rate of 17%.

THA for Crowe type IV developmental hip dysplasia is a safe and effective procedure, able to improve not only hip function but also lumbosacral and knee pain owing to a dramatic correction of static body balance. This procedure poses a wide spectrum of difficulties, however, and can represent serious risk of complications. A successful result depends on a complete preoperative assessment of the patient, attention to the details of the surgical procedure performed with an adequate prosthesis, and a reasonable selection of indications.

References

1. Charnley J, Feagin JA (1973) Low-friction arthroplasty in congenital subluxation of the hip. Clin Orthop 91:98
2. Crowe JF, Mani VJ, Ranawat C (1979) Total hip replacement in congenital dislocation and dysplastia of the hip. J Bone Joint Surg [Am] 61:15
3. Eftekhar NS (1978) Principles of total hip arthroplasty. Mosby, St. Louis

4. Hartofilakidis G, Stamos K, Karachalios T, et al (1996) Congenital hip disease in adults: classification of acetabular deficiencies and operative treatment with acetabuloplasty combined with total hip arthroplasty. J Bone Joint Surg [Am] 78:683
5. Harris WH, Crothers O, Oh I (1977) Total hip replacement and femoral-head bone-grafting for severe acetabular deficiency in adults. J Bone Joint Surg [Am] 59:752
6. Kerboull M (1996) Arthroplastie totale de hanche sur luxation congénitale. In: Encyclopédie médico-chirurgicale. Editions techniques orthopédie traumatologie. Elsevier, Amsterdam, pp 44–665B
7. Merle d'Aubigné 0 (1970) Cotation chiffrée de la fonction de la hanche. Rev Chir Orthop 56:481
8. Harris WH (1969) Traumatic arthritis of the hip after dislocation and acetabular fractures: treatment by mold arthroplasty: an end-result study using a new method of result evaluation. J Bone Joint Surg [Am] 51:737
9. De Lee J, Charnley J (1976) Radiological demarcation of cemented sockets in total hip replacement. Clin Orthop 121:20
10. Livermore J, Ilstrup D, Morrey B (1990) Effect of femoral head size on wear of the polyethylene acetabular component. J Bone Joint Surg [Am] 72:518
11. Johnston RC, Fitzgerald RH Jr, Harris WH, et al (1990) Clinical and radiographic evaluation of total hip replacement: a standard system of terminology fort reporting results. J Bone Joint Surg [Am] 72:161
12. Brooker AF, Bowerman JW, Robinson RA, et al (1973) Ectopic ossification following total hip replacement: incidence and method of classification. J Bone Joint Surg [Am] 55:1629
13. Glassman AH, Engh CA, Bobyn JD (1987) A technique of extensile exposure for total hip arthroplasty. J Arthroplasty 2:11
14. Masri BA, Campbell DG, Garbuz DS, et al (1998) Seven specialized exposures for revision hip and knee replacement. Orthop Clin N Am 29:229
15. Mercati E, Guary A, Myquel C, et al (1972) Une voie d'abord postero-externe de la hanche: intérêt de la réalisation d'un muscle digastrique. J Chir (Paris) 103:499
16. Yasgur DJ, Stuchin SA, Adler EM, et al (1997) Subtrochanteric femoral shortening osteotomy in total hip arthroplasty for high-riding developmental dislocation of the hip. J Arthroplasty 12:880
17. Cameron HU, Botsford DJ, Park YS (1996) Influence of the Crowe rating on the outcome of total hip arthroplasty in congenital hip dysplasia. J Arthroplasty 11:582
18. Kumar A, Shair AB (1997) An extended iliofemoral approach for total arthroplasty in late congenital dislocation of the hip: a case report. Int Orthop 21:265
19. Dunn HK, Hess WE (1976) Total hip reconstruction in chronically dislocated hips. J Bone Joint Surg [Am] 58:838
20. Hesse WE, Umber JS (1978) Total hip arthroplasty in chronically dislocated hips: follow-up study on the protrusio socket technique. J Bone Joint Surg [Am] 60:948
21. Gerber SD, Harris WH (1986) Femoral head autografting to augment acetabular deficiency in patients requiring total hip replacement: a minimum five-year and an average seven-year follow-up study. J Bone Joint Surg [Am] 68:1241
22. Mulroy RJ, Harris WH (1990) Failure of acetabular autogenous grafts in total hip arthroplasty: increasing incidence. A follow-up note. J Bone Joint Surg [Am] 72:1536
23. Kerboull M, Mathieu M, Sauzieres P (1987) Total hip replacement for congenital dislocation of the hip. In: Postel M, Kerboull M, Evrard J, et al (eds) Total hip replacement. Springer, New York, p 51
24. Kerboull M (1989) Implantation of a total prosthesis in the deformed hip-exemplified by congenital hip dislocation. Orthopade 18:397
25. Morsi E, Garbuz D, Stockley I, et al (1996) Total hip replacement in dysplastic hips using femoral head shelf autografts. Clin Orthop 324:164

26. Rodriguez JA, Huk OL, Pellicci PM, et al (1995) Autogenous bone grafts from the femoral head for the treatment of acetabular deficiency in primary total hip arthroplasty with cement: long-term results. J Bone Joint Surg [Am] 77:1227
27. Morsi E, Garbuz D, Gross AE (1996) Total hip arthroplasty with shelf grafts using uncemented cups: a long-term follow-up study. J Arthroplasty 11:81
28. Kerboull M, Hamadouche M, Kerboull L (2001) Total hip arthroplasty for Crowe type IV developmental hip dysplasia. J Arthroplasty 16:170
29. Hartofilakidis G, Stamos K, Karachalios T (1998) Treatment of high dislocation of the hip in adults with total arthroplasty. Operative technique and long-term clinical results. J Bone Joint Surg 80A:510–517
30. Numair J, Joshi AB, Murphy JCM, et al (1997) Total hip arthroplasty for congenital dysplasia or dislocation of the hip: survivorship analysis and long-term results. J Bone Joint Surg [Am] 79:1352

Total Hip Arthroplasty for High Congenital Dislocation of the Hip: Report of Cases Treated with New Techniques

Muroto Sofue[1] and Naoto Endo[2]

Summary. High congenital dislocation of the hip joint causes biomechanical instability around the hip. In most cases of high dislocation, the true acetabulum is small and the upwardly displaced femur is dysplastic with a narrow medullary canal, a small head and an anteverted neck. A joint-preserving procedure is not recommended for patients with this condition. Total hip arthroplasty is the most suitable procedure for responding to the needs of the present-day patient by providing a pain-free and mobile hip. The surgeon should keep in mind that the choice of components is directly related to postsurgery durability. To satisfying this requirement, the authors [1] have developed two new techniques. Herein authors report the cases that were treated with these techniques.

Key words. High dislocation of the hip, Crowe classification of the dysplastic hip, Enlargement of the true acetabulum, Enlargement of the medullary canal of the femur, Total hip arthroplasty

Introduction

Among patients with osteoarthritis secondary to congenital dislocation of the hip, those with high dislocations show poor ambulation with severe limping and usually experience a dull pain at the lumbar and pelvic region rather than pain of the hip joint itself. However, it is a known fact that symptoms and functional impairments caused by high dislocations increase with age and that conservative treatment alone is insufficient for middle-aged or older patients.

In high congenital dislocation of the hip, Crowe group III or IV [2], the femoral head is entirely outside the original acetabulum. A joint-preserving procedure is not recommended for patients with this condition. However, recent techniques of total hip arthroplasty have been established, and a certain degree of confidence has been acquired with regard to the lasting effectiveness of these techniques. Thus, painlessness, ability for weight-bearing, and mobility can be regained simultaneously by

[1] Department of Orthopaedic Surgery, Nakajo Central Hospital, 12-1 Nishihoncho, Tainai, Niigata 959-2656, Japan
[2] Division of Orthopedic Surgery, Niigata University Graduate School of Medical and Dental Sciences, 1-757 Asahimachi-dori, Niigata 951-8510, Japan

appropriate surgery, and such treatments are the most suitable for responding to the needs of the present-day patient.

In most cases of high dislocation, the true acetabulum is usually small, porotic, and triangularly shaped. The upwardly displaced femur is also dysplastic with a narrow medullary canal, a small head, and an anteverted neck, but of normal length (Fig. 1).

Initial attempts to reconstruct a high dislocation Crowe group III or IV [2], using a secondary acetabulum with formed osteophytes, have been performed in two cases. In these patients, however, poor ambulation persisted and a biomechanically stable joint could not be obtained, resulting in loosening of the acetabular cup at an early postoperative stage.

Figure 2A–C shows a case with these processes. These experiences suggest a necessity to improve the biomechanical relationship between the femoral head and the pelvis by implanting the artificial joint at the level of the original acetabulum. This necessity has also been stated in the literature by Eftekhar [4], Arcq [5], Azuma [6], and Yamamuro [7]. A second attempt to reconstruct the high dislocation, using a small-sized cup in the true acetabulum, had been performed, but this technique had a risk of abrasion of the high density polyethylene (HDP) and breakage of the component. Figure 2D–F shows a case in which the small-cup component was used, which

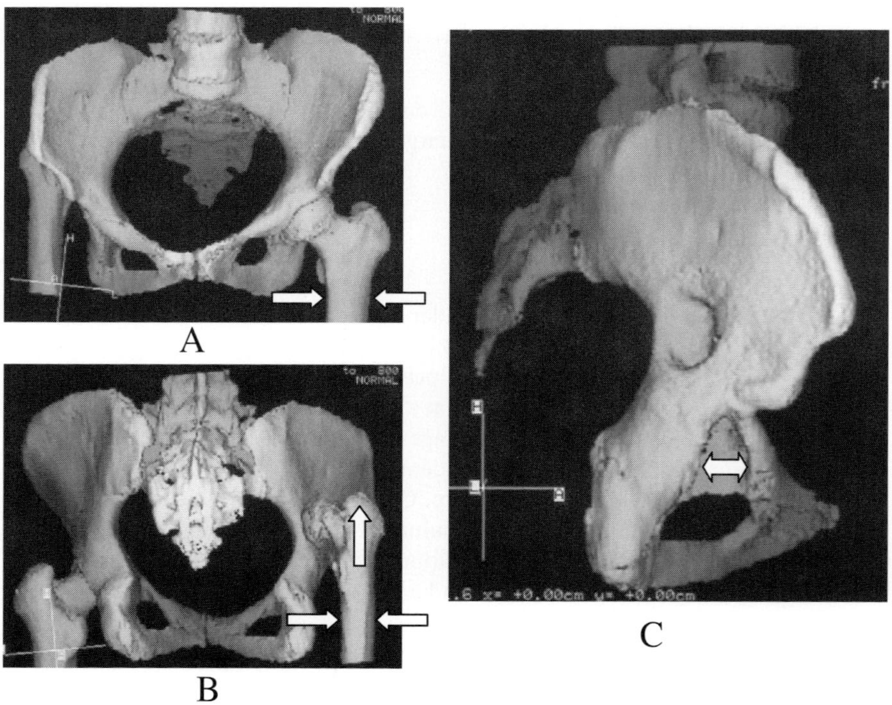

Fig. 1. A 62-year-old woman: three-dimensional (3D) computed tomography (CT) findings of right hip, Crowe group IV. **A** Anteroposterior (ap): left normal femur (*arrows*). **B** Posteroanterior (pa): right upper displaced slender femur (*arrows*). **C** Right lateral: narrow true acetabulum and pressure mark of the femoral head on iliac bone wall (*double-headed arrow*)

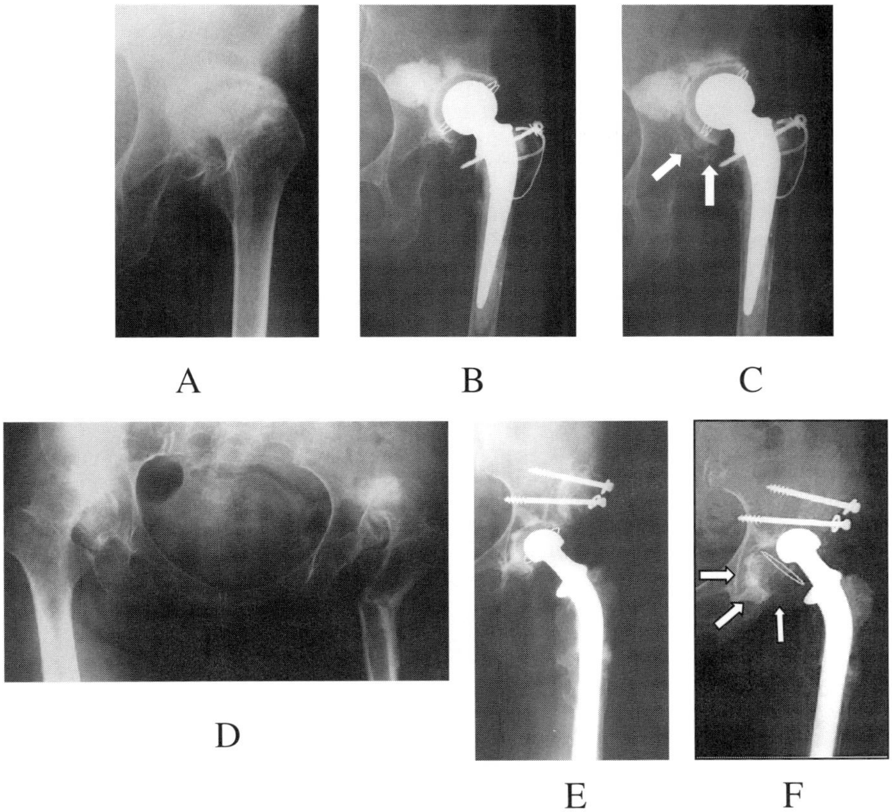

Fig. 2. **A–C** Upper case. **A** A 69-year-old woman with Crowe group III [2]. **B** Total hip replacement (THR) in the secondary acetabulum. **C** Upward migration (*arrow*) of the cup in a short period (2 years) after surgery. **D–F** Lower case. **D** A 52-year-old woman with left Crowe group IV [2]. **E** THR using a small cup. **F** Breakdown of the cup (*arrow*) in a short period (2 years) after surgery

resulted in a breakdown of the cup in a short period after surgery. If at all possible, a normal-sized component should be used.

These failures taught us that we should reconstruct a biomechanically stable condition around the hip by implanting the component in an anatomically correct position and keep in mind that using a normal-sized component is also of importance.

Original Technique

To satisfy this requirement, authors [1] developed two new techniques: the first one is for the acetabular side and the second one is for the femoral side.

In the first technique, to treat this narrow acetabulum, enlargement of its width is needed (see Fig. 4). Figure 3 shows the acetabulum in the normal and dislocated hip.

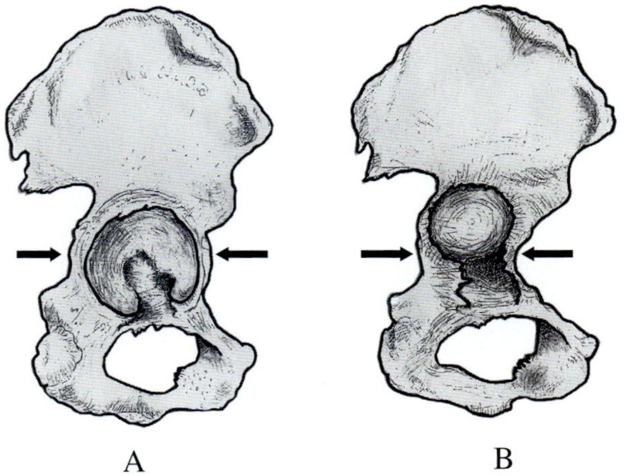

FIG. 3. Acetabulum in the normal (**A**) and dislocated (**B**) hip

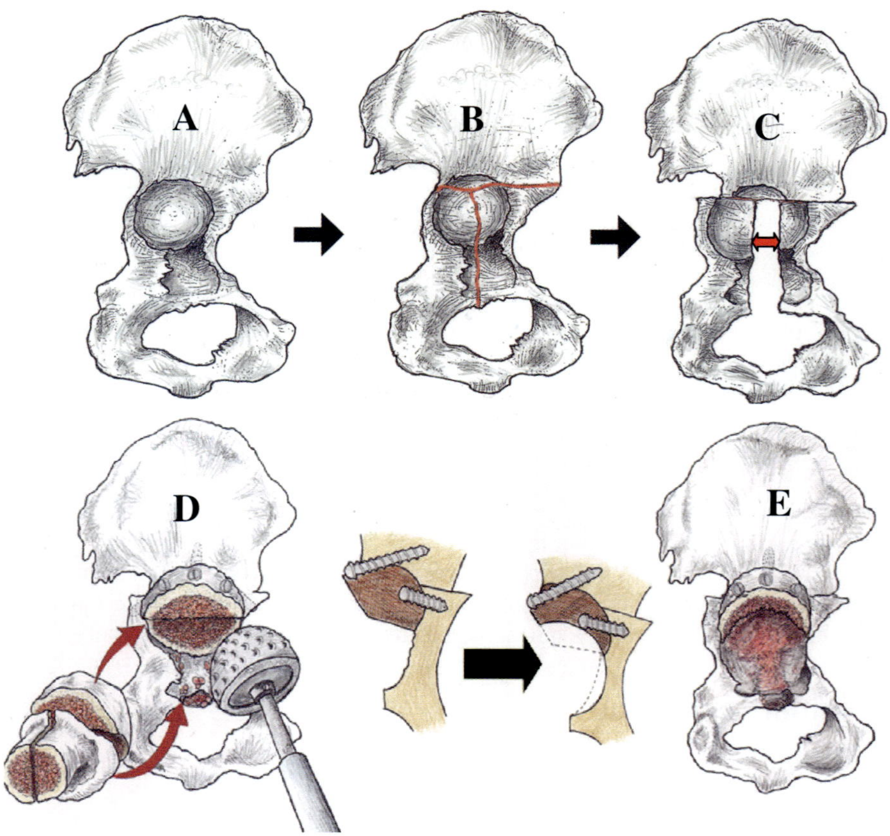

FIG. 4. Treatment of narrow acetabulum (1). **A** Narrow true acetabulum. **B** T-shaped osteotomy. **C** Enlargement. **D** Bone graft and reaming of the true acetabulum. **E** After reaming

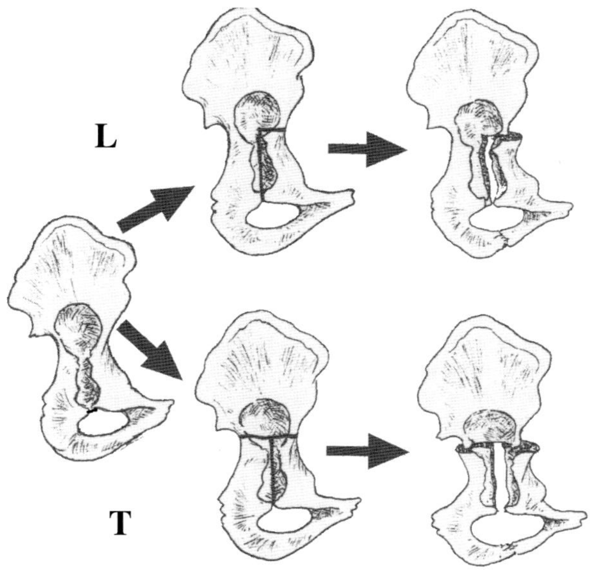

FIG. 5. Treatment of narrow acetabulum (2). *L*- or *T*-osteotomy

In the dislocated hip, in addition to the narrow true acetabulum the pelvic bone at the true acetabular level is narrow, especially in the anteroposterior direction. First, a T-shaped osteotomy is performed in the true acetabulum (Fig. 4B). Next, the osteotomized portion is enlarged while preserving the anterior and posterior walls (Fig. 4C). Then, bone grafting is done at the superior portion of the acetabulum and in the bone defect that is produced by the enlargement (Fig. 4D). Finally, reaming of the true acetabulum is performed (Fig. 4E).

If a very large enlargement is not needed, a L-shaped osteotomy is available (Fig. 5). After enlargement, the metal shell component with multiple screw holes should be implanted. The screws stabilize the shell, while at the same time stabilizing the enlarged portion (see Figs. 8B, 17B, 19B).

Case Reports

Patient 1

A 60-year-old woman with a bilateral hip dislocation, Crowe group IV [2], is shown in Fig. 6. The CT scan shows a narrow true acetabulum but a normal medullary canal of the femur on both sides (Fig. 7).

Surgery for the right side was performed in two stages. After enlargement of the true acetabulum, the metal shell was implanted in the first stage of the operation (Fig. 8B). The right leg was pulled down by skeletal traction while the patient was conscious. After adjusting the femur down to the expected level (Fig. 8C), the second procedure of implanting the femoral prosthesis and reducing the femoral head in the acetabulum was completed (Fig. 8D). For the left side, the same two-stage procedure was performed, and the total hip arthroplasty was successfully finished (Fig. 9).

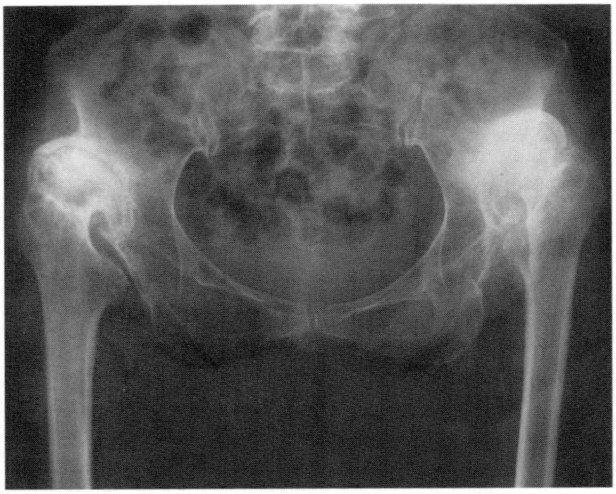

FIG. 6. A 60-year-old woman, bilateral hips with Crowe group IV

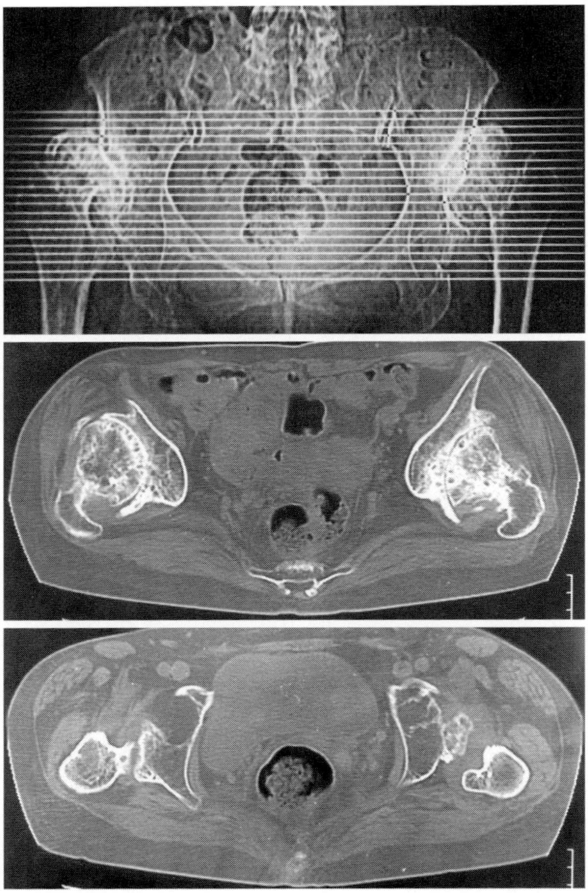

FIG. 7. Preoperative CT findings: narrow true acetabulum and normal medullary canal of the femur

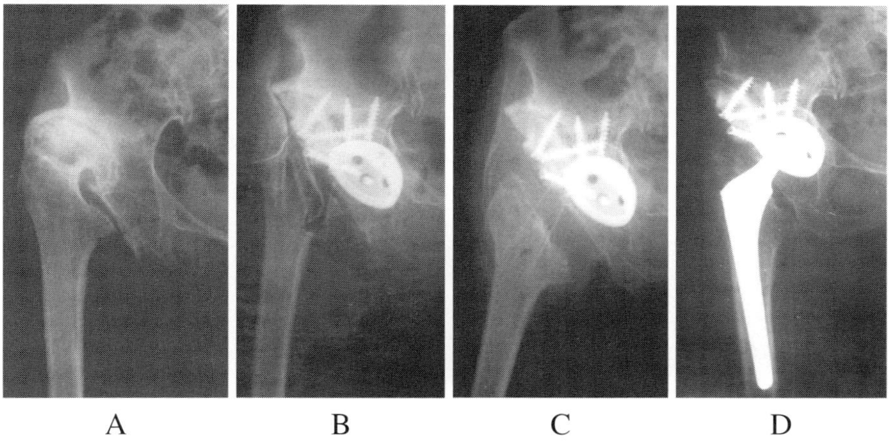

FIG. 8. Progression of the procedure for right hip. **A** Preoperative. **B** First stage of operation. **C** After traction. **D** Second state of operation

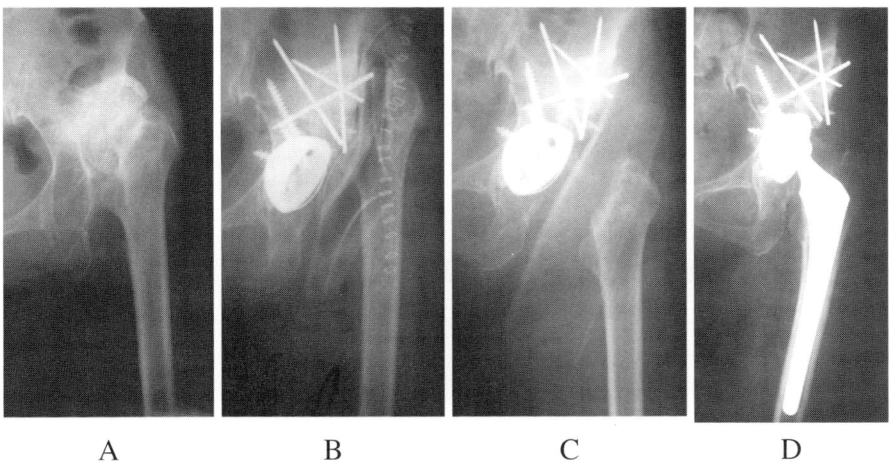

FIG. 9. Progression of the procedure for left hip. **A** Preoperative. **B** First stage of operation. **C** After traction. **D** Second stage of operation

Figure 10 show the findings at 1 month (A) and at 15 years (B) after surgery. The patient is now 75 years old, and X-ray findings show slight wear of the HDP cup component on the left side, which indicates the process should be carefully followed up.

Patient 2

A 50-year-old woman with Crowe group III [2] dysplasia of the right hip is shown in Fig. 11. After the enlargement of the true acetabulum, the patient received a

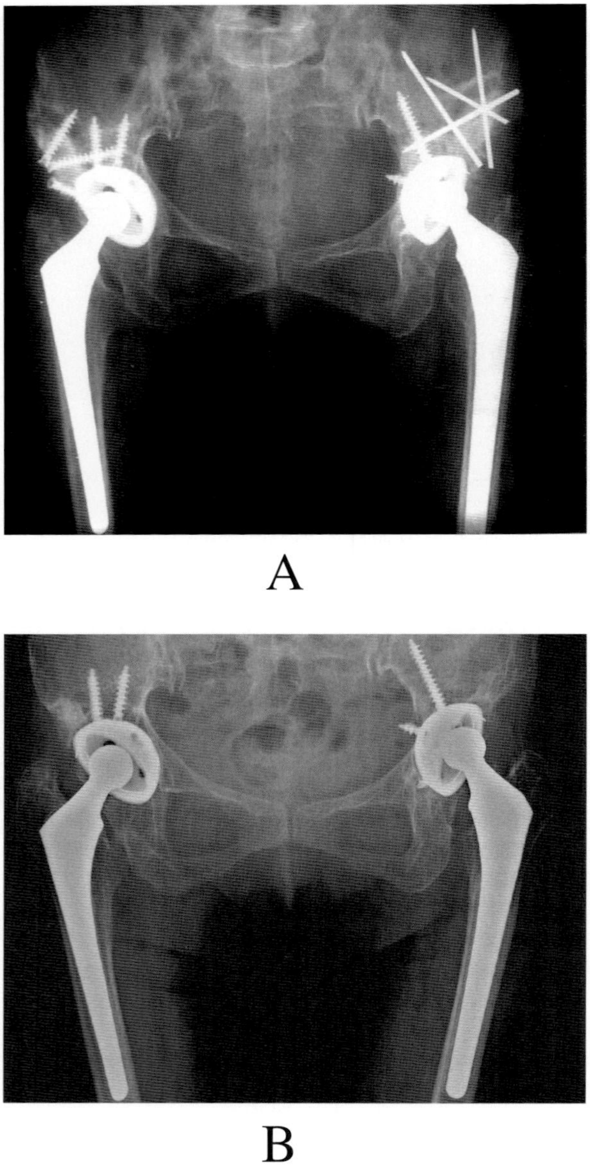

Fig. 10. X-ray findings at 1 month (**A**) and 15 years postoperative (**B**)

bipolar-type prosthesis, which showed central migration over a short period (Fig. 12). The bipolar prosthesis was revised and converted to a total hip prosthesis. Thirteen years after the conversion to total prosthesis, the hip is in good condition (Fig. 13). In this case, the total hip prosthesis would have been a better choice than the bipolar prosthesis at the first surgery.

Fig. 11. A 50-year-old woman, right hip, Crowe group III

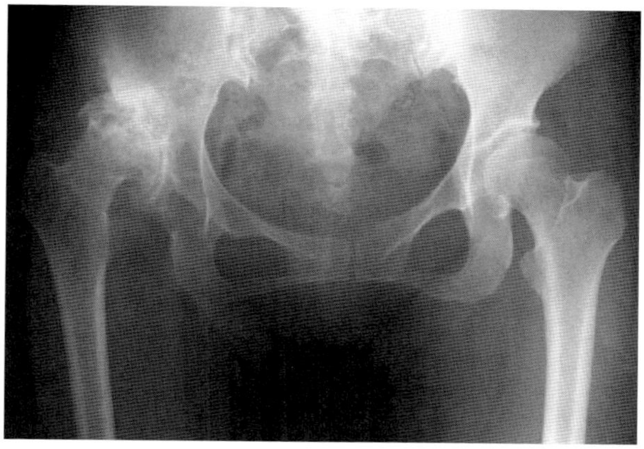

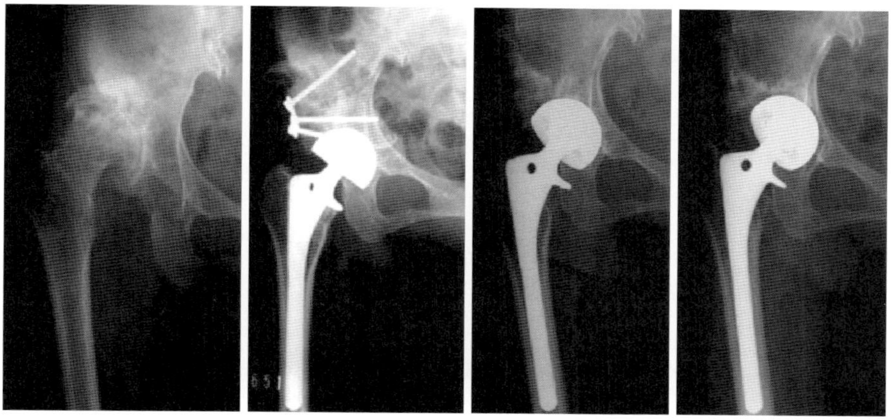

A B C D

Fig. 12. Bipolar prosthesis shows central migration in a short period after surgery. **A** Preoperative. **B** Operative with bipolar. **C** Two years postoperative. **D** Three years postoperative with migration

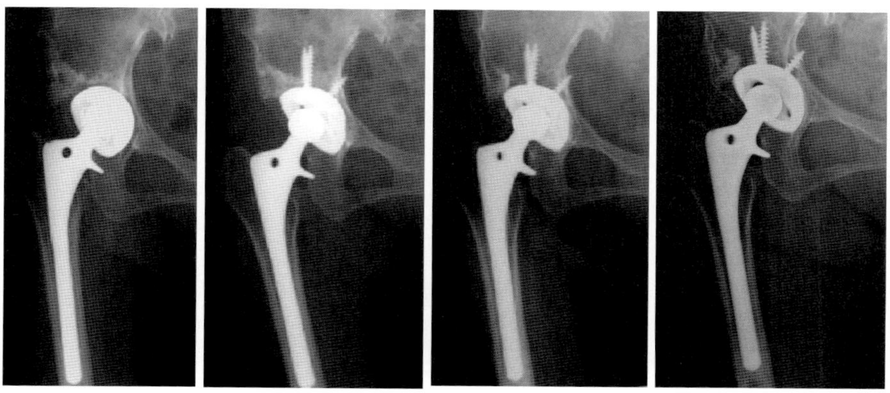

A B C D

Fig. 13. Bipolar prosthesis converted to THA. **A** Bipolar postoperative 3 years with migration (same as Fig. 12D). **B** Converted to THA. **C** Seven years after conversion. **D** Thirteen years after conversion

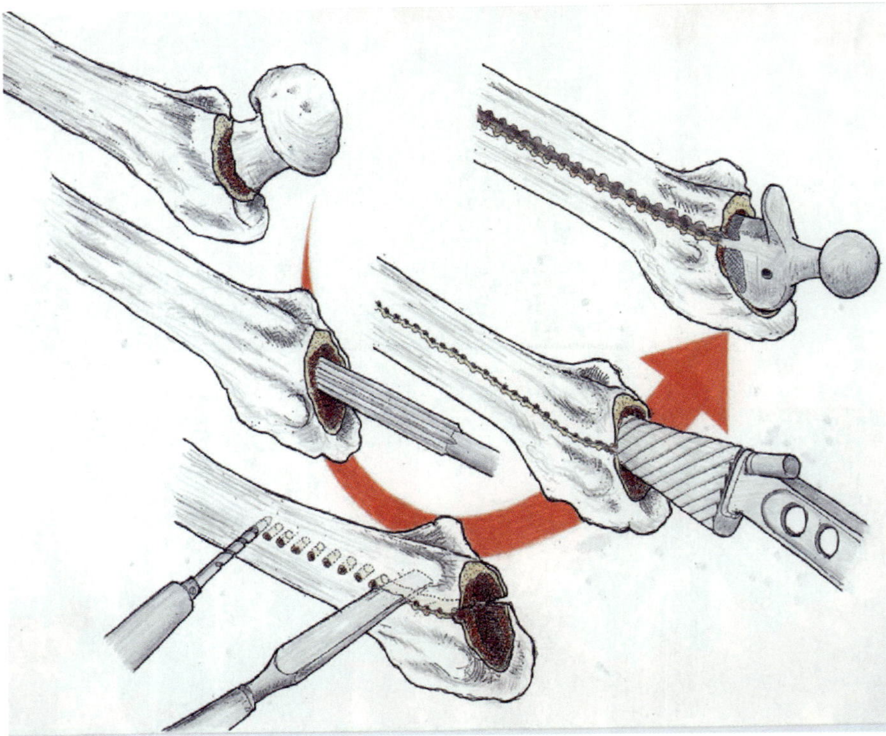

FIG. 14. Enlargement of the medullary canal of the femur

In the second technique, to treat the slender femur, enlargement of the medullary canal (Fig. 14) is performed. After femoral osteotomy at the base of the neck, multiple drill holes are made in the femur shaft in the anteroposterior direction 5 mm apart for 25 cm distally. A longitudinal osteotomy is made with an osteotome to split the femur along these holes. A rasp is used to enlarge the medullary canal to fit the selected stem size. Then, a cementless femoral component is implanted. After implantation of the prosthesis stem, four or five cerclage wires are wound around the femoral bone to stabilize the osteotomized portion (Fig. 15B; see Fig. 17D,E).

Patient 3

A 57-year-old woman with left unilateral high hip dislocation, Crowe group IV [2], is shown in Fig. 15A. In the CT scan, the upwardly displaced, slender femur and the narrow true acetabulum can be confirmed (Fig. 16A, B).

A two-stage operation was planned. In the first stage of the operation, enlargement of the true acetabulum and implantation of the metal shell were performed (Fig. 17B).

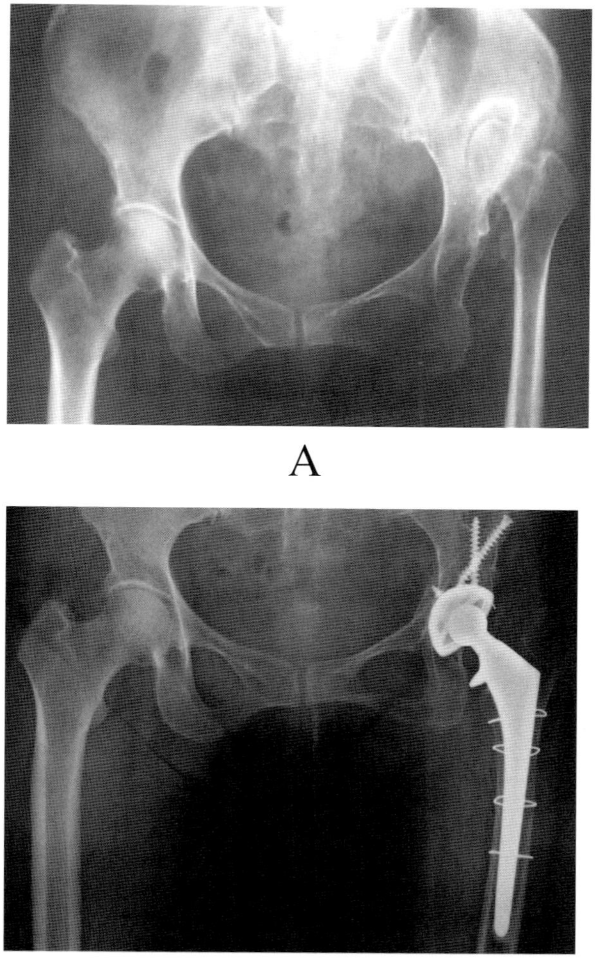

A

B

FIG. 15. A woman with high dislocation of left hip, Crowe group IV [2]. X-ray findings at 57 years of age, preoperative (**A**), and at 72 years of age, 15 years postoperative (**B**)

After the first stage of the operation was completed, the leg was pulled distally and the adjusting down of the femur was accomplished (Fig. 17C). In the second stage of the procedure, enlargement of the femoral medullary canal and implanting of the stem prosthesis were performed. After stabilizing the enlarged femur by cerclage wire, the femoral head was reduced and arthroplasty was completed (Fig. 17D, E). Figure 15B shows the 15-year postoperative X-ray finding.

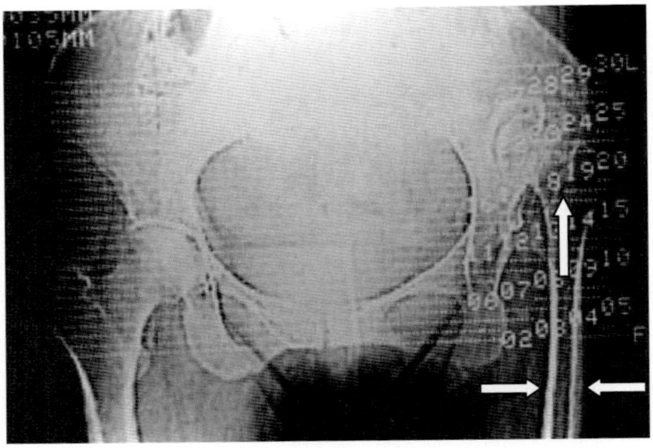

A

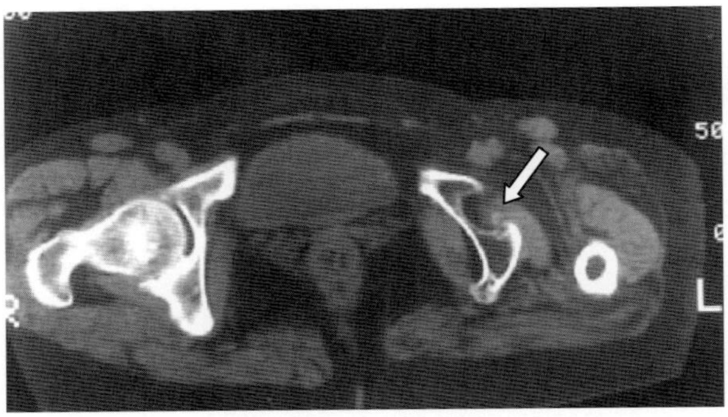

B

FIG. 16. CT findings (*arrows*): upward displaced slender femur (**A**) and small acetabulum (**B**)

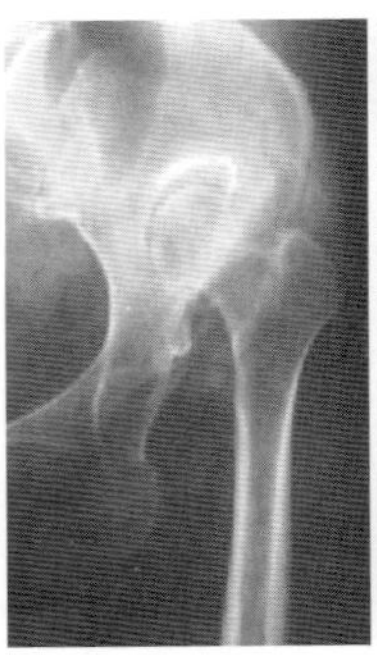

A

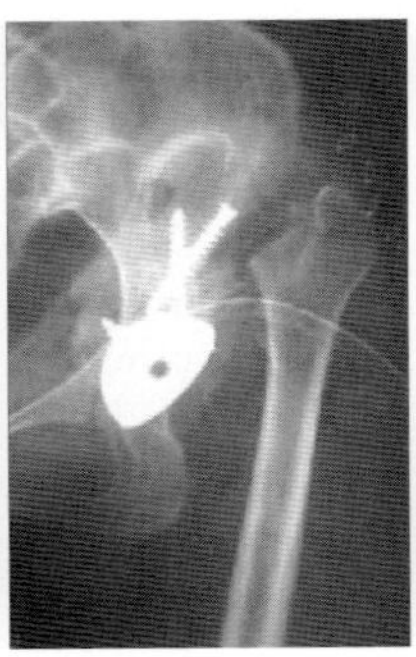

B

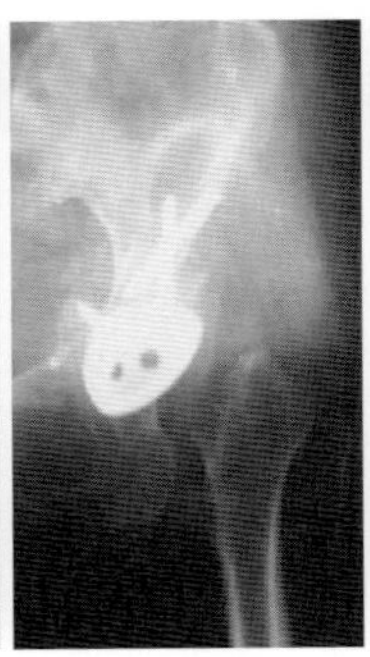

C

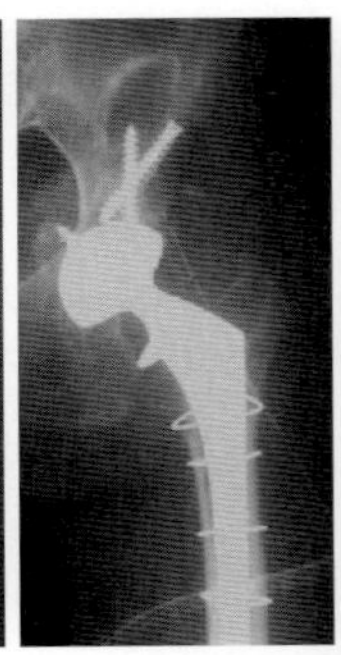

D

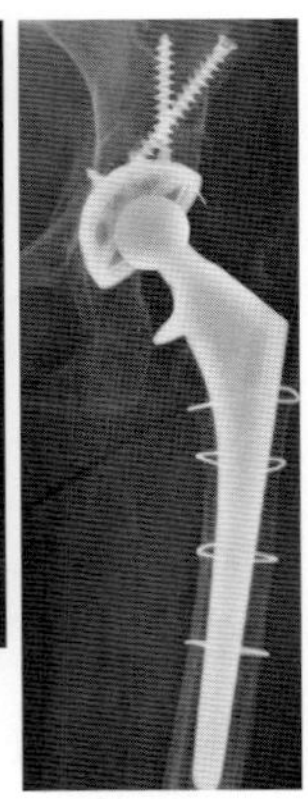

E

FIG. 17. Progression of the procedure: preoperative (**A**); first stage of operation (**B**); adjusting the femur downward by traction (**C**); second stage of operation (**D**); and 10 years after surgery (**E**)

Materials

Since 1987 we have treated 36 cases, 45 joints, with the above-described technique (Tables 1, 2). The age of patients at the time of surgery was from 40 to 69 years old. The majority were in their fifties, with 22 cases; the mean age was 57.2 years old. Ten cases were bilateral dislocations. Of 25 unilateral cases, 16 of the contralateral hips were in a low dislocation, Crowe group I or II, and 9 hips were normal.

Except for the two bipolar-type prosthetic joints, 43 joints of the cementless-type prosthesis with multiholed metal cup and straight stem were implanted. One-stage operations were done in 18 joints and two-stage operations were done in 27 joints. Enlargement of the acetabular side was done in 45 joints and of the femoral side in 4 joints. The size of acetabular component used was from 50 to 54 mm outside diameter. The size of femoral prosthesis used was number 7 or 8 from Stryker, or 10 or 11 mm from Zimmer.

TABLE 1. Cases of dysplastic hip, Crowe III and IV, treated with enlargement in 1987 to 2003

Number of cases:	36 (1 male, 35 female)
Number of joints:	45
Age (in years):	40 to 69 (mean: 57.2)
In forties:	8 cases
In fifties:	22 cases
In sixties:	6 cases
Side:	10 bilateral
	25 unilateral
Contralateral hip:	
OA:	16 cases (Crowe I or II [2])
Normal:	9 cases

OA, osteoarthritis

TABLE 2. Cases of dysplastic hip, Crowe III and IV, treated with enlargement in 1987 to 2003

Prosthesis:	
Bipolar:	2 joints
Cementless THR:	43 joints
Operation stage:	
1 stage:	18 joints
2 stages:	27 joints
Enlargement:	
True acetabulum:	45 joints
Femur:	4 joints
Size of acetabular cup:	50 to 54 mm
Size of femoral prosthesis:	
Nr 7 to 8 (Stryker)	
10 to 11 mm (Zimmer)	

THR, total hip replacement

Results

Preoperative limb shortening ranged from 20 to 70 mm with an average of 44.8 mm. Limb shortening was corrected after surgery in all cases to less than 10 mm. Follow-up time ranges from 2 to 17 years with the average being 10.7 years. The 10-year survival rate is 84.5% (Tables 3, 4).

The preoperative hip score, according to the Japanese Orthopaedic Association (JOA), was 34.5 points of a possible 100 points. The postoperative score improved to 83.6 points. In the pain category, the preoperative score was 5.8 points of a possible 40 points, and the postoperative score was 37.5 points.

Trendelenburg's sign [3] was clearly positive in all 45 preoperative joints. After surgery, 17 joints improved into negative and 20 joints showed a decrease of pelvic inclination. Eight joints remained in positive as before surgery.

Twelve cases of nerve palsy were observed. Of 7 cases of peroneal nerve palsy, 5 cases completely recovered in 6 months and slight paresthesia remained in 2 cases. 5 cases of femoral nerve palsy recovered completely in less than 1 month after the

TABLE 3. Cases of dysplastic hip, Crowe III and IV, treated with enlargement in 1987 to 2003

Limb shortening (preoperative):		20 to 70 mm (mean: 44.8 mm)
Limb shortening (postoperative):		<10 mm
Follow-up:		2–17 years (mean: 10.7 years)
10-year survival rate:		84.5%
JOA score:	Preoperative 34.5 to postoperative 83.6 (pain: preoperative 5.8 to postoperative 37.5)	
Trendelenburg's sign:		
Preoperative:		(+) all 45 joints
Postoperative:		(−) 17 joints
		(±) 20 joints
		(+) 8 joints

JOA, Japanese Orthopaedic Association

TABLE 4. Complications in cases of dysplastic hip, Crowe III and IV, treated with enlargement in 1987 to 2003

Nerve palsy:	12 cases
Peroneal nerve:	7 cases (5: fully recovered, 2: paraesthesia)
Femoral nerve:	5 cases (all fully recovered)
Dislocation:	7 cases
Closed reduction:	4 cases
Open reduction:	1 case
Converted to consrained type:	2 cases
Loosening:	9 cases
Acetabular side:	8 cases
Bipolar → cementless THR:	2 cases (within 3 years postoperative)
Cementless THR:	6 cases
Larger cementless:	4 cases
Supportring with bone cement:	2 cases
Femur side:	1 case → revision cementless stem

procedure. Seven dislocations were experienced. In 4 cases, closed reduction was performed under intravenous anesthesia and no further episodes were observed. In 1 case, an open reduction was necessary and no further episodes were seen. Because of the recurrent dislocations, it was necessary to convert to the constrained-type prosthesis in 2 cases. Loosening of the component was observed in 9 cases. 8 cases were at the acetabular side. Two bipolar cases were converted to cementless total hip arthroplasty. Among 6 cases of cementless total hip arthroplasty, 4 cases were revised by using the larger cementless cups and 2 cases had to be revised by using the cup supporter with bone cement. One case of femoral side loosening was revised by using the cementless type of revision prosthesis.

Discussion

In patients with poor acetabular bone stock, superior coverage of the acetabulum can be achieved by performing a horizontal osteotomy at the margin of the acetabulum, or by femoral head grafting as proposed by Harris et al. [8], Nagai et al. [9], Buchholz et al. [10], Matsuno [11], and Paavilainen et al. [12]. However, these techniques cannot improve anteroposterior bone deficiency, and extensive reaming of the acetabulum may lead to additional bone loss of anteroposterior osseous support.

Furthermore, it is not possible to remedy the thin femur and narrow femoral medullary canal solely with bone grafting. For treating a narrow medullary canal, the use of a narrow stem has been described by Charnley and Feagin [13], Buchholz et al. [10], and Eftekhar [4]. However, using a small component for the acetabulum or the femur has a greater risk of breakage or loosening. Therefore, the surgical methods described above were developed for the purpose of enlarging both acetabulum and femoral medullary canal. These methods permit inserting a normal-sized components into a small original acetabulum and into a narrow femoral canal without further wear of the bone stock.

Our first choice was a cementless bipolar-type prosthesis for patients in their forties. However, as can be seen in patient 2 (Fig. 12), the stability of the osteotomized acetabulum was insufficient. It is safer to use the multiholed metal outer shell and its screws to stabilize the shell, while at the same time stabilizing the osteotomized portion. After this experience, we decided the component for the acetabular side should be a multiholed metal cup.

To bring down the femur, which is necessary to implant the acetabular cup into the original true acetabulum, both the one-stage procedure (Kinoshita and Harana [13]; Kuroki et al. [14]) and the two-stage procedure (Kerboull et al. [16]; Inoue [17]; Arcq [5]) have been proposed. According to these authors, to adjust down the femur sufficiently and to enclose a gentle reduction, the two-stage procedure is employed for patients who require lengthening of more than 3 cm. Figure 18 shows the relationship between the distance of adjusting down and paralysis in our cases. Paralysis was observed in a case that required 2.5 cm pulling down distally. Because of this experience, we decided that the limit of adjusting down for the first stage should be less than 2.5 cm. In a case that requires more than 2.5 cm downward adjusting, we divide the surgery into two stages. When the surgery is divided into two stages, an acetabular cup is placed in the first stage and the soft tissue release is done. The adjusting is then performed while the patient is conscious to check for paralysis.

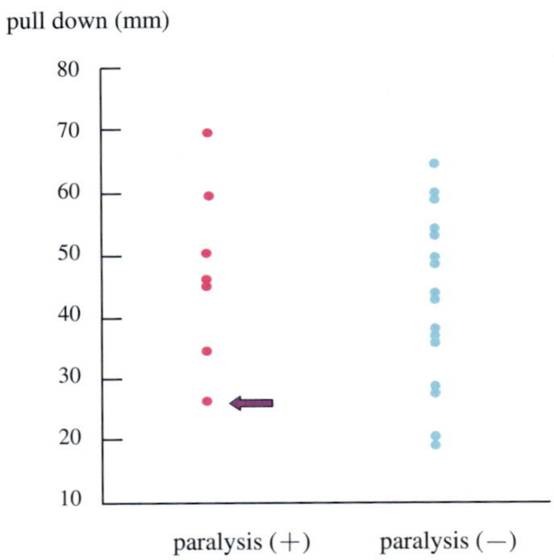

FIG. 18. Relationship between the distance pulled down and paralysis

Pulling down of the femur could be done quantitatively by using an external fixator. After the femur is pulled down to the level of the original acetabulum, the femoral prosthesis is implanted in the second stage and the joint is reduced. To avoid intra-operative nerve damage under anesthesia, monitoring of the spinal cord potential (SCP) is recommended. At each step of the operative procedure, the shape and the height of the SCP waves are checked. If there is no change in the waves, the surgery is advanced to the next step.

Patient 4

A 61-year-old woman with right side high dislocation, Crowe group IV, is shown in Fig. 19A. The SCP was checked in the first-stage operation (Fig. 19B). At each step, no change of the wave was observed (Fig. 19C), and no paralysis was found after the first-stage operation. After adjusting down the femur to the expected level (Fig. 20A), the second stage of the operation was performed while monitoring in the same way as the first stage (Fig. 20B), and the arthroplasty was successfully completed (Fig. 20C).

In general, not all patients with high dislocation of the hip joint require treatment with the method reported in this chapter. When, on the basis of preoperative CT scans, the original acetabulum and the femur are estimated to be narrow for normal-sized components and when the volume of the surrounding bone stock remaining after reaming is judged to be insufficient, this technique is utilized. Furthermore, if a conventional procedure can effectively be applied to a patient with high dislocation, it is not necessary to perform this method.

Conclusion

1. Total hip arthroplasty is recommended even for patients with high dislocation of the hip joint and aims at providing patients with a pain-free, stable, and mobile hip.

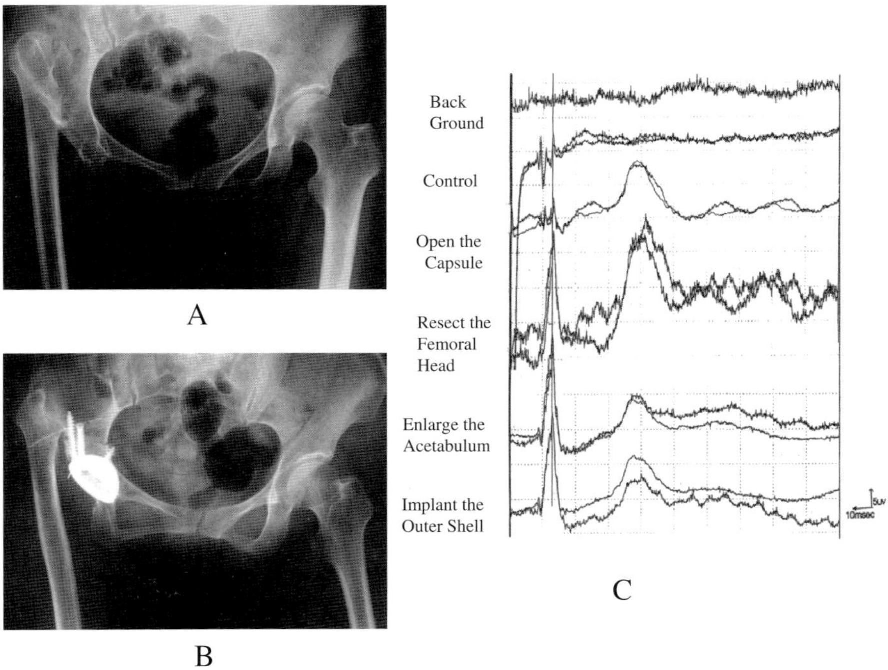

FIG. 19. A 61-year-old woman undergoing first stage of operation with spinal cord potential (SCP) monitoring: preoperative (**A**); after first stage of operation (**B**); SCP monitor findings in first stage of operation (**C**)

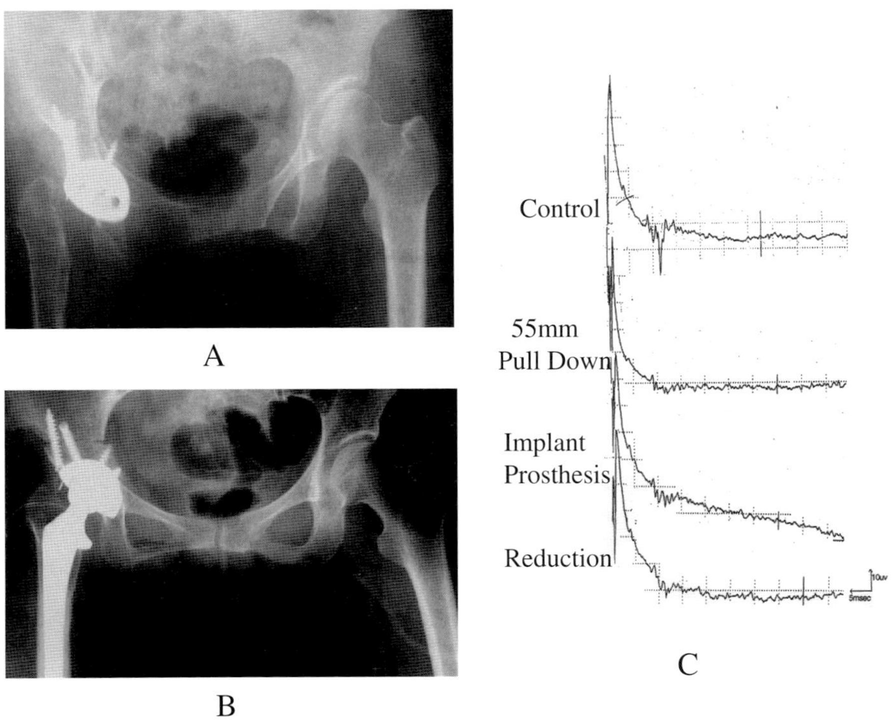

FIG. 20. Second stage of operation (same patient as in Fig. 19) with SCP monitoring: adjusting femur downward (**A**); after second stage of operation (**B**); SCP monitoring in second stage of operation (**C**) (continuation of Fig. 19)

2. In such patients, implantation of the component at the level of the original acetabulum is recommended, while equalizing leg length through the improvement of static body balance. For patients with an extremely narrow acetabulum and slender femur, a technique for enlarging the hypoplastic structure with subsequent use of normal-sized components is advantageous.

3. The method mentioned in this chapter is not suitable for all patients with a high dislocation of the hip joint, but it is indicated when preoperative CT scanning indicates the need for enlargement of the acetabulum and of the medullary canal. Selective enlargement of only the acetabulum or femoral side can be performed in selected instances.

References

1. Sofue M, Dohmae Y, Endo N, et al (1989) Total hip arthroplasty for secondary osteoarthritis due to congenital dislocation of the hip (in Japanese). Hip Joint 15:267–274
2. Crowe JF, Mani J, Ranawat CS (1979) Total hip replacement in congenital dislocation and dysplasia of the hip. J Bone and Joint Surg 61-A:15–23
3. Trendelenburg F (1985) Ueber Gang bei angeborener Hueftgelenkluxation. Dtsch Med Wochenschr 21–24
4. Eftekhar NS (1993) Congenital dysplasia and dislocation in total hip arthroplasty. Mosby, St. Louis, pp 925–963
5. Arcq M (1980) Einbau der Judet-Prothese bei einer hohen Hueftluxation. Z Orthop 118:265–269
6. Azuma T (1985) Preparation of the acetabulum to correct severe acetabular deficiency for total hip replacement—with special reference to stress distribution of periacetabular region after operation (in Japanese). J Jpn Assoc 59:269–283
7. Yamamuro T (1982) Total hip arthroplasty for high dislocation of the hip (in Japanese). J Jpn Joint Surg 1:23–35
8. Harris WH, Crothers O, Indong AO, et al (1977) Total hip replacement and femoral-head bone-grafting for severe acetabular deficiency in adults. J Bone Joint Surg 59A:752–759
9. Nagai J, Ito T, Tanaka S, et al (1975) Combined acetabuloplasty for the socket stability by the total hip replacement in dislocated hip arthrosis (in Japanese). Proc Jpn Res Assoc Replace Arthroplasty 5:23–24
10. Buchholz HW, Baars G, Dahmen G (1985) Frueherfahrungen mit der Mini-Hueftgelenkstotalendoprothese (Modell "St Georg-Mini") bei Dysplasie-Coxarthrose. Z Orthop 123:829–836
11. Matsuno T (1989) Long-term follow-up study of total hip replacement with bone graft. Arch Orthop Trauma Surg 108:14–21
12. Paavilainen T, Hoikka V, Solonen KA (1990) Cementless replacement for severely dysplastic or dislocated hip. J Bone Joint Surg 72B:205–211
13. Charnley J, Feagin JA (1973) Low-friction arthroplasty in congenital subluxation of hip. Clin Orthop 91:98–113
14. Kinoshita I, Hirano N (1985) Some problems about indication of total arthroplasty for secondary coxarthrosis (in Japanese). Cent Jpn J Orthop Trauma 18:328–330
15. Kuroki Y (1986) Total hip arthroplasty for high dislocation of the hip joint (in Japanese). Surgery (St. Louis) 40:1353–1358
16. Kerboull M, Hamadouche M, Kerboull L (2001) Total hip arthroplasty for Crowe type IV developmental hip dysplasia. J Arthroplasty 16:170–176
17. Inoue S (1983) Total hip arthroplasty for painful high dislocation of the hip in the adult (in Japanese). In: Congenital dislocation of the hip. Kanehara, Tokyo, pp 257–266

A Biomechanical and Clinical Review: The Dall–Miles Cable System

Desmond M. Dall

Summary. The Dall–Miles Cable System (Stryker Orthopaedics, Mahwah, NJ, USA) has been in clinical use since 1983. It was initially developed for reattachment of the greater trochanter in low-friction arthroplasty of the hip. The clinical uses have evolved considerably over the years. It is now used largely as a cerclage system, particularly in revision total hip arthroplasty (THA). A biomechanical review includes a comparison of the mechanical strength of different cerclage systems. The strength of wire and cable fastening systems is examined. The importance of fatigue strength is presented and discussed. The relationship between tensile strength and fatigue performance is analyzed, and comparative data are presented. A review of the clinical use of cable cerclage is presented, including fixation of the greater trochanter in various trochanteric osteotomy approaches to the hip, the use of the system in revision THA, femoral allografts, its use in fixation of periprosthetic fractures of the femur in THA, and the use of the system in augmentation of other forms of fracture fixation, emphasizing its value in the treatment of fractures in soft bone.

Key words. Dall–Miles, Cable, Biomechanical, Clinical

Introduction

Cerclage systems have been used in many clinical situations, mainly to provide, or assist in, fixation of bony fragments and occasionally of long bones. Materials have included stainless steel, chrome cobalt, titanium alloy, and nylon. Monofilament wires or bands have been used for many decades, but it was not until the late 1970s that Dall and Miles were the first to use multifilament cable in the fixation of the greater trochanter when osteotomized as an approach to the hip in total hip arthroplasty. Our early results were first published in 1983 [1].

Emeritus Professor of Clinical Orthopaedics, University of Southern California, Los Angeles, CA, USA

The Strength of Cerclage Systems

It is important to appreciate that the stress–strain curves of different cerclage systems (e.g., monofilament versus multifilament) will be the same if the cerclage systems are made of the same material. However, the load-deflection curves will be different because of the structural differences even in the same material. Thus, yield and breaking loads are the most useful measurement of mechanical strength. The other important aspect of strength in cerclage systems is that of fatigue strength, which I discuss later. Figure 1a shows the comparative yield and ultimate tensile strengths of different systems in the same material, and Fig. 1b illustrates the comparative yield and ultimate tensile strength of different geometric systems in different materials.

Strength of Fastening Methods in Different Cerclage Systems

There are great variations in the method of fastening used in cerclage systems. There is also great variation in the measurements used, and these could include measurements of displacement, slip or yield, and failure loads. There is also a great variation

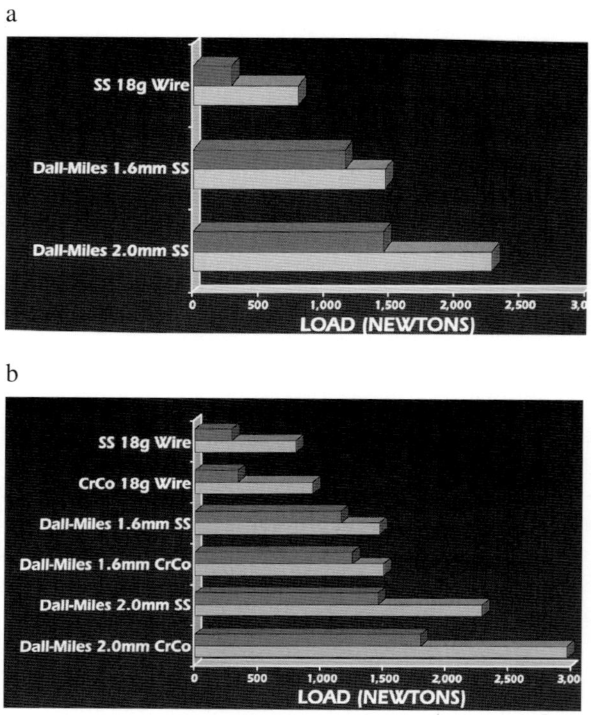

FIG. 1. Comparative yield and ultimate tensile strength of different geometric structures made of the same materials (**a**) and different geometric structures made of different materials (**b**). *Dark gray bars* represent yield strength; *light gray bars* represent ultimate strength

a

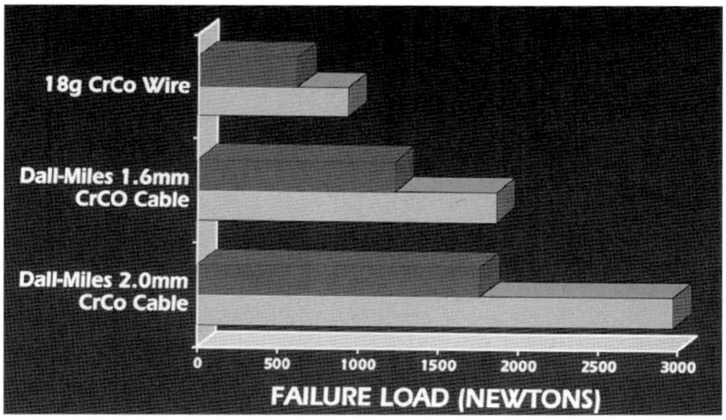

b

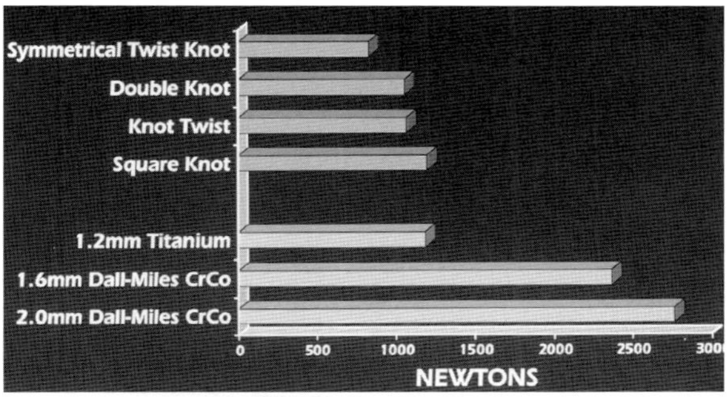

FIG. 2. **a** Comparative strength of fastening methods (*darker bars*) and cerclage material (*lighter bars*). **b** Comparative strengths of various wire fastening methods (*top, darker bars*) and cable fastening methods (*bottom, lighter bars*)

in test protocols: metal pulleys, bone cylinders, and split metal cylinders have all been used. There is therefore a plethora of comparative data, sometimes comparing apples with oranges. We have tended to use the split metal cylinder to measure the strength of fastening by measuring the amount of displacement in the split at varying loads. We believe this is the most reproducible and clinically relevant method.

Whatever the cerclage system and whatever the fastening method, the strength of any fastening method is always significantly weaker than the strength of the material used in a cerclage system (Fig. 2a). Nevertheless, there are significant differences in the strength of various fastening systems in different materials (Fig. 2b).

Clinical Performance of Dall–Miles Trochanter Cable Grip System

In a series of 595 hips (many of which were revisions), we reported a non-union rate of 2.8% with broken cables occurring in 5% of cases [2]. McCarthy et al. [3], in a series of 251 difficult revisions of whom 43% had had previous trochanteric osteotomy, reported very satisfactory results. They reported on a non-union rate of 5%, of which half had been attached to cement or allograft. Their cable breakage rate was 9%, with a high incidence occurring in lateral anchor holes.

However, the following two articles reported less satisfactory results. Ritter et al. [4] reported a very high cable breakage and non-union rate, 32.5% and 37.5%, respectively. In their discussion, they state that this failure rate might have been contributed by stainless steel cable contact with the titanium prosthesis. They reported better results with chrome cobalt cables.

Silverton et al. [5] reported on 68 trochanteric osteotomies fixed with the Dall–Miles system with a 20% trochanteric migration rate, and 12% of cases had evidence of fragmentation with deposits of cable debris. In my opinion, some of the case illustrations demonstrated splaying of the cut end of the cable, rather than fragmentation.

A further report of poor results using a 1.5-mm chrome cobalt cable manufactured by Zimmer was published by Kelley and Johnson [6], who reported cable debris and a high incidence of acetabular loosing. However, their cable was not fastened by a crimping technique; it was fastened by knotting.

Causes of Failure

There are a number of reasons why monofilament wire can fail as a cerclage material. Kinking is more likely to occur, and stress risers can easily be produced at the time of fastening of the wire with the various knotting and twisting techniques. Multifilament cable has overcome these two problems to a large extent.

However, failure of multifilament cable systems can still occur and could be the result of poor surgical technique (especially inadequate maintenance of instruments), biological factors such as poor bone bed (sometimes the trochanter is reattached to metal or cement rather than bone), and failure of the cerclage system itself. What are the contributory factors resulting in failure of a multifilament cerclage system?

Tension

There is always controversy as to whether tension in a cerclage system should be measured. Protagonists like to have a number that should be achieved. Personally, I believe that measuring tension is of no value if the strength of the bone is unknown. The cerclage system could even cut into the bone while attempting to reach a certain level of tension. I would rather rely on my own feeling in judging the amount of tension required—rather like putting a screw into bone when one can sense that if you tighten it any more it will strip the bone. The ideal level of initial tension is therefore dependent on the strength of the bone and on tensioning to below the level at which the cable will cut through it.

The other important consideration is that there is a definite tendency to overtension cables. Cable is strong and the tensioners are powerful instruments, and thus it is very easy for the surgeon to overtension a cerclage construct. It is also important to realize that a high initial tension will leave less reserve strength in the cable.

Figure 3 illustrates a load-deflection curve of a cerclage construct with an arbitrary level of pretension. The reserve strength of this construct is the difference between

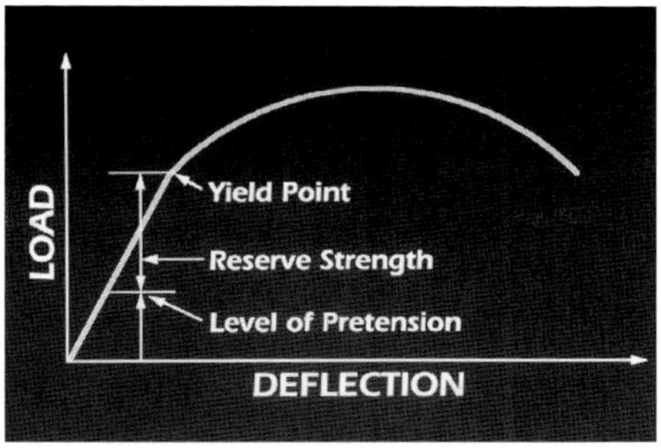

FIG. 3. Load-deflection curve of a cerclage construct with an arbitrary level of pretension

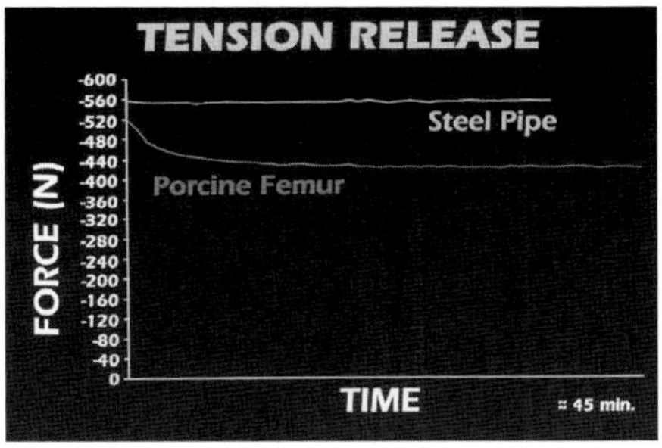

FIG. 4. Tension release in a cerclage construct around a steel pipe versus one around the porcine femur over a period of time

the yield point and the level of pretension. In other words, the higher the level of pretension, the lower the reserve strength. Furthermore, it should be realized that in tensioning cerclage constructs, after fastening there is always some loss of tension due to the viscoelastic properties of bone (Fig. 4).

The site of failure usually occurs at potential stress risers. For example, it often occurs at knots or twists in monofilament wire or where kinking has occurred. It is particularly inclined to occur at acute exit or entry points into the bone or fixation devices, or at sharp corners producing stress risers in both monofilament wires and multifilament cables (Fig. 5).

It is important to realize that in the clinical situation there is always cyclic loading of a cerclage construct as it is subjected to dynamic forces. Therefore, the failure mode is most likely going to be in fatigue. We were able to illustrate this in the majority of retrieved specimens.

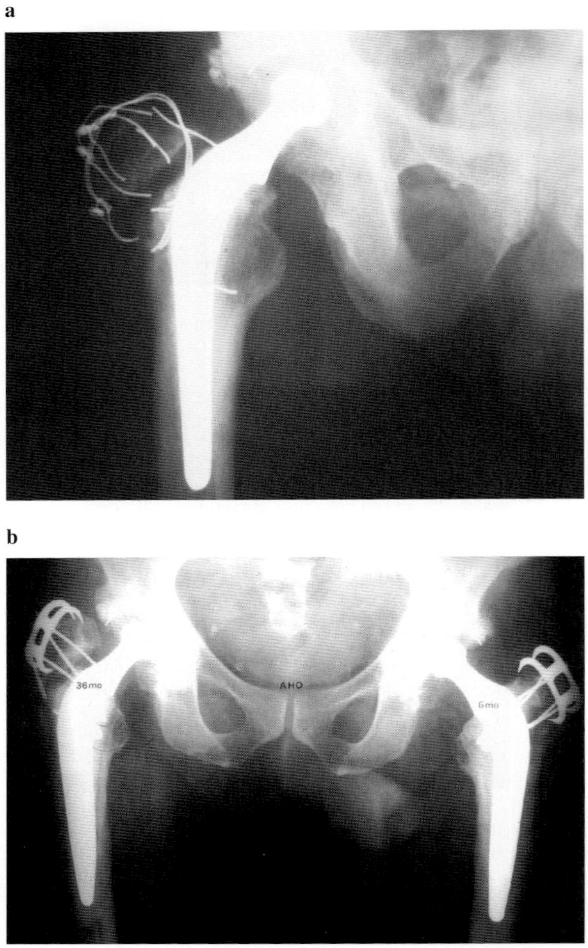

FIG. 5. Failure of fixation of the greater trochanter frequently occurs at stress risers such as acute exit points from bone. **a** Wires **b** Cables

Fatigue Strength

For these reasons we have come to realize how important fatigue strength is in any cerclage system. It is interesting that there have been no defined standards for fatigue testing of wire or cable. The first protocol for testing multifilament cables was developed in 1994 by Schmotzer [7] (Fig. 6a, b).

It is a well known fact that fatigue strength is related to the toughness of the material (Fig. 7a). Changes in design and manufacturing technique can result in huge gains in fatigue strength for a small sacrifice in tensile strength (Fig. 7b). As a result of these studies and through changes in filament design and manufacturing techniques, Stryker has been able to substantially increase the fatigue strength of the Dall–Miles cables.

a

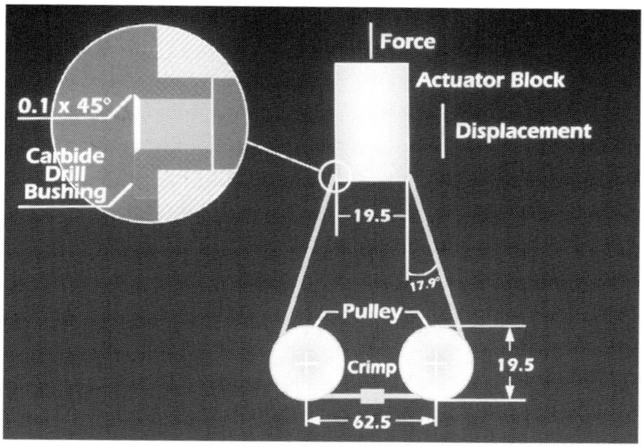

b

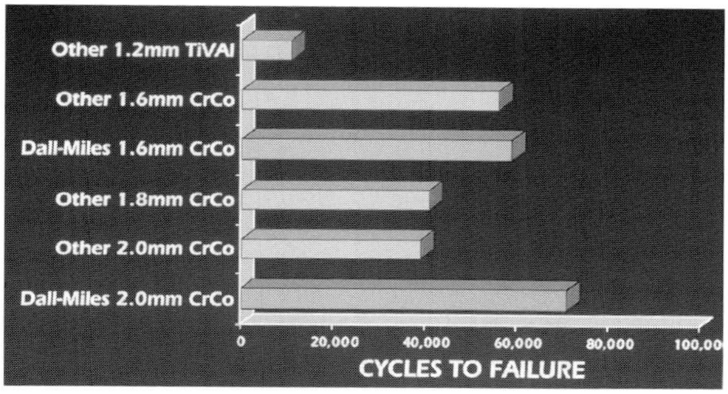

FIG. 6. **a** The fatigue test protocol designed by Schmotzer in 1994 for comparative fatigue tests on different multifilament cables. **b** Comparative fatigue data based on accelerated fatigue tests illustrating the difference in fatigue strength between Dall–Miles cables and other manufacturers

Clinical Applications of Cable Cerclage

Fixation of the Greater Trochanter

Using the grip, the Dall–Miles Cable System can be applied to fixation of the greater trochanter in a variety of situations:

- Primary hip arthroplasty
- Revision hip arthroplasty
- Detached trochanters with non-unions
- Advancement of the trochanter for recurrent dislocation or developmental coxa vara

The trochanter grip is also useful in reattaching the greater trochanter in partial trochanteric osteotomy approaches, such as the anterior partial trochanteric osteotomy described by Dall [8]. It has also proved to be very useful in extended osteotomy

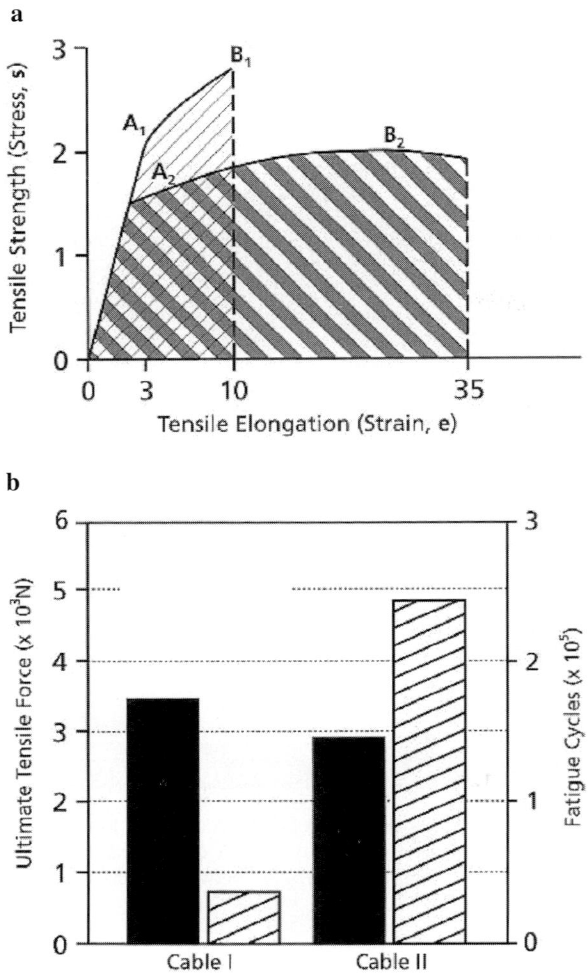

FIG. 7. **a** Comparison of stress–strain curves in materials of different toughness. A_1/B_1: *thin black-hatched curve* represents low-toughness material; A_2/B_2: *thick black-hatched curve* represents high-toughness material. A_1 and A_2 represent the yield points; B_1 and B_2 represent the ultimate tensile strength; *cross-hatched areas* represent the material toughness. **b** Relationship of tensile and fatigue performance. Significant gains in fatigue strength can be obtained for a small sacrifice in tensile strength. Tensile performance represented by *solid columns*; fatigue performance represented by *hatched columns*

approaches and should be combined with distal cerclage cables in these approaches. A trochanter grip plate is currently being developed to be used for extended trochanteric osteotomy fixation.

Allograft Fixation

Cortical allografts have proved to be very useful in a variety of situations in revision total hip arthroplasty. Cerclage cable fixation is ideal in cortical allograft struts. Prophylactically, these are particularly indicated when severe cortical thinning has occurred, a cortical window or perforation is present, and in any situation where there is a significant risk of fracture. A longer stem should always be considered in addition to supportive allograft struts. They can also be used to support very thin femoral cortices when impaction grafting is the method of choice in revision arthroplasties. The cerclage cable can be applied around supporting mesh and/or supporting cortical allograft struts.

Periprosthetic Fracture Fixation in Total Hip Arthroplasty

Cable cerclage is particularly useful for primary or adjunctive fixation of periprosthetic fractures. Intraoperative proximal fractures can be well controlled with cerclage cable. If a postoperative fracture is present in the proximal or middle stem regions and the stem is well fixed, cortical allograft struts fixed with cerclage cables can be used in the fixation of selected fractures.

Chandler et al. [9] reported on 19 cases with periprosthetic fractures around or below a well-fixed femoral stem treated by open reduction and internal fixation using massive cortical allograft struts and cerclage wires or cables. Seventeen patients united their fractures and returned to their preoperative functional status at an average of 4.5 months. There were 2 non-unions, requiring further surgery.

Distal fractures can be controlled with a Dall–Miles plate, cerclage cables, and screws, but in the majority of cases additional cortical allograft struts should be used to strengthen the construct. Periprosthetic fractures associated with loose stems require revision of the stem (frequently to a long stem femoral component) with or without supportive cortical allograft struts (Fig. 8a, b).

Treatment of Fractures

Cerclage cables can be useful in a variety of situations, usually as an augmentation to fixation of primary fractures. The fixation of proximal femoral fractures can sometimes usefully be augmented by cerclage cable. This use could apply to head–neck replacements, gamma nails, and dynamic hip screws.

Distal femoral fractures fixed with Zichel nails or blade-plates can also be augmented in certain cases with cerclage cables. Cables can be used for olecranon and patella fracture fixation.

a

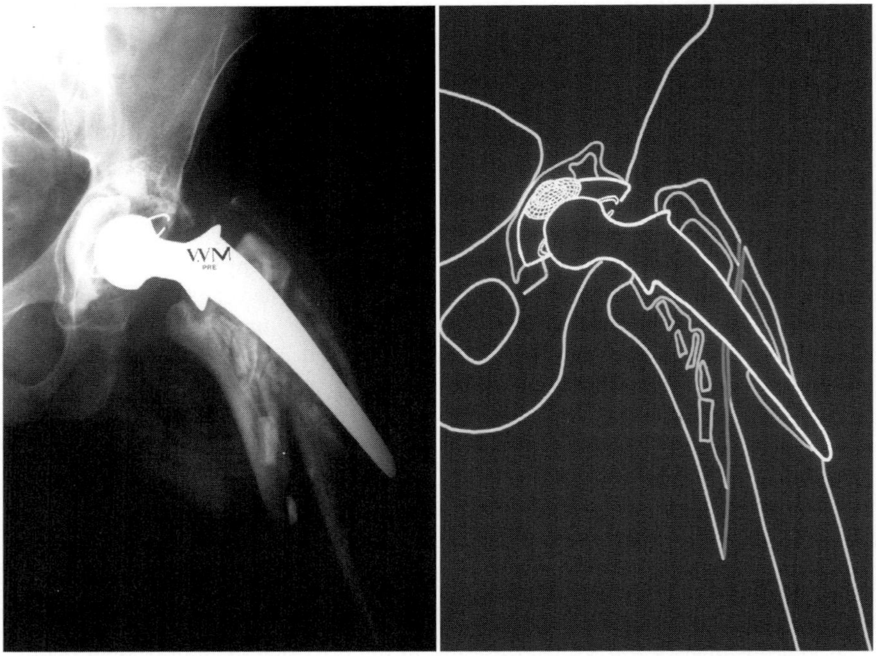

b

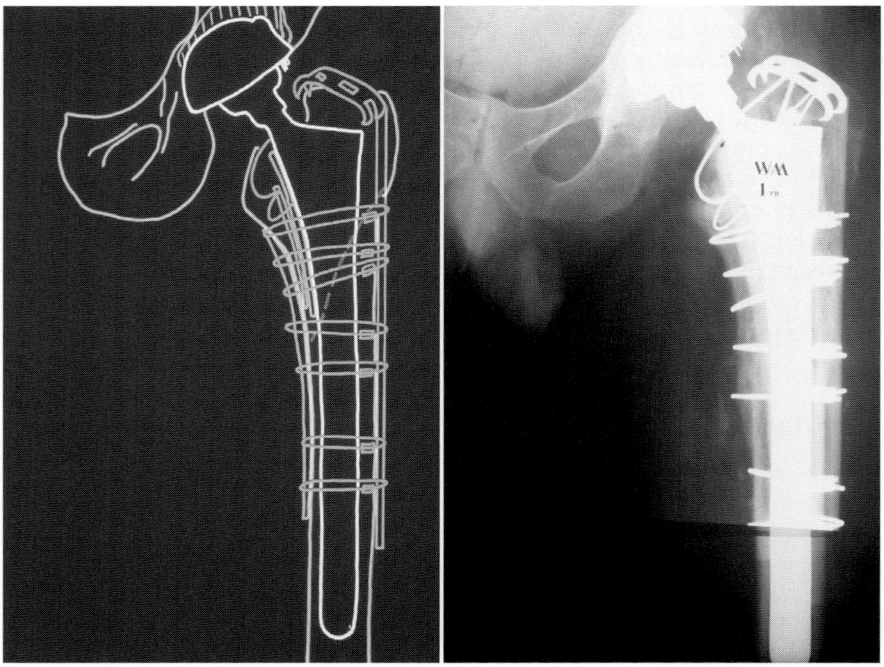

FIG. 8. **a** Preoperative X-ray (*left*) and a descriptive diagram (*right*) of a periprosthetic fracture around the middle region of a loose stem. **b** *Left:* a schematic representation of the repair using a long cementless stem augmented with a cable grip, cortical allograft struts, and cerclage cables. The X-ray on the *right* shows appearance at 1 year postoperative

a

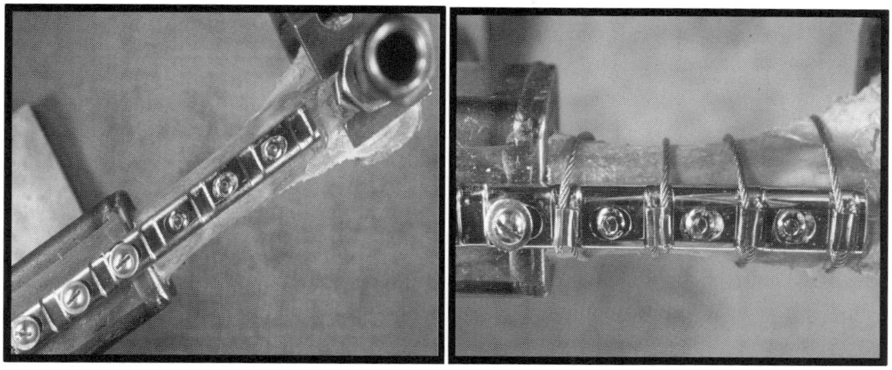

b

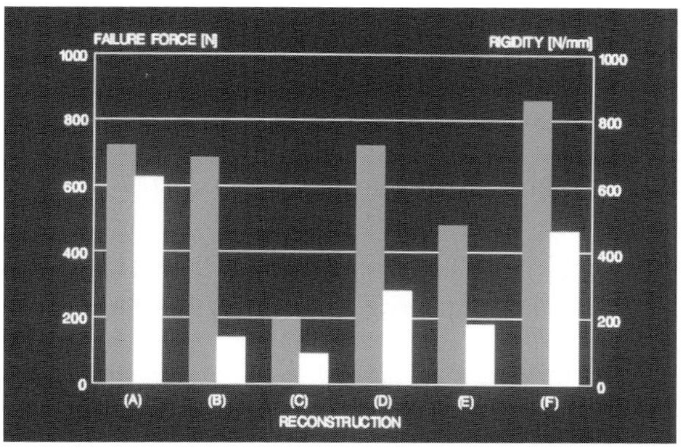

FIG. 9. **a** Bench study setup to examine the improvement of fixation when cerclage cables are used to augment unicortical screw fixation or bicortical screw fixation in soft bone. **b** Results of bench study and the considerable improvement in strength of fixation when cerclage cables are used to augment unicortical screws or biocortical screws in soft bone. *Gray columns* show force required to produce failure of fixation; *white columns* show rigidity of fixation. (**A**) Bicortical screws, (**B**) cerclage cables, (**C**) unicortical screws and (**D**) unicortical screws augmented by cable fixation, in good bone. (**E**) Bicortical screws and (**F**) bicortical screws augmented by cerclage cable fixation in soft bone

Augmentation of Screw Fixation in Soft Bone

In a bench study by Schmotzer et al. [10], the increase in fixation strength provided by a cerclage cable augmenting either unicortical screw or bicortical screw fixation in soft bone was clearly demonstrated (Fig. 9a, b). The cerclage cable therefore becomes a very useful adjunct to screw or screw-plate fixation in patients with osteopenia or osteoporosis.

References

1. Dall DM, Miles AW (1983) Re-attachment of the greater trochanter. J Bone Joint Surg 65B:55–59
2. Dall DM, Miles AW (1990) Results of fixation of the greater trochanter using the Dall–Miles Cable Grip System. Presented as a scientific exhibit, SICOT, September 9–14, 1990 Montreal
3. McCarthy JC, Bono JV, Turner RH, et al (1999) The outcome of trochanteric reattachment in revision total hip arthroplasty with a Cable Grip System: mean 6-year follow-up. J Arthroplasty 14(7):810–814
4. Ritter MA, Eizember LE, Keating EM, et al (1991) Trochanteric fixation by cable grip in hip replacement. J Bone Joint Surg 73B:580–581
5. Silverton CD, Jacobs JJ, Rosenberg AG, et al (1996) Complications of a cable grip system. J Arthroplasty 11(4):400–404
6. Kelley SS, Johnson RC (1992) Debris from cobalt-chrome cable may cause acetabular loosening. Clin Orthop Relat Res 285:140–146
7. Schmotzer H (1994) Protocol for determining fatigue strength of multifilament cable. USC Orthopaedic Research Laboratory, Los Angeles. Test data on file at Stryker Orthopaedics
8. Dall DM (1986) Exposure of the hip by anterior osteotomy of the greater trochanter. J Bone Joint Surg 68B:382–386
9. Chandler HP, King D, Limbird R, et al (1993) The use of cortical allograft struts for fixation of fractures associated with well-fixed total joint prostheses. Semin Arthroplasty 4(2):99–107
10. Schmotzer H, Tchejayan G, Richardson S, et al (1994) Augmentation of screw fixation using cerclage cables. USC Orthopaedic Laboratory, Los Angeles. Test data on file at Stryker Orthopaedics

Index